| WHILE THE WORLD SLEEPS |

EDITED BY

CHRIS BULL

| WHILE THE |
WORLD SLEEPS

Writing from the First Twenty Years of the Global AIDS Plague

THUNDER'S MOUTH PRESS
NEW YORK

While the World Sleeps:
Writing from the First Twenty Years of the Global AIDS Plague

Published by
Thunder's Mouth Press
An Imprint of Avalon Publishing Group Incorporated
161 William Street, 16th Floor
New York, NY 10038

Library of Congress Cataloging-In-Publication Data is available.

ISBN 1-56025-439-4

9 8 7 6 5 4 3 2 1

Designed by Pauline Neuwirth, Neuwirth & Associates, Inc.

Printed in the United States of America
Distributed by Publishers Group West

CONTENTS

3 | COMING TO TERMS

4 | GOING GLOBAL

ACKNOWLEDGMENTS

Thanks to all the folks at Avalon, including my editor Dan O'Connor and his assistant Michael O'Connor for backing this anthology and putting in the long hours to make it possible. Michael Bronski and Jeffrey Escoffier contributed many insights and suggestions as did Lawrence Mass and Andrew Holleran. Larry Kramer came up with the title and generously provided the foreword. To all the terrific contributors included here—and many talented writers who are not—your work gives us hope.

FOREWORD

LARRY KRAMER

I don't know why I am writing an introduction to this book. I dislike most of the pieces in it, including mine.

But it's important that you read this book. And try to figure out why I have such misgivings about its contents. It's important that you figure out for yourself why. Because this is a very important book.

There is a daily newspaper in Johannesburg called the *Mail & Guardian* that, at the beginning of every month, publishes the number of "estimated worldwide HIV infections."

As I write this, this number is over fifty million. It goes up real fast.

This total does not include the twenty-five million people who have already died from AIDS.

When I first heard about this shit in 1981 there were forty-one cases of some strange disease. Twenty-five years later there have been over seventy-five million cases of an outright worldwide plague.

Not that anyone anywhere has ever or now calls it a plague.

In twenty-five years it has been impossible to mount a careful, thoughtful, thorough, concerted effort to stop this plague.

Year after year no one in authority has done very much to stop a worldwide plague.

Not one President in office, not one head of any country, not one government, not one major newspaper, not one major network, not one big-deal magazine has done all that much to stop a worldwide plague.

No one has kept the pressure on day-by-day and rubbed the world's noses in the overwhelming day-by-day, non-stop shit of this plague so that people in authority would have no choice but to do something.

Too-late promises from President Bush and too-late chastisement by President Clinton? Too late. Too late to do any good. Too late.

Does this not tell you how much the world hates, loathes, despises homosexuals and people of color? It's happening to lots of other people now, of course, but with AIDS it's always been, continues to be, first come first served.

Does this not say something about a callousness on everyone's part that is equal to outright complicity in genocide?

The few meek voices crying out for help have been ignored.

Since 1981 not very many people have gotten angry. That's amazing to me now and has been since the beginning. It is perhaps one of the single most amazing things that I have witnessed in my life. There have been so many quiet victims.

Why hasn't there been more anger? Why hasn't there been more volume? Why haven't there been protests akin to revolutions?

Nothing anybody did was good enough.

This collection is full of people trying to reason why what's happening is happening.

There is no reason in the world that is good enough to explain why what is happening is happening.

There is no longer any useful reason to reason why.

For it has all happened already. It is here and it can no longer be stopped.

AIDS tells us about the worst of America and the world. It tells us that people don't care about others. It shows us over and over again that people can be allowed to die.

This is a book of genocide. It should break your heart to read over and over again these awful instances of man's inhumanity to man. But it won't break your heart. I'll bet it won't even make you angry.

The words in this book are the words of people lying down and dying or of people who have watched people lying down and dying.

These were not the responses that this dire plague required.

You will notice there are no pieces in this volume by (to cite only a few) Arthur Miller, Norman Mailer, William Styron, Philip Roth, John Updike, Elizabeth Hardwick, Nora Ephron, Martin Amis, A.S. Byatt, Oriana Fallaci, Harold Pinter, Martin Scorsese, Steven Spielberg, Tom Stoppard, David Hare, Caryl Churchill, Michael Holyroyd, Joyce Carol Oates, Toni

Morrison, Carlos Fuentes, Ursula Le Guin, Barbara Tuchman, Thomas Sanchez, Cynthia Ozick, Doris Kearns Goodwin, Robert Caro, Michael Crichton, Scott Turow, John Grisham, Tom Clancy, Danielle Steel, Umberto Eco, Milan Kundera, Bob Woodward, Patricia Cornwell, Michael Beschloss, Tom Brokaw, Pat Conroy, Robert Redford, Jonathan Franzen, Alice Munro, David McCullough, Salman Rushdie, Elmore Leonard, George Plimpton, Michael Jackson, Mick Jagger, Gabriel García Márquez, David Halberstam, Kurt Vonnegut, August Wilson . . . none of whom, to my knowledge, has written one word about this plague. They and many others just as famous have abrogated the primary responsibility of a writer: to be a witness to his and her times.

Evil. That is the word I live with more than any other. It is evil—not only for governments and drug companies but for all of us with voices and brains—to possess a means of saving lives and then not provide it to the people who need it most. I cannot comprehend a world in which such harsh evil is allowed to become the standard of life. What kind of hideous people have we all become?

I suppose people will read these pieces and say, how sad, isn't it awful, why didn't anybody do anything, why isn't anybody doing anything. But that is my point, isn't it? You are the anybody who isn't doing anything. You have been the anybody all along, since the beginning of this hideous plague.

None of us has really done much of anything or else we wouldn't have arrived here in this time of no hope.

For a bunch of years there was hope. For some deluded souls there probably still is hope. They are wrong. There no longer is hope.

We've failed. All of us. Everything we did and have done and are doing has failed. These fifty million and counting people are going to die. They are going to join the twenty-five million people already dead. There is nothing that is going to save them now. Nothing. It's too late now. We had our chance and we blew it.

We have failed.

Can't you see that? Don't you know that?

But then I don't know what you know anymore. I don't know what anyone knows anymore. I don't recognize what anyone believes in anymore, all that love and God and charity shit that is supposed to be overflowing in our hearts. The milk of human kindness? Where did that expression come from? Do unto others? Ditto. We live by such false meaningless mouthfuls of garbaged words, long since disenfranchised from real meaning in the real world.

We have failed mightily.
This book should show you how.
That is why this is a very important book.

January 2003

INTRODUCTION

CHRIS BULL

As the American media chronicled the war on terrorism in January 2002, a shocking wire report appeared on the back pages of major dailies: "AIDS Set to Surpass Black Death."

Epidemiologists were predicting the toll of the pandemic, which had already claimed more than thirty seven million lives, would soon surpass the forty million who perished in the plague that ravaged Asia and Europe in the fourteenth century. If HIV is allowed to continue its relentless march across the globe, the experts concluded, it one day could dwarf it. AIDS has become the leading cause of death in Africa; the fourth largest killer worldwide.

Sure enough, by the end of 2002, the United Nations was reporting that 38.6 million adults are living with HIV, with five million new infections in the course of the year alone. For the first time, men and women were infected equally, at nearly twenty million cases each. The caseload had gone from forty-one in July of 1981 to fifty million in January 2003.

To the uninitiated reader, such monstrous pronouncements might seem as inconceivable as the pre-September 11 notion that terrorists could crash jumbo jets into the Word Trade Center and Pentagon. Surely, more than twenty years into the crisis, the moment when science would vanquish AIDS—like polio and smallpox before it—was just around the corner. Weren't effective vaccines in the pipeline? Weren't the storm clouds parting?

The consequences of that failure are but the leading edge of the cataclysm of famine, poverty, and armed conflict. Like alarm bells in the night, the writings collected here constitute some of the sharpest and astute warnings of that havoc since this distinctive constellation of immune-system-related symptoms gained a name in 1981. Three more years elapsed until the virus at its root was isolated.

The best exposés, essays, and calls to action often appeared outside the mainstream press, which showed little interest in the looming health crisis. Larry Kramer's 1983 article "1,112 and Counting" appeared in the *New York Native*, a gay and lesbian newspaper. Mark Schoofs's seven-part series "The Agony of Africa" ran in the alternative weekly the *Village Voice* in 1999.

The editorial voice of such compositions frequently stepped out of the conventional bounds between advocacy and journalism, between "we" and "they." "If this article doesn't scare the shit out of you, we're in real trouble," Kramer declared in his galvanizing broadside. "Our continued existence depends on just how angry you get."

Kramer was addressing gay men, some of whom reacted with apathy or denial to early reports comprising the majority of early deaths in the U.S. and despite the appalling linkage forged between their community and the disease in its early provisional moniker: Gay-Related Immunity Deficiency, or GRID.

Kramer assailed the government and medical establishment's response in equally forceful terms, accusing each of "genocide." Yet it took years before Kramer was embraced as the Paul Revere of AIDS journalism. And it was not before Schoofs won the Pulitzer Prize for his series that the *Wall Street Journal* hired him to cover the AIDS beat.

The power and limits of AIDS reportage are recurrent themes of this anthology. These prescient scribes have laid out the human cost as well as urgency of combatting the virus on every front. Who could dismiss Schoofs's heart-rending depiction of the seventeen-year-old Arthur Chinaka's suffering? AIDS-related complications had wiped out nearly every adult in his family. "The most horrifying part of this story," Schoofs relates, "is that it's not unique."

Yet since the early days of the plague, there's been a yawning gap between these exhortations and the government's response. Part of the problem, of course, is politics. The coincidence of AIDS's emergence in America and the advent of the Reagan Administration was nothing less than disastrous. The president was busy rewarding for his margin of victory such conservative activists as Moral Majority founder Jerry Falwell, who proclaimed that "AIDS is God's judgment on a society that does not live by His rules."

Gary Bauer, a sworn enemy of gay and lesbian civil rights, served as a domestic policy advisor. Margaret Heckler's Department of Health and Human Services responded more aggressively to an outbreak of Legionnaire's disease than the sexually transmitted virus. In Congress, right-wingers Jesse Helms and William Dannemeyer worked to assure the federal response to AIDS would not be commensurate with its severity.

These were bitter, frightening times for those most affected by the disease. For authors and journalists, the question was one of the moral culpability. In his 1993 *New York Times Magazine* essay, "Whatever Happened to AIDS?" reporter Jeffrey Schmalz, who would die from the disease just two years later, angrily predicts his own demise: "Now, 12 years after it was first recognized as a new disease, AIDS has become normalized, part of the landscape. It is everywhere and nowhere, the leading cause of death among young men nationwide, but little threat to the core of American political power, the white heterosexual suburbanite. . . . The world is moving on, uncaring, frustrated and bored, leaving by the roadside those of us who are infected."

In the 1987 academic treatise "Is the Rectum a Grave?" Leo Bersani compares the Reagan administration's response to the "millions of fine Germans who never participated in the murder of Jews (and homosexuals), but who *failed to find the idea of the holocaust unbearable*."

Bersani resorts to hyperbole. But he is right to say that history is rarely kind to the powerful who fail to comprehend and to respond accordingly. Instead of Kramer—or intrepid chroniclers Lawrence Mass, or Randy Shilts, author of 1987's *And the Band Played On*—the White House took its cues from right-wing propagandists. "The poor homosexuals, they have declared war upon nature, and now nature is extracting awful retribution," former Nixon speechwriter and Reagan advisor Pat Buchanan opined.

Having based his career on antipathy to minority groups, Buchanan's views were entirely predictable. And the problem was not only Buchanan's implicit homophobia. It was also the notion that the nation was powerless to respond. Why bother to respond when God had rendered the ultimate verdict? The fact that even in 1985, when Buchanan wrote these words, the virus was also spreading through opposite-sex contact did not cost Buchanan and his ilk any sleep.

"AIDS is a particularly potent symbol for the hard-line radical right because it is evidence of sin, God's disfavor, and an ultimate solution: it is both a sign and a punishment embodied in one of the groups targeted for political decimation long before AIDS," writes Cindy Patton in *Sex & Germs*.

In the 1989 book *The Myth of Heterosexual AIDS*, Michael Fumento reassured the world that the "general population" was safe. Based on the notion that heterosexual transmission was inefficient, he ridiculed former Secretary of Health and Human Services Otis Bowen for contending, in 1987, that AIDS could one day make the Black Death "pale by comparison." Fumento—and the many who championed this demonstrably false thesis—have faced few hard questions as the predatory swath of the disease has put the lie to their rhetoric at that no-so-long-ago pep rally for indifference.

As Susan Sontag points out in *AIDS and Its Metaphors*, inexact parallels can be numbing rather than enlightening. "A proliferation of reports of unreal (that is, ungraspable) doomsday eventualities tends to produce a variety of reality-denying responses," she writes.

Nevertheless, some metaphors, judiciously employed, are on the money. The Black Death analogy turned out to be eerily accurate. Here is the incontrovertible truth: same-sex transmission has steadily declined as an overall percentage of the total caseload. Of the estimated one million Americans infected with HIV, fewer than fifty percent are among men who have sex with men. On a global basis, the disparity is far greater. (Same-sex transmission accounts for a fraction one percent of the total.) The vast majority of cases are caused by intravenous needles or unprotected vaginal intercourse. The creative protected sex techniques, promoted by Michael Callen in "How to Have Sex in an Epidemic," are still the exception to the rule in many parts of the globe. As Helen Epstein and Lincoln Chen point out in their 2002 "Can AIDS Be Stopped?" "reliable supplies of condoms" are still not "easily and cheaply available everywhere."

A few powerful government officials were able to shake off apathy and look beyond ideology. C. Everett Koop, a conservative Christian, assumed the Surgeon General's office in 1983 with a reputation for quoting scripture and scorning homosexuality. But in preparing the nation's first federal AIDS report, he began reading the gay press and listening to people with AIDS. As Stephen Chapple and David Talbot write in *Burning Desires: Sex in America—A Report from the Field*, Koop the "wrathful moralist was giving way to the compassionate physician." The result was a candid call for AIDS education "at the lowest grade possible," including "information about heterosexual and homosexual relationships."

It was a rare victory in the early battle against HIV. But the war had only just begun. Faced with indifference and resistance to their demands, advocates for people with AIDS turned to the streets. In 1987, Kramer founded the

AIDS Coalition to Unleash Power (Act Up), one of the nation's most vital modern activist movements. This organization, which at its peak drew thousands to chapter meetings across the country, inspired many of the contributions to this volume.

Gradually, ACT UP's arguments broke down resistance, at least on the domestic front, vanquishing deniers like Buchanan and Fumento to the fringes of American politics where they belonged. Douglas Crimp and Adam Rolston's "Sell Welcome, Free AZT" describes a typically audacious 1989 demonstration at the New York Stock Exchange to protest the high price of AZT, produced by the pharmaceutical company Wellcome.

The activists "walked up to the VIP balcony overlooking the trading floor, chained themselves to a banister, and just as the opening bells went off, dropped a huge banner that said SELL WELCOME," they write. "They then drowned out the traders with the piercing sound of marine foghorns, successfully stopping transactions on the exchange for five minutes—a historic first."

Today's muted reaction to the continued AIDS toll makes ACT UP's early aggressiveness all the more inspiring. It was a far more confrontational time. In a typical piece of agitprop that's rarely seen today, David Wojnarowicz's *Seven Deadly Sins* blamed AIDS on prominent politicians, church leaders, and health officials who did nothing. "Finds the human body, itself, obscene," Wojnarowicz writes dryly in his entry for Jesse Helms, the North Carolina Republican who retired in 2002 after thirty years in the Senate.

While the disease brought out the worst in a few Americans, it brought out the best in many more. The most draconian initiatives failed, from concentration camps to branding of people with AIDS (suggested in a column by *National Review* editor William F. Buckley, Jr.), to mandatory HIV testing. The 1988 Ryan White Care Act, which brought billions of dollars to the areas of the country most afflicted, is one of the few bipartisan triumphs of Congress in the last two decades.

But the gap between comprehension and action threatens to widen again. Just as a new Republican administration, along with the glacial sexual purity advocated by its religious right base, was assuming power in 2000, the international caseload was spiking exponentially.

Is the White House prepared for the new challenge? The early signs were not entirely encouraging. President George W. Bush's AIDS council is dominated by conservatives and led by Tom Coburn, a physician and former congressman who believes that homosexuality is immoral and that sex education should be replaced by abstinence lectures. The C. Everett Koop of the Bush Administration has yet to emerge.

The federal government still only contributes twenty percent—$500 million—to the global AIDS fund, already pitifully under-funded. During his 2003 State of the Union speech, the president pledged fifteen billion dollars over five years to fight the disease worldwide. This is a good first step. But foreign aid is marred by restrictions on funding for family planning agencies that provide abortion and contraceptive services.

September 11, 2001 changed everything. Other than a flurry of coverage of World AIDS Day in December, the few mentions of AIDS since find it subsumed beneath the equally critical mission to quash and quell terrorism. The White House often appears concerned about HIV only to the extent that it both emboldens terrorists and complicates efforts to bring them to justice. The Pentagon is spending several million dollars per year to help Angola and other African nations to slow the spread of HIV, which is taking a toll on military readiness in the fight against terror.

In his dealings with terrorism and Iraq, Bush has extolled the virtues of pre-emptive strikes to ward off suddenly ubiquitous "weapons of mass destruction." If only the new administration would apply the same aggressive philosophy to this equally deadly scourge, which has already killed more than all the wars of the twentieth century combined.

"I don't know if I will live to finish this," Paul Monette begins his 1998 AIDS memoir, *Borrowed Time*. Worried about their own mortality and caring for dying friends and lovers, few American writers felt comfortable taking it to the streets. Many who have written about AIDS adopted a more reflective tone, dealing with the everyday aspects of grief and loss.

In *The Absence of Anger*, Andrew Holleran elucidates the tension between activism and care. Visiting a sick friend in New York City before heading to an ACT UP meeting, he writes: "Sorrow is a sort of immobilizing emotion. It requires stillness, removal, withdrawal from the world. We sat in the dark loft while the Four Last Songs of Strauss played (*How can he bear this?* I wondered) and talked about books, friends, fate, as we watched the city sky darken and the lighted towers of Wall Street become as sharp as diamonds."

The AIDS quilt exemplifies this sentiment. *In Stitching a Revolution: The Making of An Activist*, Cleve Jones describes his 1985 vision for the AIDS memorial quilt, which would one day cover the National Mall, displayed in front of the Capitol Building. "At the time, HIV was seen as the product of aggressive gay male sexuality, and it seemed that the homey image and familial associations of a warm quilt would counter that."

The quilt boasts a political dimension, however, bringing Americans together across racial and sexual divides. Reprinted in *A Promise to Remember: The Names Project Book of Letters*, the text of Paul McCarthy's quilt panel dedicated to Roy Cohn, the anti-Communist and anti-gay crusader, sums up the merciless nature of the disease this way: "Roy Cohn died of AIDS. He was ashamed to be gay, and I'm ashamed he was one of us. He was a bully, yes. A coward, yes. He was also a victim of this horrible disease."

The father-son relationship forms the basis of Judith Valente's detailed "Love Story," published in the *Wall Street Journal* in 1991. "With so much written, said and filmed about AIDS, the toll on fathers remains largely an untold story," she writes. "In many cases, dads who had hoped their sons would follow in their footsteps are forced to deal at once with the shock of their son's sexuality and the ugly specter of AIDS."

It is never easy to fully assimilate a crisis in the middle of it. For those on the inside, it's hard to absorb the magnitude of loss. For those on the outside, it's easy to deny AIDS by looking the other way. Even thirty years after the end of Vietnam, Americans are only beginning to come to terms with the war's ruin, which took more than 55,000 American lives and many thousands more Vietnamese.

When it comes to AIDS, as the writers collected here suggest, past is prologue. Having already ravaged entire populations, the plague is exploding all over again, especially in Southeast Asia and landlocked African nations easy for the West to ignore.

But there is hope to be found in these writings, sometimes in unexpected places. In his 2001 article "India's Plague," Michael Specter profiles Yusuf K. Hamied, a wealthy Indian businessman who took on the drug companies in order to make previously unaffordable HIV and increasingly effective treatments widely available in his country, which has more HIV infections than any other.

After witnessing the horror of September 11, "Hamied went out and started a revolution," writes Specter in the *New Yorker*. "Thanks to [his company] Cipla, a year's worth of crucial AIDS-medication that until recently sold in America for more than fifteen thousand dollars is now available in many parts of the Third World for three hundred and fifty dollars. Multinational pharmaceutical giants condemned Hamied. 'Stealing ideas is not how one provides good health care,' Shannon Herzfeld, a spokeswoman for the American pharmaceutical industry, said last year."

Hamied is hardly the only one to get a wake up call, albeit a late one. In 1995 Jesse Helms, an anti-gay zealot who had blocked federally funded AIDS education programs for years, voiced opposition to HIV/AIDS funding because he said that HIV-positive people "got sick as a result of 'deliberate, disgusting, revolting conduct.'"

In February 2002, Helms sent a radically different message. Noting the explosion of the plague overseas, Helms told hundreds of Christian AIDS activists gathered for a conference in Washington, D.C., "I have been too lax too long in doing something really significant about AIDS," he intoned. "I'm not going to lay it aside on my agenda for the remaining months I have" in office. Then he admitted to "embarrassment" at his own negligence.

Helms later felt compelled to clarify that was not softening his condemnation of homosexuality, the very prejudice that had caused him to downplay the wreckage of the plague in the first place. Perhaps it was simply too much for Helms to admit that the last twenty years of his political career had been counterproductive.

It would also be a mistake to excuse Helms' negligence on the basis of a convenient retirement conversion. The point, however, is not to pin blame on any single leader. As the writers collected here suggest, it is more productive to draw attention to uncomfortable truths, in the hope of finding receptive audiences anywhere and everywhere.

As Mark Schoofs writes of the millions of Africans dead or infected, ". . . An old African proverb has new relevance: 'Something with horns cannot be hidden.' The sick and dead are forcing South Africans to confront the disease, themselves, and their brutal history."

Those fighting the disease across the globe can only hold out a similar hope.

March 2003

1

ORIGINS

RARE CANCER SEEN IN 41 HOMOSEXUALS

LAWRENCE K. ALTMAN

from The New York TImes

| **July 3, 1981** |

Doctors in New York and California have diagnosed among homosexual men forty-one cases of a rare and often rapidly fatal form of cancer. Eight of the victims died less than twenty-four months after the diagnosis was made.

The cause of the outbreak is unknown, and there is as yet no evidence of contagion. But the doctors who have made the diagnoses, mostly in New York City and the San Francisco Bay area, are alerting other physicians who treat large numbers of homosexual men to the problem in an effort to help identify more cases and to reduce the delay in offering chemotherapy treatment.

The sudden appearance of the cancer, called Kaposi's sarcoma, has prompted a medical investigation that experts say could have as much scientific as public health importance because of what it may teach about determining the causes of more common types of cancer.

FIRST APPEARS IN SPOTS

Doctors have been taught in the past that the cancer usually appeared first in spots on the legs and that the disease took a slow course of up to ten years. But these recent cases have shown that it appears in one or more violet-colored spots anywhere on the body.

The spots generally do not itch or cause other symptoms, often can be mistaken for bruises, sometimes appear as lumps, and can turn brown after a period of time. The cancer often causes swollen lymph glands, and then kills by spreading throughout the body.

Doctors investigating the outbreak believe that many cases have gone undetected because of the rarity of the condition and the difficulty even dermatologists may have in diagnosing it.

In a letter alerting other physicians to the problem, Dr. Alvin E. Friedman-Kien of New York University Medical Center, one of the investigators, described the appearance of the outbreak as "rather devastating."

Dr. Friedman-Kien said in an interview yesterday that he knew of forty-one cases collated in the last five weeks, with the cases themselves dating to the past thirty months. The federal Centers for Disease Control in Atlanta is expected to publish the first description of the outbreak in its weekly report today, according to a spokesman, Dr. James Curran. The report notes twenty-six of the cases—twenty in New York and six in California.

There is no national registry of cancer victims, but the nationwide incidence of Kaposi's sarcoma in the past had been estimated by the Centers for Disease Control to be less than six-one-hundredths of a case per 100,000 people annually, or about two cases in every three million people. However, the disease accounts for up to 9 percent of all cancers in a belt across equatorial Africa, where it commonly affects children and young adults.

In the United States, it has primarily affected men older than fifty years. But in the recent cases, doctors at nine medical centers in New York and seven hospitals in California have been diagnosing the condition among younger men, all of whom said in the course of standard diagnostic interviews that they were homosexual. Although the ages of the patients have ranged from twenty-six to fifty-one years, many have been under forty, with the mean at thirty-nine.

Nine of the forty-one cases known to Dr. Friedman-Kien were diagnosed in California, and several of those victims reported that they had been in New York in the period preceding the diagnosis. Dr. Friedman-Kien said that his colleagues were checking on reports of two victims diagnosed in Copenhagen, one of whom had visited New York.

VIRAL INFECTIONS INDICATED

No one medical investigator has yet interviewed all the victims, Dr. Curran said. According to Dr. Friedman-Kien, the reporting doctors said that most cases had involved homosexual men who have had multiple and frequent sexual encounters with different partners, as many as ten sexual encounters each night up to four times a week.

Many of the patients have also been treated for viral infections such as herpes, cytomegalovirus and hepatitis B as well as parasitic infections such as amebiasis and giardiasis. Many patients also reported that they had used drugs such as amyl nitrite and LSD to heighten sexual pleasure.

Cancer is not believed to be contagious, but conditions that might precipitate it, such as particular viruses or environmental factors, might account for an outbreak among a single group.

The medical investigators say some indirect evidence actually points away from contagion as a cause. None of the patients knew each other, although the theoretical possibility that some may have had sexual contact with a person with Kaposi's sarcoma at some point in the past could not be excluded, Dr. Friedman-Kien said.

Dr. Curran said there was no apparent danger to nonhomosexuals from contagion. "The best evidence against contagion," he said, "is that no cases have been reported to date outside the homosexual community or in women."

Dr. Friedman-Kien said he had tested nine of the victims and found severe defects in their immunological systems. The patients had serious malfunctions of two types of cells called T and B cell lymphocytes, which have important roles in fighting infections and cancer.

But Dr. Friedman-Kien emphasized that the researchers did not know whether the immunological defects were the underlying problem or had developed secondarily to the infections or drug use.

The research team is testing various hypotheses, one of which is a possible link between past infection with cytomegalovirus and development of Kaposi's sarcoma.

1,112 AND COUNTING

LARRY KRAMER

from The New York Native

| **March 1983** |

If this article doesn't scare the shit out of you, we're in real trouble. If this article doesn't rouse you to anger, fury, rage, and action, gay men may have no future on this earth. Our continued existence depends on just how angry you can get.

I am writing this as Larry Kramer, and I am speaking for myself, and my views are not to be attributed to Gay Men's Health Crisis.

I repeat: Our continued existence as gay men upon the face of this earth is at stake. Unless we fight for our lives, we shall die. In all the history of homosexuality we have never before been so close to death and extinction. Many of us are dying or already dead.

Before I tell you what we must do, let me tell you what is happening to us.

There are now 1,112 cases of serious acquired immune deficiency syndrome. When we first became worried, there were only forty-one. In only twenty-eight days, from January 13 to February 9 [1983], there were 164 new cases—and seventy-three more dead. The total death tally is now 418. Twenty percent of all cases were registered this January alone. There have been 195 dead in New York City from among 526 victims. Of all serious AIDS cases, 47.3 percent are in the New York metropolitan area.

These are the serious cases of AIDS, which means Kaposi's sarcoma, *Pneumocystis carinii* pneumonia, and other deadly infections. These numbers do not include the thousands of us walking around with what is also being called AIDS: various forms of swollen lymph glands and fatigues that doctors don't know what to label or what they might portend.

The rise in these numbers is terrifying. Whatever is spreading is now spreading faster as more and more people come down with AIDS.

And, for the first time in this epidemic, leading doctors and researchers are finally admitting they don't know what's going on. I find this terrifying too—as terrifying as the alarming rise in numbers. For the first time, doctors are saying out loud and up front, "I don't know."

For two years they weren't talking like this. For two years we've heard a different theory every few weeks. We grasped at the straws of possible cause: promiscuity, poppers, back rooms, the baths, rimming, fisting, anal intercourse, urine, semen, shit, saliva, sweat, blood, blacks, a single virus, a new virus, repeated exposure to a virus, amoebas carrying a virus, drugs, Haiti, voodoo, Flagyl, constant bouts of amebiasis, hepatitis A and B, syphilis, gonorrhea.

I have talked with the leading doctors treating us. One said to me, "If I knew in 1981 what I know now, I would never have become involved with this disease." Another said, "The thing that upsets me the most in all of this is that at any given moment one of my patients is in the hospital and something is going on with him that I don't understand. And it's destroying me because there's some craziness going on in him that's destroying him." A third said to me, "I'm very depressed. A doctor's job is to make patients well. And I can't. Too many of my patients die."

After almost two years of an epidemic, there are still no answers. After almost two years of an epidemic, the cause of AIDS remains unknown. After almost two years of an epidemic, there is no cure.

Hospitals are now so filled with AIDS patients that there is often a waiting period of up to a month before admission, no matter how sick you are. And, once in, patients are now more and more being treated like lepers as hospital staffs become increasingly worried that AIDS is infectious.

Suicides are now being reported of men who would rather die than face such medical uncertainty, such uncertain therapies, such hospital treatment, and the appalling statistics that 86 percent of all serious AIDS cases die after three years' time.

If all of this had been happening to any other community for two long years, there would have been, long ago, such an outcry from that community and all its members that the government of this city and this country would not know what had hit them.

Why isn't every gay man in this city so scared shitless that he is screaming for action? Does every gay man in New York *want* to die?

Let's talk about a few things specifically.

- Let's talk about which gay men get AIDS.

No matter what you've heard, there is no single profile for all AIDS victims. There are drug users and non–drug users. There are the truly promiscuous and the almost monogamous. There are reported cases of single-contact infection.

All it seems to take is the one wrong fuck. That's not promiscuity—that's bad luck.

- Let's talk about AIDS happening in straight people.

We have been hearing from the beginning of this epidemic that it was only a question of time before the straight community came down with AIDS, and that when that happened AIDS would suddenly be high on all agendas for funding and research and then we would finally be looked after and all would then be well.

I myself thought, when AIDS occurred in the first baby, that would be the breakthrough point. It was. For one day the media paid an enormous amount of attention. And that was it, kids.

There have been no confirmed cases of AIDS in straight, white, non-intravenous-drug-using, middle-class Americans. The only confirmed straights struck down by AIDS are members of groups just as disenfranchised as gay men: intravenous drug users, Haitians, eleven hemophiliacs (up from eight), black and Hispanic babies, and wives or partners of IV drug users and bisexual men.

If there have been—and there may have been—any cases in straight, white, non-intravenous-drug-using, middle-class Americans, the Centers for Disease Control isn't telling anyone about them. When pressed, the CDC says there are "a number of cases that don't fall into any of the other categories." The CDC says it's impossible to fully investigate most of these "other category" cases; most of them are dead. The CDC also tends not to believe living, white, middle-class male victims when they say they're straight, or female victims when they say their husbands are straight and don't take drugs.

Why isn't AIDS happening to more straights? Maybe it's because gay men don't have sex with them.

Of all serious AIDS cases, 72.4 percent are in gay and bisexual men.

- Let's talk about "surveillance."

The Centers for Disease Control is charged by our government to fully monitor all epidemics and unusual diseases.

To learn something from an epidemic, you have to keep records and statistics. Statistics come from interviewing victims and getting as much information from them as you can. Before they die. To get the best information, you have to ask the right questions.

There have been so many AIDS victims that the CDC is no longer able to get to them fast enough. It has given up. (The CDC also had been using a questionnaire that was fairly insensitive to the lives of gay men, and thus the data collected from its early study of us have been disputed by gay epidemiologists. The National Institutes of Health is also fielding a very naïve questionnaire.)

Important, vital case histories are now being lost because of this cessation of CDC interviewing. This is a woeful waste with as terrifying implications for us as the alarming rise in case numbers and doctors finally admitting they don't know what's going on. As each man dies, as one or both sets of men who had interacted with each other come down with AIDS, yet more information that might reveal patterns of transmissibility is not being monitored and collected and studied. We are being denied perhaps the easiest and fastest research tool available at this moment.

It will require at least $200,000 to prepare a new questionnaire to study the next important question that must be answered: *How* is AIDS being transmitted? (In which bodily fluids, by which sexual behaviors, in what social environments?)

For months the CDC has been asked to begin such preparations for continued surveillance. The CDC is stretched to its limits and is dreadfully underfunded for what it's being asked, in all areas, to do.

• Let's talk about various forms of treatment.

It is very difficult for a patient to find out which hospital to go to or which doctor to go to or which mode of treatment to attempt.

Hospitals and doctors are reluctant to reveal how well they're doing with each type of treatment. They may, if you press them, give you a general idea. Most will not show you their precise number of how many patients are doing well on what and how many failed to respond adequately.

Because of the ludicrous requirements of the medical journals, doctors are prohibited from revealing publicly the specific data they are gathering from their treatments of our bodies. Doctors and hospitals need money for research, and this money (from the National Institutes of Health, from cancer research funding organizations, from rich patrons) comes based on the performance of their work (i.e., their tabulations of their results of their treatment of our bodies); this performance is written up as "papers" that must be submitted to and accepted by such "distinguished" medical publications as the *New England Journal of Medicine*. Most of these "distinguished" publications, however, will not publish anything that has been spoken of, leaked, announced, or intimated publicly in advance. Even after acceptance, the doctors must hold their tongues until the article is actually published. Dr. Bijan Safai of Sloan-Kettering has been waiting over six months for the *New England Journal,* which has accepted his interferon study, to publish it. Until that happens, he is only permitted to speak in the most general terms of how interferon is or is not working.

Priorities in this area appear to be peculiarly out of kilter at this moment of life or death.

• Let's talk about hospitals.

Everybody's full up, fellows. No room in the inn.

Part of this is simply overcrowding. Part of this is cruel. Sloan-Kettering still enforces a regulation from pre-AIDS days that only one dermatology patient per week can be admitted to that hospital. (Kaposi's sarcoma falls under dermatology at Sloan-Kettering.) But Sloan-Kettering is also the second-largest treatment center for AIDS patients in New York. You can be near death and still not get into Sloan-Kettering.

Additionally, Sloan-Kettering (and the Food and Drug Administration) require patients to receive their initial shots of interferon while they are hospitalized. A lot of men want to try interferon at Sloan-Kettering before they try chemotherapy elsewhere.

It's not hard to see why there is such a waiting list to get into Sloan-Kettering.

Most hospital staffs are still so badly educated about AIDS that they don't know much about it, except that they've heard it's infectious. (There still have been no cases in hospital staff or among the very doctors who have been treating AIDS victims for two years.) Hence, as I said earlier, AIDS patients are often treated like lepers.

For various reasons, I would not like to be a patient at the Veterans Administration Hospital on East Twenty-fourth Street or at New York Hospital. (Incidents involving AIDS patients at these two hospitals have been reported in news stories in the *Native*.)

I believe it falls to this city's Department of Health, under Commissioner David Spencer, and the Health and Hospitals Corporation, under

Commissioner Stanley Brezenoff, to educate this city, its citizens, and its hospital workers about all areas of a public health emergency. Well, they have done an appalling job of educating our citizens, our hospital workers, and even, in some instances, our doctors. Almost everything this city knows about AIDS has come to it, in one way or another, through Gay Men's Health Crisis, and that includes television programs, magazine articles, radio commercials, newsletters, health-recommendation brochures, open forums, and sending speakers everywhere, including—when asked—into hospitals. If three out of four AIDS cases were occurring in straight men instead of gay men, you can bet all hospitals and staff would know what was happening. And it would be this city's Health Department and Health and Hospitals Corporation who would be telling them.

• Let's talk about what gay tax dollars are buying for gay men.

Now we're arriving at the truly scandalous.

For over a year and a half the National Institutes of Health has been "reviewing" which from among some $55 million worth of grant applications for AIDS research money it will eventually fund.

It's not even a question of NIH having to ask Congress for money. It's already there. Waiting. NIH has almost $8 million already appropriated that it has yet to release into usefulness.

There is no question that if this epidemic was happening to the straight, white, non-intravenous-drug-using middle class, that money would have been put into use almost two years ago, when the first alarming signs of this epidemic were noticed by Dr. Alvin Friedman-Kien and Dr. Linda Laubenstein at New York University Hospital.

During the first *two weeks* of the Tylenol scare, the United States government spent $10 million to find out what was happening.

Every hospital in New York that's involved in AIDS research has used up every bit of the money it could find for researching AIDS while waiting for NIH grants to come through. These hospitals have been working on AIDS for up to two years and are now desperate for replenishing funds. Important studies that began last year, such as Dr. Michael Lange's at St. Luke's-Roosevelt, are now going under for lack of money. Important leads that were and are developing cannot be pursued. (For instance, few hospitals can afford plasmapheresis machines, and few patients can afford this experimental treatment either, since few insurance policies will cover the $16,600 bill.) New York University Hospital, the largest treatment center for AIDS patients in the world, has had its grant application pending at NIH for a year and a half. Even if the application is successful, the earliest time that NYU could receive any money would be late summer.

The NIH would probably reply that it's foolish just to throw money away, that that hasn't worked before. And, NIH would say, if nobody knows what's happening, what's to study?

Any good administrator with half a brain could survey the entire AIDS mess and come up with twenty leads that merit further investigation. I could do so myself. In any research, in any investigation, you have to start somewhere. You can't just not start anywhere at all.

But then, AIDS is happening mostly to gay men, isn't it?

All of this is indeed ironic. For within AIDS, as most researchers have been trying to convey to the NIH, perhaps may reside the answer to the question of what it is that causes cancer itself. If straights had more brains, or were less bigoted against gays, they would see that, as with hepatitis B, gay men are again doing their suffering for them, revealing this disease to them. They can use us as guinea pigs to discover the cure for AIDS before it hits them, which most medical authorities are still convinced will be happening shortly in increasing numbers.

(As if it had not been malevolent enough, the NIH is now, for unspecified reasons, also turning away AIDS patients from its hospital in Bethesda, Maryland. The hospital, which had been treating anyone and everyone with AIDS free of charge, now will only take AIDS patients if they fit into their current investigating protocol. Whatever that is. The NIH publishes "papers," too.)

Gay men pay taxes just like everyone else. NIH money should be paying for our research just like everyone else's. We desperately need something from our government to save our lives, and we're not getting it.

• Let's talk about health insurance and welfare problems.

Many of the ways of treating AIDS are experimental, and many health insurance policies do not cover most of them. Blue Cross is particularly bad about accepting anything unusual.

Many serious victims of AIDS have been unable to qualify for welfare because AIDS is not on the list of qualifying disability illnesses. (Immune deficiency is an acceptable determining factor for welfare among children, but not adults. Figure that one out.) There are also increasing numbers of men unable to pay their rent, men thrown out on the street with nowhere to live and no money to live with, and men who have been asked by roommates to leave because of their illnesses. And men with serious AIDS are being fired from certain jobs.

The horror stories in this area, of those suddenly found destitute, of those facing this illness with insufficient insurance, continue to mount. (One man who'd had no success on other therapies was forced to beg from his friends the $16,600 he needed to try, as a last resort, plasmapheresis.)

• Finally, let's talk about our mayor, Ed Koch.

Our mayor, Ed Koch, appears to have chosen, for whatever reason, not to allow himself to be perceived by the non-gay world as visibly helping us in this emergency.

Repeated requests to meet with him have been denied us. Repeated attempts to have him make a very necessary public announcement about this crisis and public health emergency have been refused by his staff . . .

On October 28, 1982, Mayor Koch was implored to make a public announcement about our emergency. If he had done so then, and if he was only to do so now, the following would be put into action:

1. The community at large would be alerted (you would be amazed at how many people, including gay men, still don't know enough about the AIDS danger).
2. Hospital staffs and public assistance offices would also be alerted and their education commenced.
3. The country, President Reagan, and the National Institutes of Health, as well as Congress, would be alerted, and these constitute the most important ears of all.

If the mayor doesn't think it's important enough to talk up AIDS, none of these people is going to, either.

The mayor of New York has an enormous amount of power—when he wants to use it. When he wants to help his people. With the failure yet again of our civil rights bill, I'd guess our mayor doesn't want to use his power to help us.

With his silence on AIDS, the mayor of New York is helping to kill us.

I am sick of our electing officials who in no way represent us. I am sick of our stupidity in believing candidates who promise us everything for our support and promptly forget us and insult us after we have given them our votes. Koch is the prime example, but not the only one. [Senator] Daniel Patrick Moynihan isn't looking very good at this moment, either. Moynihan was requested by gay leaders to publicly ask Margaret Heckler at her confirmation hearing for secretary of Health and Human Services if she could be fair to gays in view of her voting record of definite antigay bias. (Among other horrors, she voted to retain the sodomy law in Washington, D.C., at rectify any of what I'm writing about. Doctors—the very letters "M.D."—have enormous clout, particularly when they fight in groups. Can you imagine what gay doctors could accomplish, banded together in a network, petitioning local and federal governments, straight colleagues, and the American Medical Association. I am sick of the passivity or nonparticipation or half-hearted protestation of all the gay medical associations (American Physicians for Human Rights, Bay Area Physicians for Human Rights, Gay Psychiatrists of New York, etc., etc.), and particularly our own New York Physicians for Human Rights, a group of 175 of our gay doctors who have, as a group, done *nothing*. You can count on one hand the number of our doctors who have really worked for us.

I am sick of the *Advocate*, one of this country's largest gay publications, which has yet to quite acknowledge that there's anything going on. That newspaper's recent AIDS issue was so innocuous you'd have thought all we were going through was little worse than a rage of the latest designer flu. And their own associate editor, Brent Harris, died from AIDS. Figure that one out.

With the exception of the *New York Native* and a few, very few, other gay publications, the gay press has been useless. If we can't get our own papers and magazines to tell us what's really happening to us, and this negligence is added to the negligent noninterest of the straight press (the *New York Times* took a leisurely year and a half between its major pieces, and the *Village Voice* took a year and a half to write anything at all), how are we going to get the word around that we're dying? Gay men in smaller towns and cities everywhere must be educated, too. Has the *Times* or the *Advocate* told you that twenty-nine cases have been reported from Paris?

I am sick of gay men who won't support gay charities. Go give your bucks to straight charities, fellows, while we die. Gay Men's Health Crisis our only hope for national leadership, with its new and splendid leader, Virginia Apuzzo—which is spending more and more time fighting for the AIDS issue, is broke. Senior Action in a Gay Environment and Gay Men's Health Crisis are, within a few months, going to be without office space they can afford, and thus will be out on the street. The St. Mark's Clinic, held together by some of the few devoted gay doctors in this city who aren't interested in becoming rich, lives in constant terror of even higher rent and eviction. This community is desperate for the services these organizations are providing for it. And these organizations are all desperate for money, which is certainly not coming from straight people or President Reagan or Mayor Koch. (If every gay man within a 250-mile radius of Manhattan isn't in Madison Square Garden on the night of April 30 to help Gay Men's Health Crisis make enough money to get through the next horrible year of fighting against AIDS, I shall lose all hope that we have any future whatsoever.)

I am sick of closeted gays. It's 1983 already, guys, when are you going to come out? By 1984 you could be dead. Every gay man who is unable to come forward now and fight to save his own life is truly helping to kill the rest of us. There is only one thing that's going to save some of us, and this is *numbers* and pressure and our being perceived as united and a threat. As more and more of my friends die, I have less and less sympathy for men who are afraid their mommies will find out or afraid their bosses will find out or afraid their fellow doctors or professional associates will find out. Unless we can generate, visibly, numbers, masses, we are going to die.

I am sick of everyone in this community who tells me to stop creating a panic. How many of us have to die before *you* get scared off your ass and into action? Aren't 195 dead New Yorkers enough? Every straight person who is knowledgeable about the AIDS epidemic can't understand why gay men aren't marching on the White House. Over and over again I hear from them, "Why aren't you guys doing anything?" Every politician I have spoken to has said to me confidentially, "You guys aren't making enough noise. Bureaucracy only responds to pressure."

I am sick of people who say "it's no worse than statistics for smokers and lung cancer" or "considering how many homosexuals there are in the United States, AIDS is really statistically affecting only a very few." That would wash if there weren't 164 cases in twenty-eight days. That would wash if case numbers hadn't jumped from 41 to 1,112 in eighteen months. That would wash if cases in one city—New York—hadn't jumped to cases in fifteen countries and thirty-five states (up from thirty-four last week). That would wash if cases weren't coming in at more than four a day nationally and over two a day locally. That would wash if the mortality rate didn't start at 38 percent the first year of diagnosis and climb to a grotesque 86 percent after three years. Get your stupid heads out of the sand, you turkeys!

I am sick of guys who moan that giving up careless sex until this blows over is worse than death. How can they value life so little and cocks and asses so much? Come with me, guys, while I visit a few of our friends in Intensive Care at NYU. Notice the looks in their eyes, guys. They'd give up sex forever if you could promise them life.

I am sick of guys who think that all being gay means is sex in the first place. I am sick of guys who can only think with their cocks.

I am sick of "men" who say, "We've got to keep quiet or *they* will do such and such." *They* usually means the straight majority, the "Moral" Majority, or similarly perceived representatives of *them*. OK, you "men"—be my guests: You can march off now to the gas chambers; just get right in line.

We shall always have enemies. Nothing we can ever do will remove them. Southern newspapers and Jerry Falwell's publications are already printing editorials proclaiming AIDS as God's deserved punishments on homosexuals. So what? Nasty words make poor little sissy pansy wilt and die?

And I am very sick and saddened by every gay man who does not get behind this issue totally and with commitment—to fight for his life.

I don't want to die. I can only assume you don't want to die. Can we fight together?

For the past few weeks, about fifty community leaders and organization representatives have been meeting at Beth Simchat Torah, the gay synagogue, to prepare action. We call ourselves the AIDS Network. We come from all areas of health concern: doctors, social workers, psychologists, psychiatrists, nurses; we come from Gay Men's Health Crisis, from the National Gay Health Education Foundation, from New York Physicians for Human Rights, the St. Mark's Clinic, the Gay Men's Health Project; we come from the gay synagogue, the Gay Men's Chorus, from the Greater Gotham Business Council, SAGE, Lambda Legal Defense, Gay Fathers, the Christopher Street Festival Committee, Dignity, Integrity; we are lawyers, actors, dancers, architects, writers, citizens; we come from many component organizations of the Gay and Lesbian Community Council.

We have a leader. Indeed, for the first time our community appears to have a true leader. Her name is Virginia Apuzzo, she is head of the National Gay Task Force, and, as I have said, so far she has proved to be magnificent.

The AIDS Network has sent a letter to Mayor Koch. It contains twelve points that are urged for his consideration and action.

This letter to Mayor Koch also contains the following paragraph:

> *It must be stated at the outset that the gay community is growing increasingly aroused and concerned and angry. Should our avenues to the mayor of our city and the members of the Board of Estimate not be available, it is our feeling that the level of frustration is such that it will manifest itself in a manner heretofore not associated with this community and the gay population at large. It should be stated, too, at the outset, that as of February 25th, there were 526 cases of serious AIDS in New York's metropolitan area and 195 deaths (and 1,112 cases nationally and 418 deaths) and it is the sad and sorry fact that most gay men in our city now have close friends and lovers who have either been stricken with or died from this disease. It is against this background that this letter is addressed. It is this issue that has, ironically, united our community in a way not heretofore thought possible.*

Further, a number of AIDS Network members have been studying civil disobedience with one of the experts from Dr. Martin Luther King's old team. We are learning how. Gay men are the strongest, toughest people I know. We are perhaps shortly to get an opportunity to show it.

I'm sick of hearing that Mayor Koch doesn't respond to pressures and threats from the disenfranchised, that he walks away from confrontations. Maybe he does. But we have *tried* to make contact with him, we are *dying*, so what other choice but confrontation has he left us?

I hope we don't have to conduct sit-ins or tie up traffic or get arrested. I hope our city and our country will start to do something to help start saving us. But it is time for us to be perceived for what we truly are: an angry community and a strong community, and therefore *a threat*. Such are the realities of politics. Nationally we are twenty-four million strong, which is more than there are Jews or blacks or Hispanics in this country.

I want to make a point about what happens if we *don't* get angry about AIDS. There are the obvious losses, of course: Little of what I've written about here is likely to be rectified with the speed necessary to help the growing number of victims. But something worse will happen, and is already happening. Increasingly, we are being *blamed* for AIDS, for this epidemic; we are being called its perpetrators, through our blood, through our "promiscuity," through just being the gay men so much of the rest of the world has learned to hate. We can point out until we are blue in the face that we are not the cause of AIDS but its victims, that AIDS has landed among us first, as it could have landed among them first. But other frightened populations are going to drown out these truths by playing on the worst bigoted fears of the straight world, and send the status of gays right back to the Dark Ages. Not all Jews are blamed for Meyer Lansky, Rabbis Bergman and Kahane, or for money-lending. All Chinese aren't blamed for the recent Seattle slaughters. But all gays are blamed for John Gacy, the North American Man/Boy Love Association, and AIDS.

Enough. I am told this is one of the longest articles the *Native* has ever run. I hope I have not been guilty of saying ineffectively in five thousand words what I could have said in five: we must fight to live.

I am angry and frustrated almost beyond the bound my skin and bones and body and brain can encompass. My sleep is tormented by nightmares and visions of lost friends, and my days are flooded by the tears of funerals and memorial services and seeing my sick friends. How many of us must die before *all* of us living fight back?

I know that unless I fight with every ounce of my energy I will hate myself. I hope, I pray, I implore you to feel the same.

I am going to close by doing what Dr. Ron Grossman did at GMHC's second Open Forum last November at Julia Richman High School. He listed the names of the patients he had lost to AIDS. Here is a list of twenty dead men I knew:

Nick Rock, Rick Wellikoff, Jack Nau, Shelly, Donald Krintzman, Jerry Green, Michael Maletta, Paul Graham, Toby, Harry Blumenthal, Stephen Sperry, Brian O'Hara, Barry, David, Jeffrey Croland, Z., David Jackson, Tony Rappa, Robert Christian, Ron Doud. And one more, who will be dead by the time these words appear in print.

If we don't act immediately, then we face our approaching doom.

Volunteers Needed for Civil Disobedience

It is necessary that we have a pool of at least three thousand people who are prepared to participate in demonstrations of civil disobedience. Such demonstrations might include sit-ins or traffic tie-ups. All participants must be prepared to be arrested. I am asking every gay person and every gay organization to canvass all friends and members and make a count of the total number of people you can provide toward this pool of three thousand.

Let me know how many people you can be counted on providing. Just include the number of people; you don't have to send actual names—you keep that list yourself. And include your own phone numbers. *Start these lists now.*

EQUAL TO MURDERERS

LARRY KRAMER

from Reports from the Holocaust: The Making of an AIDS Activist

| 1989 |

11 June 1984

To:

Mr. Abe Rosenthal, *The New York Times*
Dr. Lawrence Altman, *The New York Times*
Mr. Tom Morgan, *The New York Times*
Judge Richard Failla, Gay Men's Health Crisis
Mr. Rodger McFarlane, Gay Men's Health Crisis
Mr. Paul Popham, Gay Men's Health Crisis
Ms. Virginia Apuzzo, National Gay Task Force
Dr. David Sencer, Commissioner of Health
Dr. Roger Enlow, Office of Gay and Lesbian Health
Mayor Edward Koch

I am attaching an article from last Friday's *Washington Post* entitled "AIDS Epidemic Is Expanding, Not Shrinking, Experts Say." As you can see, this was a main, featured article, appearing on page A-3. It was sent to me by Tim Westmoreland, counsel to Representative Henry Waxman, who is chairman of the House Subcommittee on Health. Tim, like me, cannot understand why there is so little information passed on to the New York community about the appalling continuation, the march of this epidemic. After all, New York is still the worst hit. There are now *over four* new cases every day in this area, but you would not know it from reading the *New York Times*, or any of the literature put out by the above offices. The worst epidemic known to modern man is happening right here in this very city, and it is one of the best-kept secrets around.

All that is asked for, from all of you, is to transmit information, to keep an endangered population informed. Why is that so difficult?

That all of you listed above continue to refuse to transmit to the public the facts and figures of what is happening *daily* makes you, in my mind, equal to murderers, with blood on your hands just as if you had used knives or bullets or poison. Because you continue to refuse to inform New York's population, the perception by the average gay man on the street is that this epidemic has disappeared or leveled off or improved. Because of false hope (owing to the announcement that a virus has been isolated) that a cure will come tomorrow, the average gay man is back to living with his head in the sand. Because the *New York Times* is not reporting this vital news, because the city's Department of Health is not disseminating these appalling statistics, because the gay community's own organizations are too cowardly to speak out and speak up—all of this perpetuates the widespread ignorance that can only make for continued contagion, infection, and—at the present rate of increase—a minimum of sixty-four thousand cases in two years' time.

In the name of God, Christ, Moses, whatever impels you to, at last, perform acts of humanity, when will you address this issue with the courage it demands?

2

RESPONSE and BACKLASH

THE NEW RIGHT

CINDY PATTON

from Sex & Germs

| 1985 |

At the beginning of its emergence in the 1970s, the New Right's social program seemed sadly out of step with the times. Although their economic agenda has received extensive analysis and strategic attention, many progressives view the New Right's regressive social agenda as a smoke screen to be taken seriously only as a *bas-relief* of the reactionary spirit hidden among more sophisticated conservatives. But to dismiss the absurdity of New Right rhetoric misses the real power that their visceral authoritarianism holds on a profoundly Calvinist nation.

The New Right's response to AIDS displays in blatant, ghastly terms what is latent in even the most sophisticated liberals. Old notions of sin, sickness, and criminality emerge in a full program aimed at suppressing difference. Skeptical that scientific "facts" are part of a liberal conspiracy, radical rightists look for physical signs that distinguish the sinful from the pure. One of the remarkable features of fundamentalist Christian and neopopulist right-wing ideologues is their obsession with matters corporeal. In ironic contrast, the U.S. Left has in recent years been more fascinated by intellectual and historical processes. This political mind/body split creates an almost unbridgeable conceptual gulf laying each open to humorous and vicious caricature in the literature of the other.

Physical control and restraint are ideologically, strategically, and symbolically significant to the New Right. Eras of rightist ascendancy are marked by legislative shifts toward more stringent physical controls—law and order, capital punishment, punishment of sexuality, more stringent pedagogical styles. Rightist ascendancy is accompanied by renewed interest in participation in organized religion, with its individual daily rituals of discipline, and its weekly collective worship.

A symbolism of physical restraint and bodily invasion translates the abstract Calvinist concepts of the right-wing ideology into a vivid and visceral reality, deeply felt by adherents and opponents alike. Using lurid descriptions and hateful edicts, propagandists ask their constituencies whether they want to expose their children to the sin and sickness of homosexuals, blacks, Jews, even "idol-worshiping" Catholics. Implicit in their rhetoric, and explicit in their policies, is a notion of racial purity and absolute community consensus that decries pluralism and abhors "mixing."

SEE NO EVIL

A political ideology that taps deep, inchoate feelings about pain and pleasure, freedom and restraint has particular potency. Profoundly morbid, yet sincerely apocalyptic, the right-wing populism terrifies individuals with stories of plots barely held in check by rituals of cleansing and constant vigilance to avert one's eyes lest one inadvertently stare pure evil in the face. Although they have gained political prominence with rhetoric about the return to traditional norms, the New Right is a profoundly countercultural movement: like the apocalyptic Left movement of the 1960s, their goal is to supplant the existing culture.

Calvinism's bizarre mix of predestination with scrutiny of acts as signs of election loses little of its paranoid force and zealotry through secularization and technocratization. Indeed, these trends reignite the Calvinist search for proof of God's supremacy over "man." New Right Calvinism accedes to a program of "Christ against culture" by allowing leaders to prove their election in symbolic or real battle with the evil forces of homosexuality, abortion, miscegenation, etc.

Their crude mix of crusading authoritarianism and religious populism allows New Right leaders to go out and do battle with the forces of perversion, sparing the innocent citizen the danger of confronting the foe him/herself. Computer-engineered direct-mail and TV evangelism are the miracle of technology in the service of Calvinism. By paying money to the various groups, the vigilant moralist can stay locked safely at home, out of danger of pollution by contact with the diseased sinners.

Yet, there is a lot of peeping between the fingers. New Right leaders prove their cause (and garner ever more funds) with tantalizing glimpses of the grotesque evils they are combating. But the propagandists and direct-mail letter writers must continually up the ante: each new cause must seem more lurid, more dangerous, more immediate than the last if they expect letters to get more support. It is less the particular information conveyed than the process of breaking taboos that repulses and tantalizes readers and contributors. The tactic turns product advertising on its head: instead of selling items which the consumer can't do without, the radical Right markets shocking and threatening images which readers can't afford to live with. A classic direct-mail fund-raising letter from the American Family Association encourages its readers with a come-on to close down homosexual establishments by signing their petition:

> Dear Family Member,
>
> Since AIDS is transmitted primarily by perverse homosexuals, your name on my national petition to quarantine all homosexual establishments is crucial to your family's health and security. . . . These disease carrying deviants wander the street unconcerned, possibly making *you* their next victim. What else can you expect from sex-crazed degenerates but selfishness?

Finally, after impressing the reader with the immediacy and magnitude of this threat, it is clear that only money will do the trick:

> Our effort to WIPE OUT AIDS will cost thousands of dollars. I have established a budget of $28,570.00 for the next 15 days' expenses. We must fight this crucial battle through the newspapers, television media and even door to door! But all this costs money. . . . I urge you to return your signed petition and generous gift to me today.
>
> P.S. Only your contribution can help us protect Americans from the "Gay Plague" and its perverted carriers. Please send your generous contribution and signed petition to me today.

Signing a petition (although they do make their way to governors and federal officials like Surgeon General Koop) is a variation on reader-participation schemes: "put the enclosed token in the slot and send $25 for your subscription to—."

Christian Family Renewal circulated a similar "petition" as a fund-raiser:

> You may soon fall victim to an irreversible, fatal disease! And it won't be your fault!
>
> But, you'll have to pay the terrible price anyway because of the promiscuous homosexuals, whose lustful life-styles have created this uncontrollable incurable plague.

They cleverly play on the euphemism of "life-style" to equate gay rights with destruction.

> And now, they've acquired their own distinct death-style, the AIDS plague, and like all their other rights, the homosexuals are forcing this painful, deadly disease on the rest of society.
>
> . . . Send the largest gift you can as if your life—and it very well may—depended on it.
>
> AIDS MUST BE STOPPED NOW! I'm trusting you realize the drastic and emergency steps we're about to take together is the only way to stop this dreaded disease.

Enclosed with this letter is a yellow petition and donation card that is bordered with the purple imprint of, presumably, healthy cells.

The Right's systematic misinformation and mind-boggling distortion of medical reports blurs the distinction between transmission of an etiological agent during sexual activity and the sexual acts themselves: homosexual acts become the *prima facie* cause of AIDS. Once the notion of a virus is dropped from the equation, the disease becomes proof of the commission of an immoral act. Death is not too great a penalty for violation of moral law. Conversely, for a "normal" or "innocent" person to die as the result of this disease is a horrible travesty, worse than the disease itself.

The ultimate corporeal threat of death or proof of election through death is important ammunition in the arsenal of radical right hate ideology. To die for a just cause (like war) ennobles life. To desecrate life (by being a homosexual or having an abortion) merits death. In Calvinist ideology, life itself is not symbolically valued except as an opportunity to demonstrate election. Death is far more valuable as a principle for organizing morality. Predestination means that no good works can produce salvation, but to doubt one's election and live as if one were destined for hell is the worst of sins. Risking death provides an opportunity to prove election by dramatically demonstrating faith. To rightists, some death is very cheap indeed, but life is even cheaper. The rightists are firmly and self-consciously apocalyptic and can strategize final solutions.

AIDS is a particularly potent symbol for the hard-line radical right because it is evidence of sin, God's disfavor, and an ultimate solution: it is both a sign and a punishment embodied in one of the groups targeted for political decimation long before AIDS. Even rightist doctors, whom one supposes might separate their science and bigotry, have fused them into pseudoscientific logic:

> If we act as empirical scientists, can we not see the implications of the data before us? If homosexuality, or even just male homosexuality, is "OK," then why the high prevalence of associated complications both in general and especially with respect to AIDS? Might not these "complications" be "consequences"? Might it be that our society's approval of homosexuality is an error and that the unsubtle words of wisdom of the Bible are frightfully correct?
>
> Indeed, from an empirical medical perspective alone, current scientific observation seems to require the conclusion that homosexuality is a pathologic condition.

SPEAK NO EVIL

Until very recently, those who had to make authoritative pronouncements on homosexuality used euphemisms that made it clear that "it" was not a fit topic of conversation. Numerous historians have catalogued the "namelessness" of this "crime" that sheds light on evolving social views of homosexuality. An Illinois judge was forced to comment on the subject in 1897, and said that the crime against nature was "not fit to be named among Christians." D'Emilio notes that "commentators composed their remarks according to a formula that discouraged further amplification."

Through the 1950s and 1960s, although lesbian/gay activists saw some increased coverage of their issues and events, homosexuality was a topic that many wanted neither to see nor hear about. An October 7, 1959, San Francisco *Progress* headline read, "Sex Deviates Make San Francisco Headquarters." The story read, "homosexualism has been allowed to flourish to a shocking extent, and under shocking circumstances." Lest the poor innocent who has never even heard of homosexualism be misled, he or she is repeatedly told that sex deviates are on the rise, and it is "shocking" but the story offers no concrete information on who these sex deviates are or what it is they do. This incipient form of social terrorism lets people know that something is happening that they are better off not knowing about. The fascist mentality that unearthed and described "spy rings" under the dubious machinations of national security invented a plot of homosexuals who were alleged to be weakening the moral fiber of U.S. citizens. Even today some rightist groups claim that homosexuality and even AIDS is a communist plot, despite the fact that communist countries and parties have generally been hostile toward homosexuality. With the homosexual plot, the government and media asked citizens to trust that there was nothing of merit to know about homosexuality except that it was being vigilantly rooted out: the less said about perversion, the better.

Even after sex became accepted as a subject of scientific study with Kinsey, Masters and Johnson, Hite, Rubin, and other less popularized reports, medical doctors, religious leaders, and media still confused scientific terms and their symbolic uses. The same San Francisco *Progress* story claimed that "this unsavory wicked situation is allowed to fester and spread like a cancerous growth on the body of San Francisco." Dr. Charles Socarides, at the June 1968 AMA convention, said homosexuality was a "dread dysfunction, malignant in character, which has risen to epidemic proportions."

Right-wing solipsists have used medical and military imagery interchangeably: reds and queers were alternately diseases and invasions. The military/disease imagery was honed in the 1950s during the extensively covered House Un-American Activities Committee (HUAC) trials. Although homosexuality was less overtly discussed (though much alluded to), communism and faggotry were well established as threats to U.S. security. Both were assaults from within U.S. culture—infiltration—by people who didn't look different to the untrained eye. The HUAC trials heightened the paranoid search for the telltale limp wrist or a certain turn of nose—signs of perversion or foreignness that became markers of guilt that needed no court.

Despite recent losses, the lesbian/gay community made a crucial, if little observed gain, which cannot be repealed along with civil rights statutes. Through increasing coverage of lesbian/gay issues in news and features, as well as the proliferation of lesbian/gay book titles and an aboveground press, homosexuality has acquired not only "a name," but a sophisticated vocabulary of distinctions. Language about homosexuality has evolved from vague, embarrassed references through the euphemistic "lifestyle" until today even very conservative politicians refer to the "lesbian and gay community" as they rail against homosexuality. "Lifestyle" has become appropriated from "me generation" jargon to indicate a consumerist neo-pluralism. While serving as editor of Boston's *Gay Community News*, I received a call asking for the "Lifestyle" editor. I was tempted to reply in my best high camp, "But darling, we *are* a lifestyle."

Media coverage surrounding lesbian/gay victories and losses accepts the existence of a lesbian/gay political force: a vote to be courted by liberals, a conspiracy to be unmasked by rightists. Mainstream media accounts of lesbian/gay political activity rubber stamped the consolidation of a lesbian/gay identity that has at least some political interests in common by admitting the existence of a constituency capable of collective action. In the New Right literature, lesbians and gay men graduated from a covert conspiracy to an audacious and open lobby.

This more open discourse on homosexuality made possible a kind of coverage of AIDS that would have been unfathomable fifteen years ago. Not only do lesbians and gay men exist, but, at least in the AIDS coverage, they are undoubtedly sexual beings. And in a second interesting shift, the actuality of gay male sex acts has reached some level of public articulation, even if more colloquial terms like "cock sucking" or "fucking" are replaced by "oral" and "anal" intercourse. Under the guise of scientific reporting, direct references to gay male sex acts moved from crime stories buried in the Help Wanted section, to the front page of the news and "living" sections. Implicitly, the idea that scientists were examining these taboo areas of the "love that dare not speak its name" both legitimized and demythologized gay male (but not lesbian) sexual practice for at least some media consumers.

A more explicit discussion of gay male sex is necessary in the New Right literature, too, if they are to capitalize on this opportunity to prove their point. Discussion of AIDS in scientific terms by right-wing doctors and lay people serves to legitimize misinformation by appearing objective and scientific while making their political agenda clear with prefaces to the "facts" that are apologies for having to tell innocent people these disgusting things. In order to cash in on the political power of science, New Right propagandists must scientologize their antisex tracts and add the litany of gay male sex acts to counter claims that homosexuality is just another kind of sex: recitation provides a vivid exposé of the "excesses" of homosexuality. It is no longer enough to allude to vague acts that "can't be named by Christians."

The laundry list of perverse acts elicits great interest among New Rightists, and a constantly increasing diet seems to be necessary to feed this horror of unleashed sexuality and sex germs. The scientific discussion of heterosexual sex that has given baby boom adults a blasé attitude toward imagery that shocked their parents has merely been extended to gay male sex (no one yet knows what lesbians do!). The list isn't nearly as frightening as the speak-no-evil rightists feared, even if the inflated numbers of "average" sexual partners is mind-boggling (it's just new math). The New Right's own revelation of perverse sexual practices has undermined its ability to shock.

RIGHTIST NEO-POPULISM

The New Right did not spring into existence full-blown merely to combat the evils of homosexuality and abortion, although U.S. activism is so often fragmented and ahistorical that it must seem that way to those activists who cut their teeth in the last two decades. Nor is the New Right a coherent monolith.

The New Right welds together bits of fundamentalist Christianity, fear of anything different, genuine frustration with leaders who don't seem to represent anyone, and a political primitivism reminiscent of the Know-Nothing party, a similar U.S. grassroots reactionism that gained prominence in the mid-nineteenth century.

At their height, the Know-Nothings elected seventy-five congressional representatives but they never passed any significant legislation. Their appeal lay in their finger-pointing: "aliens" (European immigrants, not space invaders) were the root of all social ills. They offered no concrete solution, and supported no coherent program. Like the New Right today, they became entrenched in a mentality of zealous separatism predicated on opposition to an inchoate and contradictory "other" composed of a plurality of immigrants and urbanites in the burgeoning industrialized East. The Know-Nothings are distinguished by their isolationism, populism, negativism, and attitude that the West represented the "real America." Nostalgic and anti-progressive, the Know-Nothings split over the issue of slavery, and by 1895 they had no significant federal representation and were reduced to an out-of-touch, infighting group of political incompetents.

The rift between the East and the West/South bloc of "pioneers" that spawned the Know-Nothings extends for over one hundred years of U.S. political history, and lays some of the foundation for the New Right today. The new Old West cowboy mentality of Reaganism provides a convenient symbol for the New Right's ascendancy in the 1980s, even if Reagan did not live up to the New Right's expectations in his first term by being too corporatist and centralist. Through his rhetoric of traditionalism and the sheer idiocy of his public blunders, Reagan thrives in his second term because of the zealous personality cult surrounding him. If Reagan says everyone is better off, many people are convinced, in spite of real decreases in spending power as measured by common indexes. Liberals and leftists who fail to see the power of the Calvinist undercurrent tapped by Reaganism cannot understand why economic oppression seems like moral liberation. Material conditions no longer matter to the Protestant middle and lower classes if cessation of doubt rather than worldly wealth becomes the measure of Christian election.

> It is the rich who by risking their wealth ultimately lose it, and save the economy. . . . That is the function of the rich: fostering opportunities for the classes below them in the continuing drama of creation of wealth and progress.
>
> This drama is most essentially not of measurable money and machines, aggregations and distributions, but of mind and morale.

With a brash wave of his wand, George Gilder, architect of Reagan's supply-side ethics, dismisses all materialist analysis and class antagonisms. The wealthy who engage in capitalism (not charity) are altruistic because they engender opportunities for the whole economy. The new Southern and Western rich, whose vast wealth is amassed from venture capitalist endeavors (not inheritance or trusts, like the Eastern establishment wealthy) are the elect, not because to be rich is to be saved, but rather because they command and deploy the resources which, when "lost," save the whole economy. The rugged *individual* capitalist may lose his shirt by financing the wrong business, but even this proves his election: doubting capital, and not risking it, is a grave offense and these wealthy will not enter the gates of heaven. This parable of wealth and poverty, faith and doubt gives hope to the lower classes in the most crass Horatio Algeresque sense, and tricks them into believing that their natural antagonists—the financially active rich—are really trying to help them.

THE CULTURAL BATTLE LINES

The 1970s were marked by a struggle between the New Right and two new political forces: the women's liberation and lesbian/gay liberation movements. Anti-Vietnam war forces had won the letter of their battle, though not the spirit, and the "ecology" movement seemed to be the trend, even if things were not progressing very rapidly. The prevailing mainstream mentality was labeled the "me generation," which, deserved or not, became a self-fulfilling media prophecy. Traditional notions of conservative versus liberal broke down: the 1970s mainstream was held together by shared economic and personal values, not by a coherent political spirit.

The idea of the "me generation" became an effective if subtle method for diverting the struggle for civil rights and cultural autonomy that marked lesbian/gay, women's, and ethnic groups' liberation struggles. As if to prove that the U.S. had won on the domestic front, even if it had lost abroad, the "me generation" ideology pretended to have overcome the color bar by including faces of color on ads for consumer products. A propaganda of introspection could ignore surface color and class differences as long as there was a Cuisinart in the kitchen and Le Car in the garage.

"Telling it like it is" gave way to "I am what I am." Liberal born-again moderationism sought to wash away the bad taste of both the conservative conspiracy of Watergate and the radical student and black riots. The "me generation" ideology neatly embraced an offended middle class of all colors, the unregulated rich, and to some extent the urban low-income people who had moved just above poverty with social service programs that had not yet been dismantled. There was still a Great Society ethos, although the political ideology of fairness at home and peace abroad was quietly being slipped out of the practicality back door. Optimistic liberals believed that progressive changes would remain intact, that the chaos was merely a settling-in period. The Right was drawing different conclusions: chaos was the problem, and progressive changes were the impediment to a strong U.S. In the 1984 national election, liberal fairness gave way to a concept of justice that told the traditionally disadvantaged to pull up their own bootstraps. Threat of war was only the most blatant form of terrorism, as random, state-supported violence reached paramilitary proportions.

Feminist and lesbian/gay activists were able to mobilize in the environment of the "me generation" ethos in part because sexism and homophobia made their self-consciousness seem like introspection, "getting in touch with feelings," self-expression, or acting out—1960s countercultural values that were twisted and marketed in the 1970s to promote consumerism over activism. The radical Right could ascend in this very same environment because their rhetoric alone translated the social upheaval of the 1960s and 1970s to bewildered, conservative, nonactivist citizens.

Primarily cultural critiques, all three rejected attempts to buy off a nation struggling to place in perspective a meaningless and lost war, and a sinister and lying president. Fundamentalist Christians and populist rightists were not tantalized by decadent toys and a media that increasingly promoted a sexualized consumer aesthetic. Feminists and lesbian/gay activists were not lulled by these salves to a badly bruised U.S. Women couldn't afford the toys, and at any rate, were part of the consumer package. The lesbian/gay culture, where it existed, was circumscribed from open consumption by fear of harassment or discovery. The emerging Right and the feminist and lesbian/gay movements, at least on the surface, all criticized the structure of the same institutions—family, church, sexual relations.

The battle lines were drawn dramatically between the New Right and the women's and lesbian/gay liberation movements, and between blacks and radical rightists. The various movements who stood in opposition to the radical Right would eventually meander toward the "rainbow coalition," a strategically and ideologically significant realignment of the last remnants of the New Deal coalition. Moderates stood by alternately amused by the incomprehensible demands of gays and women, and repulsed by the insanity of New Right disinformation. Moderates did not initially take either of the groups seriously and hedged their political bets by accommodating to both.

Jimmy Carter's election most aptly captures the spirit of the moderates in the 1970s. The Carter years were distinguished by "trying to answer the spiritual needs of a frightened Calvinist mainstream while courting the very people scaring them most." Carter pacified the broad mainstream with his rhetoric of moral restoration, while failing to put the lid on Pandora's box of new cultural values. The radical Right and the cultural progressives both bid for structural power in the years between Watergate/Vietnam and the first Reagan election. Liberals and moderates, perplexed by noneconomistic social programs, ceded the most important turf to the New Right—control over the body.

Reaganism has ripped off the language of grassroots activism from the left/feminist/gay movements and dismantled the federal support for community-based programs of the 1960s and 1970s. The right-wing majoritarianism threatens to replace liberal pluralism. Despite the experience of progressives in the last two decades, whose history created a belief that grassroots organizing is necessarily progressive, if the roots are planted in traditional soil the movement spawned will exhibit a rightward tropism. The similarity in progressive and right-wing rhetoric stems in part from a battle to control grassroots-style organizing.

The decentralist neo-populism of the New Right is different from leftists' socialist populism in strategy and theory. However, the right-wing populism, and some new versions of "left" populism, bear an important feature in common. Both move toward analyzing racism and sexism in economistic terms, even though Gilder is anti-Marxian and the progressives are Marxian. New Rightists blame liberal economic policies for supposedly making blacks and women dependent on the welfare state, which then multiplies the oppression of women by causing the breakdown of the family. If women can strike less of a bargain in the sexual arena, they must depend on the state rather than punish errant males by coercing them into economic support through marriage.

Neo-progressive economic reductionists insist that continued attention to race *per se* only incites racial tension. They believe that great strides have been made to remove individual prejudice and citizens must move on to address structural economic barriers which prohibit blacks from gaining equal economic clout. Both neo-populisms reject the cultural pluralist values embodied in the "rainbow coalition" by asserting that given equal access to material, everyone will "be the same."

HATE RHETORIC

A critical point of dissonance among rightists concerns the reformability of homosexuals. Some groups have bid for greater credibility (as more "conservative" homosexuals have "come out") by tempering their rhetoric. Christian groups have countered the criticisms of their hate-mongering by professing to "love the homosexual, but hate homosexuality." This logic conveniently allows that some children might grow up to be homosexuals for reasons beyond their control—hormones, bad family experiences, lack of protection from queers—and shifts the moral burden toward "making good choices," or doing what is right in the face of a bad deal. They see two categories of homosexuals: those who try not to act on their perverse urges and those who flagrantly commit homosexual acts. These groups of New Rightists seek to convert homosexuals and AIDS provides particularly fertile ground. Their logic claims that antigay campaigns are not bigoted but compassionate programs to help the homosexuals stop killing themselves.

> This pamphlet has been written for the benefit of heterosexuals and homosexuals alike. We believe that homosexual sex practices seriously threaten the

> well-being of the individual homosexual along with the well-being of our nation. Our goal is to diminish that danger for both.

Like Gilder's attack on liberal society this and other groups blame AIDS and the "spread" of homosexuality on the permissive society that allowed the lesbian/gay liberation movement to even speak its name.

> Over the last two decades, Americans have become increasingly tolerant of homosexuals and "homosexual practices." What consenting adults did in private was of no real concern at all to many of the last several generations.
>
> Now it turns out that homosexuals and their practices can threaten our lives, our families, our children, can influence whether or not we have elective surgery, eat in certain restaurants, visit a given city or take up a certain profession or career—all because a tiny minority flaunts its lifestyle and demands that an entire nation tolerate its diseases and grant it status as a privileged minority.

The New Rightists differ in their position on whether the homosexual with AIDS can relinquish "his" dangerous state of homosexuality. One group claims to be more compassionate than its farther right brethren, and purports to being committed to saving AIDS "victims" through prayer.

> I had made a silent agreement with the Lord not to wear the assigned robe, plastic gloves or any other garment required in visiting an AIDS patient. . . . I leaned closer to him and spoke very carefully, so that he would understand my words, "Charles, this is not a judgment from God but a consequence of our past lifestyles. Different people live different lifestyles. When these are out of order with God's best for us, consequences come. All of us in this room have suffered consequences and are unworthy of God's grace. . . ."
>
> I asked Charles if he would like us to pray with him for his healing. His answer was affirmative. I explained that there are two healings for which to pray. The first and most important was his spiritual healing.
>
> We prayed also for his physical restoration. The next day, we returned to take him the New Testament on tape to feed him spiritually. We were astounded at his physical progress in 24 hours time. His fever was down. . . . We believe with Charles that God is in the business of restoring and making WHOLE ALL THOSE WHO ARE STRUGGLING SPIRITUALLY OR PHYSICALLY WITH SATAN'S LIES.

It is unclear whether they think they have cured AIDS or homosexuality. This conflation of the "gay disease" with the gay person is persistent throughout the Right's AIDS literature (and everywhere else in AIDS imagery). But this lack of clarity passes unnoticed by the right-wing audience, since their real agenda is to get rid of all homosexuals one way or another.

AIDS rhetoric merely becomes a more sophisticated antigay campaign that pretends to be more enlightened. The patronizing tone of the literature varies from "we told you so" to "we tried to be nice to homosexuals, but this time they've gone too far." Antigay AIDS literature arises from the political stalemate between far right initiatives to void progressive lesbian/gay rights ordinances and the increased numbers of lesbian/gay or supportive politicians in elective and appointive offices. The right wing views AIDS as proof that even if their rhetoric and strategy was inarticulate and not wholly effective, their logic was correct: gays are a scourge to society and to themselves.

> Prayer Focus: AIDS—That God would prevent the spread of this dreaded disease to the general public, use it to expose the depravity of homosexuality and cause those who are practicing homosexuals to repent and totally reject their detestable life style. May He have mercy and bring healing to those AIDS victims who repent and turn to Him.

The Tearcatchers provide a pamphlet on counseling the gay person, maintaining that the rabid right-wing Christians have given the rest of the evangelicals a bad name. By the end of the several-page, well-produced pamphlet containing accurate information and good resources, however, the message is much the same: convert homosexuals from their sexual practice. This view that homosexual identity can't change but individuals can stop practicing gay sex has been maintained by a range of religious institutions, including the Catholic church and the relatively liberal Methodists. They concede that some homosexuals can't change (then they don't have to admit defeat when the lesbian/gay person keeps having lesbian/gay sexual desire) but they can be "ministered to" by helping them live happily with celibacy. This idea embraces the homosexual individual within the church but says, kindly leave your dirty sexual habits at the door, thank you. With the advent of AIDS, even the liberal Christian has stopped to wonder: if gays themselves are advocating safe sex (which, given the level of knowledge of most middle Americans about gay sexual practice, probably sounds like celibacy or at any rate marriage) then perhaps they were right to discourage gay sex all along. AIDS, like VD historically, is viewed as willfully contracted. One rightist medical doctor said: ". . . a logical conclusion is that AIDS is a self-inflicted disorder for the majority of those who suffer from it."

The Moral Majority began lobbying against federal AIDS funding in 1982.

> If the medical community thinks that a new drug is what is needed to combat these diseases, it is deluding itself. There is a price to pay for immorality and immoral behavior.

A little more than a year later:

> Why should the taxpayers have to spend money to cure diseases that don't have to start in the first place? Let's help the drug users who want to be helped and the Haitian people. But let's let the homosexual community do its own research. Why should the American taxpayer have to bail out these perverted people?

Tearcatchers disapproves of this compassionless approach. Not only will the Moral Majority's attitude endanger the public health by not deploying all possible resources to stop the disease, but it does not address the "real" cause of AIDS, which they claim is promiscuity. They still oppose homosexuality, not because it is in itself immoral, but because it is a symptom of the crisis of masculinity wrought by the women's movement. Shunning the homosexual in the age of AIDS is missing out on a brilliant opportunity for evangelism to people confused by progressive political movements, a sentiment echoed in the *Be Whole* letter cited above.

But the sex problem goes deeper. U.S. Protestantism is the heir of the Puritan notion that there is good sex and bad sex, good violence and bad violence. Good sex takes place in the confines of marriage and serves to weld together the family unit through procreation, or in the more liberal home, through the healthy display of intimacy within the married couple. Good violence is that exercised by the state through the military or police. The New Right advocates penalizing nonmarital, nonprocreative sex with just violence—capital punishment, quarantine, or simply letting unrepentant homosexuals kill themselves off with AIDS. Right-wing populism justifies its generally pro–legitimate violence, antisex stand as a secular version of religious redemption. Gilder makes particularly insidious connections between the economy of sex and the ideology of violence:

> The key to lower-class life in contemporary America is that unrelated individuals, as the census calls them, are so numerous and conspicuous that they set the tone for the entire community . . .
>
> . . . The lives of the poor, all too often, are governed by the rhythms of tension and release that characterize the sexual experience of young single men. Because female sexuality, as it evolved over the millennia, is psychologically rooted in the bearing and nurturing of children, women have long horizons within their very bodies, glimpses of eternity within their wombs. Civilized society is dependent upon the submission of the short-term sexuality of young men to the extended maternal horizons of women. This is what happens in monogamous marriage; the man disciplines his sexuality and extends it into the future through the womb of a woman.

NEW RIGHT AND FAMILY IDEOLOGY

The New Right appeals across class lines by creating a symbol of unity that makes no overt class reference. "The family" is the galvanizing symbol of the New Right, and engenders programs that aim to reverse the trends that are perceived to have attacked the nuclear family. The family so ardently defended is in reality a recent and predominantly white, middle-class, Anglo-American invention, and not even the dominant pattern in the U.S. As a symbol enmeshed in a politics of paranoia, the "family" neatly defines categories of people who fall outside it as intruders, anti-American. This pro-family rhetoric allows the Right to see as coherent the left, feminist, and lesbian/gay liberation movements, even though these progressive movements do not agree on a common agenda. This is the same "up-against-ness" that fueled the Know-Nothings and other antiprogressive backlashes: it is easier to define a reaction against progressive changes than to develop a coherent rightist program. Only now that the Right has achieved some structural power has it been necessary to create an umbrella of theory, but this theory only rationalizes disparate reactionisms rather than building a systematic plan from a clearly articulated critique. The New Left experienced similar cohesion problems in the seventies, with the positive result of the emerging "rainbow coalition" but the negative trend toward a pro-family left faction and economistic neo-progressives who ignore cultural and sexual oppression.

Family rhetoric is potent and sensational, like pictures of children and puppies, and it is difficult to argue against the paranoid clutching for something that is more myth than reality. Major rightist efforts have attempted to legislate a pro-family agenda. The Family Protection Act, now being resubmitted to Congress in pieces, as well as the outrageous Model Sexuality Bill (which appears in piecemeal form as an exclusion of other fair practice bills) reverse legislation which enabled greater access to social services and civil rights remedies for a wide range of people. These bills recreate the pre–civil rights structural impediments, only this time through a conscious effort.

WOMEN AND THE RIGHT

The New Right updates the script of traditional gender-based social disparity. Men are still out riding the political range, risking contact with the pagan perverts while fighting for gun ownership, national defense, law and order. New Right women protect the hearth and home through domestic politics—issues involving family, children, school, and the church. There is no contradiction between their belief that "a woman's place is in the home," and their brand of activism—women engage in public politics only on issues that are an extension of the domestic arena. The division of political labor by sex doubles the available "manpower" without creating internal splits like those experienced on the left: for example, progressive feminists organized autonomously from men after their experiences with the male-dominated Left.

Phyllis Schlafly, whose pamphlet "AIDS-ERA" epitomizes the New Right tendency toward disinformation, claims to be a single-issue leader. By subsuming abortion, lesbianism, the draft, and now AIDS under the banner of anti-ERA organizing, she claims interest in a "single issue," not a broader political (i.e., male) agenda which might, incidentally, make Schlafly's bid for power contradict her position on the ERA. Many members of her Eagle Forum disagree on the issues related to ERA but the fervor of Schlafly's rhetoric and tidy conflation prevents issue differences from emerging vocally enough to cause a split on the symbolic main issue of the ERA.

The New Right obscures the political agenda of the principal leaders by maintaining this illusion of grassroots, single-issue organizing. One of the major factors that has permitted the far Right to maintain this position is a small core of power-brokers and several computers. Where the Left has traditionally instilled a sense of political participation through direct action, the far Right creates a sense of belonging and action through letter writing, petition, and financial contribution—methods that create a sense of unity and mass without gathering people together in face-to-face discussion. The core New Right activists amass great financial resources and provoke very little opposition or call for accountability. The newsletters depend on a personal anti-intellectual style that claims its authenticity by fueling the paranoia that no one else will tell the reader the truth. This intimate experience of receiving the privileged truth at home creates a zeal which requires very little commitment of time and energy, and doesn't require the New Right masses to be politically active in a world full of dangerous people. This separatist ethos heightens individual paranoia and makes New Right followers increasingly dependent on their leaders.

The New Right has been successful in building a base of power outside big business and the two parties, traditional sources of conservative power. From their extra-party base, they have taken over the ultra-conservative wings of both parties. They promote a politics of revenge, often attacking candidates they don't like rather than offering their own. This negative strategy allows them to rally voters against candidates who favor specific issues without having to form a coalition that can agree on enough issues to elect an alternative candidate. Issues are highlighted in a domino theory format: rightists often support candidates who have the correct view on a few key issues (especially abortion, busing, and homosexuality) but have a totally different philosophy. The New Right leaders that emerge maintain an air of reluctance, and claim to be "out front followers."

The differences in the various New Right group's positions on AIDS create little conflict: the real goal is to manipulate AIDS to gain popular support. In decentralist rhetoric of community control or community standards, the community defined by the Right excludes the people to be controlled by the standards. Thus, U.S. Department of Health and Human Services secretary, Margaret Heckler, can have it both ways when she claims that AIDS is her department's number-one priority. Uncritical progressives may applaud the apparent deployment of federal resources (however scant), but the right knows that the money is going to develop blood tests and vaccines to protect "the innocent," and not primarily toward curing the sick.

THE TERRIFYING NORMALCY OF AIDS

STEPHEN JAY GOULD

from The New York Times Magazine

| **April 19, 1987** |

Disney's Epcot Center in Orlando, Florida is a technological tour de force and a conceptual desert. In this permanent World's Fair, American industrial giants have built their versions of an unblemished future. These masterful entertainments convey but one message, brilliantly packaged and relentlessly expressed: Progress through technology is the solution to all human problems. G.E. proclaims from Horizons: "If we can dream it, we can do it." AT&T speaks from on high within its giant golf ball: We are now "unbounded by space and time." United Technologies bubbles from the depths of Living Seas: "With the help of modern technology, we feel there's really no limit to what can be accomplished."

Yet several of these exhibits at the Experimental Prototype Community of Tomorrow, all predating space disaster, belie their stated message from within by using the launch of the shuttle as a visual metaphor for technological triumph. The *Challenger* disaster may represent a general malaise, but it remains an incident. The AIDS pandemic, an issue that may rank with nuclear weaponry as the greatest danger of our era, provides a more striking proof that mind and technology are not omnipotent and that we have not canceled our bond to nature.

In 1984, John Platt, a biophysicist who taught at the University of Chicago for many years, wrote a short paper for private circulation. At a time when most of us were either ignoring AIDS, or viewing it as a contained and peculiar affliction of homosexual men, Platt recognized that the limited data on the origin of AIDS and its spread in America suggested a more frightening prospect: we are all susceptible to AIDS, and the disease has been spreading in a simple exponential manner.

Exponential growth is a geometric increase. Remember the old kiddy problem: If you place a penny on square one of a checkerboard and double the number of coins on each subsequent square—two, four, eight, sixteen, thirty-two . . . —how big is the stack by the sixty-fourth square? The answer: about as high as the universe is wide. Nothing in the external environment inhibits this increase, thus giving to exponential processes their relentless character. In the real, noninfinite world, of course, some limit will eventually arise, and the process slows down, reaches a steady state, or destroys the entire system: the stack of pennies falls over, the bacterial cells exhaust their supply of nutrients.

Platt noticed that data for the initial spread of AIDS fell right on an exponential curve. He then followed the simplest possible procedure of extrapolating the curve unabated into the 1990s. Most of us were incredulous, accusing Platt of the mathematical gamesmanship that scientists call "curve fitting." After all, aren't exponential models unrealistic? Surely we are not all susceptible to AIDS. Is it not spread only by odd practices to odd people? Will it not, therefore, quickly run its short course within a confined group?

Well, hello 1987—worldwide data still match Platt's extrapolated curve. This will not, of course, go on forever. AIDS has probably already saturated the African areas where it probably originated, and where the sex ratio of afflicted people is 1-to-1, male-female. But AIDS still has far to spread, and may be moving exponentially, through the rest of the world. We have learned enough about the cause of AIDS to slow its spread, if we can make rapid and fundamental changes in our handling of that most powerful part of human biology—our own sexuality. But medicine, as yet, has nothing to offer as a cure and precious little even for palliation.

This exponential spread of AIDS not only illuminates its, and our, biology, but also underscores the tragedy of our moralistic misperception. Exponential processes have a definite time and place of origin, an initial point of "inoculation"—in this case, Africa. We didn't notice the spread at first. In a population of billions, we pay little attention when one increases to two, or eight to sixteen, but when one million becomes two million, we panic, even though the *rate* of doubling has not increased.

The infection has to start somewhere, and its initial locus may be little more than an accident of circumstance. For a while, it remains confined to those in close contact with the primary source, but only by accident of proximity, not by intrinsic susceptibility. Eventually, given the power and lability of human sexuality, it spreads outside the initial group and into the general population. And now AIDS has begun its march through our own heterosexual community.

What a tragedy that our moral stupidity caused us to lose precious time, the greatest enemy in fighting an exponential spread, by downplaying the danger because we thought that AIDS was a disease of three irregular groups: minorities of lifestyle (needle users), of sexual preference (homosexuals), and of color (Haitians). If AIDS had first been imported from Africa into a Park Avenue apartment, we would not have dithered as the exponential march began.

The message of Orlando—the inevitability of technological solutions—is wrong, and we need to understand why.

Our species has not won its independence from nature, and we cannot do all that we can dream. Or at least we cannot do it at the rate required to avoid tragedy, for we are not unbounded from time. Viral diseases are preventable in principle, and I suspect that an AIDS vaccine will one day be produced. But how will this discovery avail us if it takes until the millennium, and by then AIDS has fully run its exponential course and saturated our population, killing a substantial percentage of the human race? A fight against an exponential enemy is primarily a race against time.

We must also grasp the perspective of ecology and evolutionary biology and recognize, once we reinsert ourselves properly into nature, that AIDS represents the ordinary workings of biology, not an irrational or diabolical plague with a moral meaning. Disease, including epidemic spread, is a natural phenomenon, part of human history from the beginning. An entire subdiscipline of my profession, paleopathology, studies the evidence of ancient diseases preserved in the fossil remains of organisms. Human history has been marked by episodic plagues. More native peoples died of imported disease than ever fell before the gun during the era of colonial expansion. Our memories are short, and we have had a respite, really, only since the influenza pandemic at the end of World War I, but AIDS must be viewed as a virulent expression of an ordinary natural phenomenon.

I do not say this to foster either comfort or complacency. The evolutionary perspective is correct, but utterly inappropriate for our human scale. Yes,

AIDS is a natural phenomenon, one of a recurring class of pandemic diseases. Yes, AIDS may run through the entire population, and may carry off a quarter or more of us. Yes, it may make no *biological* difference to *Homo sapiens* in the long run: there will still be plenty of us left and we can start again. Evolution cares as little for its agents—organisms struggling for reproductive success—as physics cares for individual atoms of hydrogen in the sun. But *we* care. These atoms are our neighbors, our lovers, our children, and ourselves. AIDS is both a natural phenomenon and, potentially, the greatest natural tragedy in human history.

The cardboard message of Epcot fosters the wrong attitudes; we must both reinsert ourselves into nature and view AIDS as a natural phenomenon in order to fight properly. If we stand above nature and if technology is all powerful, then AIDS is a horrifying anomaly that must be trying to tell us something. If so, we can adopt one of two attitudes, each potentially fatal. We can either become complacent, because we believe the message of Epcot and assume that medicine will soon generate a cure, or we can panic in confusion and seek a scapegoat for something so irregular that it must have been visited upon us to teach a moral lesson.

But AIDS is not irregular. It is part of nature. So are we. This should galvanize us and give us hope, not prompt the worst of all responses: a kind of "new-age" negativism that equates natural with what we must accept and cannot, or even should not, change. When we view AIDS as natural, and when we recognize both the exponential property of its spread and the accidental character of its point of entry into America, we can break through our destructive tendencies to blame others and to free ourselves of concern.

If AIDS is natural, then there is no *message* in its spread. But by all that science has learned and all that rationality proclaims, AIDS works by a *mechanism*—and we can discover it. Victory is not ordained by any principle of progress, or any slogan of technology, so we shall have to fight like hell, and be watchful. There is no message, but there is a mechanism.

IS THE RECTUM A GRAVE?

LEO BERSANI

from October

| 1987 |

AIDS

to the memory of Robert Hagopian

These people have sex twenty to thirty times a night. . . . A man comes along and goes from anus to anus and in a single night will act as a mosquito transferring infected cells on his penis. When this is practiced for a year, with a man having three thousand sexual intercourses, one can readily understand this massive epidemic that is currently upon us.

—Professor Opendra Narayan,
The Johns Hopkins Medical School

I will leave you wondering, with me, why it is that when a woman spreads her legs for a camera, she is assumed to be exercising free will.

—Catherine A. MacKinnon

Le moi *est haïssable....*

—Pascal

There is a big secret about sex: most people don't like it. I don't have any statistics to back this up, and I doubt (although since Kinsey there has been no shortage of polls on sexual behavior) that any poll has ever been taken in which those polled were simply asked, "Do you like sex?" Nor am I suggesting the need for any such poll, since people would probably answer the question as if they were being asked, "Do you often feel the need to have sex?" and one of my aims will be to suggest why these are two wholly different questions. I am, however, interested in my rather irresponsibly announced findings of our nonexistent poll because they strike me as helping to make intelligible a broader spectrum of views about sex and sexuality than perhaps any other single hypothesis. In saying that most people don't like sex, I'm not arguing (nor, obviously, am I denying) that the most rigidly moralistic dicta about sex hide smoldering volcanoes of repressed sexual desire. When you make this argument, you divide people into two camps, and at the same time you let it be known to which camp you belong. There are, you intimate, those who can't face their sexual desires (or, correlatively, the relation between those desires and their views of sex), and those who know that such a relation exists and who are presumably unafraid of their own sexual impulses. Rather, I'm interested in something else, something both camps have in common, which may be a certain *aversion*, an aversion that is not the same thing as a repression and that can coexist quite comfortably with, say, the most enthusiastic endorsement of polysexuality with multiple sex partners.

The aversion I refer to comes in both benign and malignant forms. Malignant aversion has recently had an extraordinary opportunity both to express (and to expose) itself, and, tragically, to demonstrate its power. I'm thinking of course of responses to AIDS—more specifically, of how a public health crisis has been treated like an unprecedented sexual threat. The signs and sense of this extraordinary displacement are the subject of an excellent book just published by Simon Watney, aptly entitled *Policing Desire*. Watney's premise is that "AIDS is not only a medical crisis on an unparalleled scale, it involves a crisis of representation itself, a crisis over the entire framing of knowledge about the human body and its capacities for sexual pleasure." *Policing Desire* is both a casebook of generally appalling examples of this crisis (taken largely from government policy concerning AIDS, as well as from press and television coverage, in England and America) and, most interestingly, an attempt to account for the mechanisms by which a spectacle of suffering and death has unleashed and even appeared to legitimize the impulse to murder.

There is, first of all, the by now familiar, more or less transparent, and ever-increasing evidence of the displacement that Watney studies. At the highest levels of officialdom, there have been the criminal delays in funding research and treatment, the obsession with testing instead of curing, the singularly unqualified members of Reagan's (belatedly constituted) AIDS commission, and the general tendency to think of AIDS as an epidemic of the future rather than a catastrophe of the present. Furthermore, "hospital policies," according to a New York City doctor quoted by Watney, "have more to do with other patients' fears than a concern for the health of AIDS patients." Doctors have refused to operate on people known to be infected with the HIV virus, schools have forbidden children with AIDS to attend classes, and recently citizens of the idyllically named town of Arcadia, Florida, set fire to the house of a family with three hemophiliac children apparently infected with HIV. Television and the press continue to confuse AIDS with the HIV virus, to speak of AIDS as if it were a venereal disease, and consequently to suggest that one catches it by being promiscuous. The effectiveness of the media as an educating force in the fight against AIDS can be measured by the results of a poll cited by Watney in which 56.8 percent of *News of the World* readers came out "in favour of the idea that 'AIDS carriers' should be 'sterilised and given treatment to curb their sexual appetite,' with a mere fifty-one percent in favour of the total recriminalisation of homosexuality." Anecdotally, there is, at a presumably high level of professional expertise, the description of gay male sex—which I quote as an epigraph to this essay—offered to viewers of a BBC *Horizon* program by one Opendra Narayan of the Johns Hopkins Medical School (background in veterinary medicine). A less colorfully expressed but equally lurid account of gay sex was given by Justice Richard Wallach of New York State Supreme Court in Manhattan when, in issuing the temporary restraining order that closed the New St. Marks Baths, he noted: "What a bathhouse like this sets up is the orgiastic behavior of multiple partners, one after the other, where in five minutes you can have five contacts." Finally, the story that gave me the greatest morbid delight appeared in the London *Sun* under the headline "I'd Shoot My Son if He Had AIDS, Says Vicar!" accompanied by a photograph of a man holding a rifle at a boy at point-blank range. The son, apparently more attuned to his father's penchant for violence than the respectable reverend himself, candidly added, "Sometimes I think he would like to shoot me whether I had AIDS or not."

All of this is, as I say, familiar ground, and I mention these few disparate items more or less at random simply as a reminder of where our analytical inquiry starts, *and* to suggest that, given the nature of that starting point, analysis, while necessary, may also be an indefensible luxury. I share Watney's interpretive interests, but it is also important to say that, morally, the only *necessary* response to all of this is rage. "AIDS," Watney writes, "is effectively being used as a pretext throughout the West to 'justify' calls for increasing legislation and regulation of those who are considered to be socially unacceptable." And the unacceptable ones in the AIDS crisis are, of course, male homosexuals and IV drug users (many of the latter are, as we know, poor blacks and Hispanics). Is it unjust to suggest that *News of the World* readers and the gun-toting British vicar are representative examples of the "general public's" response to AIDS? Are there more decent heterosexuals around, heterosexuals who don't awaken a passionate yearning not to share the same planet with them? Of course there are, but—and this is particularly true of England and the United States—*power* is in the hands of those who give every sign of being able to sympathize more with the murderous "moral" fury of the good vicar than with the agony of a terminal KS patient. It was, after all, the Justice Department of the United States that issued a legal opinion stating that employers could fire employees with AIDS if they had so much as the suspicion that the virus could be spread to other workers, regardless of medical evidence. It was the American secretary of Health and Human Services who recently urged Congress to defer action on a bill that would ban discrimination against people infected with HIV, and who also argued against the need for a federal law guaranteeing the confidentiality of HIV antibody test results.

To deliver such opinions and arguments is of course not the same thing as pointing a gun at your son's head, but since, as it has often been said, the failure to guarantee confidentiality will discourage people from taking the test and thereby make it more difficult to control the spread of the virus, the only conclusion we can draw is that Secretary Otis R. Bowen finds it more important to have the names of those who test positive than to slow the spread of AIDS into the sacrosanct "general public." To put this schematically: having the information necessary to lock up homosexuals in quarantine camps may be a higher priority in the family-oriented Reagan administration than saving the heterosexual members of American families from AIDS. Such a priority suggests a far more serious and ambitious passion for violence than what are after all the rather banal, rather normal son-killing impulses of the Reverend Robert Simpson. At the very least, such things as the Justice Department's near recommendation that people with AIDS be thrown out of their jobs suggest that if Edwin Meese would not hold a gun to the head of a man with AIDS, he might not find the murder of a gay man with AIDS (or without AIDS?) intolerable or unbearable. And this is precisely what can be said of millions of fine Germans who never participated in the murder of Jews (and of homosexuals), but who *failed to find the idea of the Holocaust unbearable*. That was the more than sufficient measure of their collaboration, the message they sent to their Führer even before the Holocaust began but when the *idea* of it was around, was, as it were, being tested for acceptability during the 1930s by less violent but nonetheless virulent manifestations of anti-Semitism, just as our leaders, by relegating the protection of people infected with HIV to local authorities, are telling those authorities that anything goes, that the federal government does not find the idea of camps—or perhaps worse—intolerable.

We can of course count on the more liberal press to editorialize against Meese's opinions and Bowen's urgings. We can, however, also count on that same press to give front-page coverage to the story of a presumably straight health worker testing positive for the HIV virus and—at least until recently—almost no coverage at all to complaints about the elephantine pace at which various drugs are being tested and approved for use against the virus. Try keeping up with AIDS research through TV and the press, and you'll remain fairly ignorant. You will, however, learn a great deal from the tube and from your daily newspaper about heterosexual anxieties. Instead of giving us sharp investigative reporting—on, say, "60 Minutes"—on research inefficiently divided among various uncoordinated and frequently competing private and public centers and agencies, or on the interests of pharmaceutical companies in helping to make available (or helping to keep unavailable) new antiviral treatments and in furthering or delaying the development of a vaccine, TV treats us to nauseating processions of yuppie women announcing to the world that they will no longer put out for their yuppie boyfriends unless these boyfriends agree to use a condom. Thus hundreds of thousands of gay men and IV drug users, who have reason to think that they may be infected with HIV, or who know that they are (and who therefore live in daily terror that one of the familiar symptoms will show up), or who are already suffering from an AIDS-related illness, or who are dying from one of these illnesses, are asked to sympathize with all those yuppettes agonizing over whether they're going to risk losing a good fuck by taking the "unfeminine" initiative of interrupting the invading male in order to insist that he practice safe sex. In the face of all that, the shrillness of a Larry Kramer can seem like the simplest good sense. The danger of not exaggerating the hostility to homosexuality "legitimized" by AIDS is that, being "sensible," we may soon find ourselves in situations where exaggeration will be difficult, if not impossible. Kramer has recently said that "if AIDS does not spread out widely into the white non-drug-using heterosexual population, as it may or may not do, then the white non-drug-using population is going to hate us even more—for scaring them, for costing them a fucking fortune, for our 'lifestyle,' which they say caused this." What a morbid, even horrendous, yet perhaps sensible suggestion: only when the "general public" is threatened can whatever the opposite of a general public is hope to get adequate attention and treatment.

Almost all the media coverage of AIDS has been aimed at the heterosexual groups now minimally at risk, as if the high-risk groups were not part of the audience. And in a sense, as Watney suggests, they're not. The media targets "an imaginary national family unit which is both white and heterosexual." This doesn't mean that most TV viewers in Europe and America are *not* white and heterosexual and part of a family. It does, however, mean, as Stuart Hall argues, that representation is very different from reflection: "It implies the active work of selecting and presenting, of structuring and shaping: not merely the transmitting of already-existing meaning, but the more active labour of *making things mean*." TV doesn't make the family, but it makes the family *mean* in a certain way. That is, it makes an exceptionally sharp distinction between the family as a biological unit and as a cultural identity, and it does this by teaching us the attributes and attitudes by which people who thought they were already in a family actually only *begin to qualify* as belonging to a family. The great power of the media, and especially of television, is, as Watney writes, "its capacity to manufacture subjectivity itself," and in so doing to dictate the shape of an identity. The "general public" is at once an ideological construct and a moral prescription. Furthermore, the definition of the family *as an identity* is, inherently, an exclusionary process, and the cultural product has no obligation whatsoever to coincide exactly with its natural referent. Thus the family identity produced on American television is much more likely to include your dog than your homosexual brother or sister.

The peculiar exclusion of the principal sufferers in the AIDS crisis from the discourse about it has perhaps been felt most acutely by those gay men who, until recently, were able to feel that they could both be relatively open about their sexuality and still be thought of as belonging to the "general public," to the mainstream of American life. Until the late 1960s and 1970s, it was of course difficult to manage both these things at the same time. There is, I believe, something salutary in our having to discover the illusory nature of that harmonious adjustment. We now know, or should know, that "gay men," as Watney writes, "are officially regarded, in our entirety, as a disposable constituency." "In our entirety" is crucial. While it would of course be obscene to claim that the comfortable life of a successful gay white businessman or doctor is as oppressed as that of a poverty-stricken black mother in one of our ghettoes, it is also true that the power of blacks *as a group* in the United States is much greater than that of homosexuals. Paradoxically, as we have recently seen in the vote of conservative Democratic senators from the South against the Bork nomination to the Supreme Court, blacks, by their sheer number and their increasing participation in the vote, are no longer a disposable constituency in those very states that have the most illustrious record of racial discrimination. This obviously doesn't mean that blacks have made it in white America. In fact, some political attention to black interests has a certain tactical utility: it softens the blow and obscures the perception of a persistent indifference to the always flourishing economic oppression of blacks. Nowhere is that oppression more visible, less disguised, than in such great American cities as New York, Philadelphia, Boston, and Chicago, although it is typical of the American genius for politically displaced thought that when white liberal New Yorkers (and white liberal columnists such as Anthony Lewis) think of racial oppression, they probably always have images of South Africa in mind. Yet, some blacks are needed in positions of prominence or power, which is not at all true for gay people. Straights can very easily portray gays on TV, while whites generally can't get away with passing for black and are much less effective than blacks as models in TV ads for fast-food chains targeted at the millions of blacks who don't have the money to eat anywhere else. The more greasy the product, the more likely some black models will be allowed to make money promoting it. Also, the country obviously needs a Civil Rights Commission, and it just as obviously has to have blacks on that commission, while there is clearly no immediate prospect for a federal commission to protect and promote gay ways of life. There is no longer a rationale for the oppression of blacks in America, while AIDS has made the oppression of gay men seem like a moral imperative.

In short, a few blacks will always be saved from the appalling fate of most blacks in America, whereas there is no political need to save or protect any homosexuals at all. The country's discovery that Rock Hudson was gay changed nothing: nobody needs actors' votes (or even actors, for that matter) in the same way Southern senators need black votes to stay in power. In those very cities where white gay men could, at least for a few years, think of themselves as decidedly more white than black when it came to the distribution of privileges in America, cities where the increasingly effective ghettoization of blacks progresses unopposed, the gay men who have had as little trouble as their straight counterparts in accepting this demographic and economic segregation must now accept the fact that, unlike the underprivileged blacks all around them whom, like most other whites, they have developed a technique for not seeing, they—the gays—have no claims to power at all. Frequently on the side of power, but powerless; frequently affluent, but politically destitute; frequently articulate, but with *nothing but a moral argument*—not even recognized as a moral argument—to keep themselves in the protected white enclaves and out of the quarantine camps.

On the whole, gay men are no less socially ambitious, and, more often than we like to think, no less reactionary and racist than heterosexuals. To want sex with another man is not exactly a credential for political radicalism—a fact both recognized and denied by the gay liberation movement of the late 1960s and early 1970s. Recognized to the extent that gay liberation, as Jeffrey Weeks has put it, proposed "a radical separation . . . between homosexuality, which was about sexual preference, and 'gayness,' which was about a subversively political way of life." And denied in that this very separation was proposed by homosexuals, who were thereby at least implicitly arguing for homosexuality itself as a privileged locus or point of departure for a political-sexual identity not "fixed" by, or in some way traceable to, a specific sexual orientation. It is no secret that many homosexuals resisted, or were simply indifferent to, participation in "a subversively political way of life," to being, as it were, de-homosexualized in order to join what Watney describes as "a social identity defined not by notions of sexual 'essence,' but in oppositional relation to the institutions and discourses of medicine, the law, education, housing and welfare policy, and so on." More precisely—and more to the point of an assumption that radical sex means or leads to radical politics—many gay men could, in the late 1960s and early 1970s, begin to feel comfortable about having "unusual" or radical ideas about what's OK in sex without modifying one bit their proud middle-class consciousness or even their racism. Men whose behavior at night at the San Francisco Cauldron or the New York Mineshaft could win five-star approval from the (mostly straight) theoreticians of polysexuality had no problem being gay slumlords during the day and, in San Francisco for example, evicting from the Western Addition black families unable to pay the rents necessary to gentrify that neighborhood.

I don't mean that they *should* have had a problem about such combinations in their lives (although I obviously don't mean that they should have felt comfortable about being slumlords), but I do mean that there has been a lot of confusion about the real or potential political implications of homosexuality. Gay activists have tended to deduce those implications from the status of homosexuals as an oppressed minority rather than from what I think are (except perhaps in societies more physically repressive than ours has been) the more crucially operative continuities between political sympathies on the one hand and, on the other, fantasies connected with sexual pleasure. Thanks to a system of gliding emphases, gay activist rhetoric has even managed at times to suggest that a lust for other men's bodies is a by-product or a decision consequent upon political radicalism rather than a given point of departure for a whole range of political sympathies. While it is indisputably true that sexuality is always being politicized, the ways in which *having sex* politicizes are highly problematical. Right-wing politics can, for example, emerge quite easily from a sentimentalizing of the armed forces or of blue-collar workers, a sentimentalizing which can itself prolong and sublimate a marked sexual preference for sailors and telephone linemen.

In short, to put the matter polemically and even rather brutally, we have been telling a few lies—lies whose strategic value I fully understand, but which the AIDS crisis has rendered obsolescent. I do not, for example, find it helpful to suggest, as Dennis Altman has suggested, that gay baths created "a sort of Whitmanesque democracy, a desire to know and trust other men in a type of brotherhood far removed from the male bondage of rank, hierarchy, and competition that characterise much of the outside world." Anyone who has ever spent one night in a gay bathhouse knows that it is (or was) one of the most ruthlessly ranked, hierarchized, and competitive environments imaginable. Your looks, muscles, hair distribution, size of cock, and shape of ass determined exactly how happy you were going to be during those few hours, and rejection, generally accompanied by two or three words at most, could be swift and brutal, with none of the civilizing hypocrisies with which we get rid of undesirables in the outside world. It has frequently been suggested in recent years that such things as the gay-macho style, the butch-fem lesbian couple, and gay and lesbian sadomasochism, far from expressing unqualified and uncontrollable complicities with a brutal and misogynous ideal of masculinity, or with the heterosexual couple permanently locked into a power structure of male sexual and social mastery over female sexual and social passivity, or, finally, with fascism, are in fact subversive parodies of the very formations and behaviors they appear to ape. Such claims, which have been the subject of lively and often intelligent debate, are, it seems to me, totally aberrant, even though, in terms probably unacceptable to their defenders, they can also—indeed, must also—be supported.

First of all, a distinction has to be made between the possible effects of these styles on the heterosexual world that provides the models on which they are based, and their significance for the lesbians and gay men who perform them. A sloganesque approach won't help us here. Even Weeks, whose work I admire, speaks of "the rise of the macho-style amongst gay men in the 1970s . . . as another episode in the ongoing 'semiotic guerilla warfare' waged by sexual outsiders against the dominant order," and he approvingly quotes Richard Dyer's suggestion that "by taking the signs of masculinity and eroticizing them in a blatantly homosexual context, much mischief is done to the security with which 'men' are defined in society, and by which their power is secured." These remarks deny what I take to be wholly nonsubversive intentions by conflating them with problematically subversive effects. It is difficult to know how "much mischief" can be done by a style that straight men see—if indeed they see it at all—from a car window as they drive down Folsom Street. Their security as males with power may very well not be threatened at all by that scarcely traumatic sight, because nothing forces them to see any relation between the gay-macho style and their image of their own masculinity (indeed, the very exaggerations of that style make such denials seem plausible). It may, however, be true that to the extent that the heterosexual male more or less secretly admires or identifies with motorcycle masculinity, its adoption by faggots creates, as Weeks and Dyer suggest, a painful (if passing) crisis of representation. The gay-macho style simultaneously invents the oxymoronic expression "leather queen" and denies its oxymoronic status; for the macho straight man, leather queen is intelligible, indeed tolerable, only *as* an oxymoron—which is of course to say that it must remain unintelligible. Leather and muscles are defiled by a sexually feminized body, although—and this is where I have trouble with Weeks's contention that the gay-macho style "gnaws at the roots of a male heterosexual identity"—the macho male's rejection of his representation by the leather queen can also be accompanied by the secret satisfaction of knowing that the leather queen, for all his despicable blasphemy, at least *intends* to pay worshipful tribute to the style and behavior he defiles. The very real potential for subversive confusion in the joining of female sexuality (I'll return to this in a moment) and the signifiers of machismo is dissipated once the heterosexual recognizes in the gay-macho style a *yearning* toward machismo, a yearning that, very conveniently for the heterosexual, makes of the leather queen's forbidding armor and warlike manners a *per*version rather than a *sub*version of real maleness.

Indeed, if we now turn to the significance of the macho-style for gay men, it would, I think, be accurate to say that this style gives rise to two reactions, both of which indicate a profound respect for machismo itself. One is the classic put-down: the butch number swaggering into a bar in a leather getup opens his mouth and sounds like a pansy, takes you home, where the first thing you notice is the complete works of Jane Austen, gets you into bed, and—well, you know the rest. In short, the mockery of gay machismo is almost exclusively an internal affair, and it is based on the dark suspicion that you may not be getting the real article. The other reaction is, quite simply, sexual excitement. And this brings us back to the question not of the reflection or expression of politics in sex, but rather of the extremely obscure process by which sexual pleasure *generates* politics.

If licking someone's leather boots turns you (and him) on, neither of you is making a statement subversive of macho masculinity. Parody is an erotic turn-off, and all gay men know this. Much campy talk is parodistic, and while that may be fun at a dinner party, if you're out to make someone you turn off the camp. Male gay camp is, however, largely a parody of women, which, obviously, raises some other questions. The gay male parody of a certain femininity, which, as others have argued, may itself be an elaborate social construct, is both a way of giving vent to the hostility toward women that probably afflicts every male (and which male heterosexuals have of course expressed in infinitely nastier and more effective ways) *and* could also parodoxically be thought of as helping to deconstruct that image for women themselves. A certain type of homosexual camp speaks the truth of that femininity as mindless, asexual, and hysterically bitchy, thereby provoking, it would seem to me, a violently antimimetic reaction in any female spectator. The gay male bitch desublimates and desexualizes a type of femininity glamorized by movie stars, whom he thus lovingly assassinates with his style, even though the campy parodist may himself be quite stimulated by the hateful impulses inevitably included in his performance. The gay-macho style, on the other hand, is intended to excite others sexually, and the only reason that it continues to be adopted is that it frequently succeeds in doing so. (If, especially in its more extreme leather forms, it is so often taken up by older men, it is precisely because they count on it to supplement their diminished sexual appeal.)

The dead seriousness of the gay commitment to machismo (by which I of course don't mean that all gays share, or share unambivalently, this commitment) means that gay men run the risk of idealizing and feeling inferior to certain representations of masculinity on the basis of which they are in fact judged and condemned. The logic of homosexual desire includes the potential for a loving identification with the gay man's enemies. And that is a fantasy-luxury that is at once inevitable and no longer permissible. Inevitable because a sexual desire for men can't be merely a kind of culturally neutral attraction to a Platonic Idea of the male body; the object of that desire necessarily includes a socially determined and socially pervasive definition of what it means to be a man. Arguments for the social construction of gender are by now familiar. But such arguments almost invariably have, for good political reasons, quite a different slant; they are didactically intended as demonstrations that the male and female identities proposed by a patriarchal and sexist culture are not to be taken for what they are proposed to be: ahistorical, essential, biologically determined identities. Without disagreeing with this argument, I want to make a different point, a point understandably less popular with those impatient to be freed of oppressive and degrading self-definitions. What I'm saying is that a gay man doesn't run the risk of loving his oppressor *only* in the ways in which blacks or Jews might more or less secretly collaborate with their oppressors—that is, as a consequence of the oppression, of that subtle corruption by which a slave can come to idolize power, to agree that he should be enslaved because he is enslaved, that he should be denied power because he doesn't have any. But blacks and Jews don't *become* blacks and Jews as a result of that internalization of an oppressive mentality, whereas that internalization is in part constitutive of male homosexual desire, which, like all sexual desire, combines and confuses impulses to appropriate and to identify with the object of desire. An authentic gay male political identity therefore implies a struggle not only against definitions of maleness and of homosexuality as they are reiterated and imposed in a heterosexist social discourse, but also against those very same definitions so seductively and so faithfully reflected by those (in large part culturally invented and elaborated) male bodies that we carry within us as permanently renewable sources of excitement.

There is, however, perhaps a way to explode this ideological body. I want to propose, instead of a denial of what I take to be important (if politically unpleasant) truths about male homosexual desire, an arduous representational discipline. The sexist power that defines maleness in most human cultures can easily survive social revolutions; what it perhaps cannot survive is a certain way of assuming, or taking on, that power. If, as Weeks puts it, gay men "gnaw at the roots of a male heterosexual identity," it is not because of the parodistic distance that they take from that identity, but rather because, from within their nearly mad identification with it, *they never cease to feel the appeal of its being violated*.

To understand this, it is perhaps necessary to accept the pain of embracing, at least provisionally, a homophobic representation of homosexuality. Let's return for a moment to the disturbed harmonies of Arcadia, Florida, and try to imagine what its citizens—especially those who set fire to the Rays' home—actually saw when they thought about or looked at the Rays' three boys. The persecuting of children or of heterosexuals with AIDS (or who have tested positive for HIV) is particularly striking in view of the popular description of such people as "innocent victims." It is as if gay men's "guilt" were the real agent of infection. And what is it, exactly, that they are guilty of? Everyone agrees that the crime is sexual, and Watney, along with others, defines it as the imagined or real promiscuity for which gay men are so famous. He analyzes a story about AIDS by the science correspondent of the *Observer* in which the "major argument, supported by 'AIDS experts in America,' [is] against 'casual sexual encounters.'" A London doctor does, in the course of the article, urge the use of condoms in such encounters, but "the main problem . . . is evidently 'promiscuity,' with issues about the kinds of sex one has pushed firmly into the background." But the kinds of sex involved, in quite a different sense, may in fact be crucial to the argument. Since the promiscuity here is homosexual promiscuity, we may, I think, legitimately wonder if what is being done is not as important as how many times it is being done. Or, more exactly, the act being represented may itself be associated with insatiable desire, with unstoppable sex.

Before being more explicit about this, I should acknowledge that the argument I wish to make is a highly speculative one, based primarily on the exclusion of the evidence that supports it. An important lesson to be learned from a study of the representation of AIDS is that the messages most likely to reach their destination are messages already there. Or, to put this in other terms, representations of AIDS have to be X-rayed for their fantasmatic logic; they document the comparative irrelevance of information in communication. Thus the expert medical opinions about how the virus cannot be transmitted (information that the college-educated mayor of Arcadia and his college-educated wife have heard and refer to) is at once rationally discussed and occulted. SueEllen Smith, the Arcadia mayor's wife, makes the unobjectionable comment that "there are too many unanswered questions about this disease," only to conclude that "if you are intelligent and listen and read about AIDS you get scared when it involves your own children, because you realize all the assurances are not based on solid evidence." In strictly rational terms, this can of course be easily answered: there are indeed "many unanswered questions" about AIDS, but the assurances given by medical authorities that there is no risk of the HIV virus being transmitted through casual contact among schoolchildren is in fact based on "solid evidence." But what interests me most about the *New York Times* interview with the Smiths from which I am quoting (they are a genial, even disarming couple: "I know I must sound like a country jerk saying this," remarks Mr. Smith, who really never does sound like a country bumpkin) is the evidence that they have in fact received and thoroughly assimilated quite different messages about AIDS. The mayor said that "a lot of local people, including himself, believed that powerful interests, principally the national gay leaders, had pressured the government into refraining from taking legitimate steps to help contain the spread of AIDS." Let's ignore the charming illusion that "national gay leaders" are powerful enough to pressure the federal government into doing anything at all, and focus on the really extraordinary assumption that those belonging to the group hit most heavily by AIDS want nothing more intensely than to see it spread unchecked. In other words, those being killed are killers. Watney cites other versions of this idea of gay men as killers (their behavior is seen as the cause and source of AIDS), and he speaks of "a displaced desire to kill them all—the teeming deviant millions." Perhaps; but the presumed original desire to kill gays may itself be understandable only in terms of the fantasy for which it is offered as an explanation: homosexuals are killers. But what is it, exactly, that makes them killers?

The public discourse about homosexuals since the AIDS crisis began has a startling resemblance (which Watney notes in passing) to the representation of female prostitutes in the nineteenth century "as contaminated vessels, conveyancing 'female' venereal diseases to 'innocent' men." Some more light is retroactively thrown on those representations by the association of gay men's murderousness with what might be called the specific sexual heroics of their promiscuity. The accounts of Professor Narayan and Judge Wallach of gay men having sex twenty to thirty times a night, or once a minute, are much less descriptive of even the most promiscuous male sexuality than they are reminiscent of male fantasies about women's multiple orgasms. The Victorian representation of prostitutes may explicitly criminalize what is merely a consequence of a more profound or original guilt.

Promiscuity is the social correlative of a sexuality physiologically grounded in the menacing phenomenon of the nonclimactic climax. Prostitutes publicize (indeed, sell) the inherent aptitude of women for uninterrupted sex. Conversely, the similarities between representations of female prostitutes and male homosexuals should help us to specify the exact form of sexual behavior being targeted, in representations of AIDS, as the criminal, fatal, and irresistibly repeated act. This is of course anal sex (with the potential for multiple orgasms having spread from the insertee to the insertor, who, in any case, may always switch roles and be the insertee for ten or fifteen of those thirty nightly encounters), and we must of course take into account the widespread confusion in heterosexual *and* homosexual men between fantasies of anal and vaginal sex. The realities of syphilis in the nineteenth century and of AIDS today "legitimate" a fantasy of female sexuality as intrinsically diseased; and promiscuity in this fantasy, far from merely increasing the risk of infection, is the *sign of infection*. Women and gay men spread their legs with an unquenchable appetite for destruction. This is an image with extraordinary power; and if the good citizens of Arcadia, Florida, could chase from their midst an average, law-abiding family, it is, I would suggest, because in looking at three hemophiliac children they may have seen—that is, unconsciously represented—the infinitely more seductive and intolerable image of a grown man, legs high in the air, unable to refuse the suicidal ecstasy of being a woman.

But why "suicidal"? Recent studies have emphasized that even in societies in which, as John Boswell writes, "standards of beauty are often predicated on male archetypes" (he cites ancient Greece and the Muslim world) and, even more strikingly, in cultures that do not regard sexual relations between men as unnatural or sinful, the line is drawn at "passive" anal sex. In medieval Islam, for all its emphasis on homosexual eroticism, "the position of the 'insertee' is regarded as bizarre or even pathological," and while for the ancient Romans, "the distinction between roles approved for male citizens and others appears to center on the giving of seed (as opposed to the receiving of it) rather than on the more familiar modern active-passive division," to be anally penetrated was no less judged to be an "indecorous role for citizen males." And in Volume II of *The History of Sexuality*, Michel Foucault has amply documented the acceptance (even glorification) *and* profound suspicion of homosexuality in ancient Greece. A general ethical polarity in Greek thought of self-domination and a helpless indulgence of appetites has, as one of its results, a structuring of sexual behavior in terms of activity and passivity, with a correlative rejection of the so-called passive role in sex. What the Athenians find hard to accept, Foucault writes, is the authority of a leader who as an adolescent was an "object of pleasure" for other men; there is a legal and moral incompatibility between sexual passivity and civic authority. The only "honorable" sexual behavior "consists in being active, in dominating, in penetrating, and in thereby exercising one's authority."

In other words, the moral taboo on "passive" anal sex in ancient Athens is primarily formulated as a kind of hygienics of social power. *To be penetrated is to abdicate power*. I find it interesting that an almost identical argument—from, to be sure, a wholly different moral perspective—is being made today by certain feminists. In an interview published a few years ago in *Salmagundi*, Foucault said, "Men think that women can only experience pleasure in recognizing men as masters"—a sentence one could easily take as coming from the pens of Catherine MacKinnon and Andrea Dworkin. These are unlikely bedfellows. In the same interview from which I have just quoted, Foucault more or less openly praises sadomasochistic practices for helping homosexual men (many of whom share heterosexual men's fear of losing their authority by "being under another man in the act of love") to "alleviate" the "problem" of feeling "that the passive role is in some way demeaning." MacKinnon and Dworkin, on the other hand, are of course not interested in making women feel comfortable about lying under men, but in changing the distribution of power both signified and constituted by men's insistence on being on top. They have had quite a bit of bad press, but I think that they make some very important points, points that—rather unexpectedly—can help us to understand the homophobic rage unleashed by AIDS. MacKinnon, for example, argues convincingly against the liberal distinction between violence and sex in rape and pornography, a distinction that, in addition to denying what should be the obvious fact that violence *is* sex for the rapist, has helped to make pornography sound merely sexy, and therefore to protect it. If she and Dworkin use the word *violence* to describe pornography that would normally be classified as nonviolent (for example, porno films with no explicit sadomasochism or scenes of rape), it is because they define as violent the power relation that they see inscribed in the sex acts pornography represents. Pornography, MacKinnon writes, "eroticizes hierarchy"; it "makes inequality into sex, which makes it enjoyable, and into gender, which makes it seem natural." Not too differently from Foucault (except, of course, for the rhetorical escalation), MacKinnon speaks of "the male supremacist definition of female sexuality as lust for self-annihilation." Pornography "institutionalizes the sexuality of male supremacy, fusing the eroticization of dominance and submission with the social construction of male and female." It has been argued that even if such descriptions of pornography are accurate, they exaggerate its importance: MacKinnon and Dworkin see pornography as playing a major role in constructing a social reality of which it is really only a marginal reflection. In a sense—and especially if we consider the size of the steady audience for hard-core pornography—this is true. But the objection is also something of a cop-out, because if it is agreed that pornography eroticizes—and thereby celebrates—the violence of inequality itself (and the inequality doesn't have to be enforced with whips to be violent: the denial to blacks of equal seating privileges on public buses was rightly seen as a form of racial violence), then legal pornography is legalized violence.

Not only that: MacKinnon and Dworkin are really making a claim for the realism of pornography. That is, whether or not we think of it as constitutive (rather than merely reflective) of an eroticizing of the violence of inequality, pornography would be the most accurate description and the most effective promotion of that inequality. Pornography can't be dismissed as less significant socially than other more pervasive expressions of gender inequality (such as the abominable and innumerable TV ads in which, as part of a sales pitch for cough medicine and bran cereals, women are portrayed as slaves to the normal functioning of their men's bronchial tubes and large intestines), because only pornography tells us why the bran ad is effective: the slavishness of women is erotically thrilling. The ultimate logic of MacKinnon's and Dworkin's critique of pornography—and, however parodistic this may sound, I really don't mean it as a parody of their views—would be *the criminalization of sex itself until it has been reinvented*. For their most radical claim is not that pornography has a pernicious effect on otherwise nonpernicious sexual relations, but rather that so-called normal sexuality is already pornographic. "When violence against women is eroticized as it is in this culture," MacKinnon writes, "it is very difficult to say that there is a major distinction in the level of sex involved between being assaulted by a penis and being assaulted by a fist, especially when the perpetrator is a man." Dworkin has taken this position to its logical extreme: the rejection of intercourse itself. If, as she argues, "there is a relationship between intercourse per se and the low status of women," and if intercourse itself "is immune to reform," then there must be no more penetration. Dworkin announces: "In a world of male power—penile power—fucking is the essential sexual experience of power and potency and possession; fucking by mortal men, regular guys." Almost everybody reading such sentences will find them crazy, although in a sense they merely develop the implicit *moral* logic of Foucault's more detached and therefore more respectable formulation: "Men think that women can only experience pleasure in recognizing men as masters." MacKinnon, Dworkin, and Foucault are all saying that a man lying on top of a woman assumes that what excites her is the idea of her body being invaded by a phallic master.

The argument against pornography remains, we could say, a liberal argument as long as it is assumed that pornography violates the natural conjunction of sex with tenderness and love. It becomes a much more disturbingly radical argument when the indictment against pornography is identified with an indictment against sex itself. This step is usually avoided by the positing of pornography's violence as either a sign of certain fantasies only marginally connected with an otherwise essentially healthy (caring, loving) form of human behavior, or the symptomatic by-product of social inequalities (more specifically, of the violence intrinsic to a phallocentric culture). In the first case, pornography can be defended as a therapeutic or at least cathartic outlet for those perhaps inescapable but happily marginal fantasies, and in the second case pornography becomes more or less irrelevant to a political struggle against more pervasive social structures of inequality (for once the latter are dismantled, their pornographic derivatives will have lost their raison d'être). MacKinnon and Dworkin, on the other hand, rightly assume the immense power of sexual images to orient our imagination of how political power can and should be distributed and enjoyed, and, it seems to me, they just as rightly mistrust a certain intellectual sloppiness in the catharsis argument, a sloppiness that consists in avoiding the question of how a center of presumably wholesome sexuality ever produced those unsavory margins in the first place. Given the public discourse around the center of sexuality (a discourse obviously not unmotivated by a prescriptive ideology about sex), the margins may be the only place where the center becomes visible.

Furthermore, although their strategies and practical recommendations are unique, MacKinnon's and Dworkin's work could be inscribed within a more general enterprise, one which I will call the *redemptive reinvention of sex*. This enterprise cuts across the usual lines on the battlefield of sexual politics, and it includes not only the panicky denial of childhood sexuality, which is being "dignified" these days as a nearly psychotic anxiety about child abuse, but also the activities of such prominent lesbian proponents of S & M sex as Gayle Rubin and Pat Califia, neither of whom, to put it mildly, share the political agenda of MacKinnon and Dworkin. The immense body of contemporary discourse that argues for a radically revised imagination of the body's capacity for pleasure—a discursive project to which Foucault, Weeks, and Watney belong—has as its very condition of possibility a certain refusal of sex as we know it, and a frequently hidden agreement about sexuality as being, in its essence, less disturbing, less socially abrasive, less violent, more respectful of "personhood" than it has been in a male-dominated, phallocentric culture. The mystifications in gay activist discourse on gay male machismo belong to this enterprise; I will return to other signs of the gay participation in the redemptive sex project. For the moment, I want to argue, first of all, that MacKinnon and Dworkin have at least had the courage to be explicit about the profound *moral revulsion* with sex that inspires the entire project, whether its specific program be antipornography laws, a return to the arcadian mobilities of childhood polysexuality, the S & M battering of the body in order to multiply or redistribute its loci of pleasure, or, as we shall see, the comparatively anodyne agenda (sponsored by Weeks and Watney) of sexual pluralism. Most of these programs have the slightly questionable virtue of being indubitably saner than Dworkin's lyrical tribute to the militant pastoralism of Joan of Arc's virginity, but the pastoral impulse lies behind them all. What bothers me about MacKinnon and Dworkin is not their analysis of sexuality, but rather the pastoralizing, redemptive intentions that support the analysis. That is—and this is the second, major point I wish to argue—they have given us the reasons why pornography must be multiplied and not abandoned, and, more profoundly, the reasons for defending, for cherishing the very sex they find so hateful. Their indictment of sex—their refusal to prettify it, to romanticize it, to maintain that fucking has anything to do with community or love—has had the immensely desirable effect of publicizing, of lucidly laying out for us, the inestimable value of sex as—at least in certain of its ineradicable aspects—anticommunal, antiegalitarian, antinurturing, antiloving.

Let's begin with some anatomical considerations. Human bodies are constructed in such a way that it is, or at least has been, almost impossible not to associate mastery and subordination with the experience of our most intense pleasures. This is first of all a question of positioning. If the penetration necessary (until recently . . .) for the reproduction of the species has most generally been accomplished by the man's getting on top of the woman, it is also true that being on top can never be just a question of a physical position—either for the person on top or for the one on the bottom. (And for the woman to get on top is just a way of letting her play the game of power for awhile, although—as the images of porn movies illustrate quite effectively—even on the bottom, the man can still concentrate his deceptively renounced aggressiveness in the thrusting movement of his penis.) And, as this suggests, there is also, alas, the question of the penis. Unfortunately, the dismissal of penis envy as a male fantasy rather than a psychological truth about women doesn't really do anything to change the assumptions behind that fantasy. For the idea of penis envy describes how men feel about having one, and, as long as there are sexual relations between men and women, this can't help but be an important fact *for women*. In short, the social structures from which it is often said that the eroticizing of mastery and subordination derive are perhaps themselves derivations (and sublimations) of the indissociable nature of sexual pleasure and the exercise or loss of power. To say this is not to propose an "essentialist" view of sexuality. A reflection on the fantasmatic potential of the human body—the fantasies engendered by its sexual anatomy and the specific moves it makes in taking sexual pleasure—is not the same thing as an a priori, ideologically motivated, and prescriptive description of the essence of sexuality. Rather, I am saying that those effects of power which, as Foucault has argued, are inherent in the relational itself (they are immediately produced by "the divisions, inequalities and disequilibriums" inescapably present "in every relation from one point to another") can perhaps most easily be exacerbated, and polarized into relations of mastery and subordination, in sex, and that this potential may be grounded in the shifting experience that every human being has of his or her body's capacity, or failure, to control and to manipulate the world beyond the self.

Needless to say, the ideological exploitations of this fantasmatic potential have a long and inglorious history. It is mainly a history of male power, and by now it has been richly documented by others. I want to approach this subject from a quite different angle, and to argue that a gravely dysfunctional aspect of what is, after all, the healthy pleasure we take in the operation of a coordinated and strong physical organism is the temptation to deny the perhaps equally strong appeal of powerlessness, of the loss of control. Phallocentrism is exactly that: not primarily the denial of power to women (although it has obviously also led to that, everywhere and at all times), but above all the denial of the *value* of powerlessness in both men and women. I don't mean the value of gentleness, or nonaggressiveness, or even of passivity, but rather of a more radical disintegration and humiliation of the self. For there is finally, beyond the fantasies of bodily power and subordination that I have just discussed, a transgressing of that very polarity which, as Georges Bataille has proposed, may be the profound sense of both certain mystical experiences and of human sexuality. In making this suggestion I'm also thinking of Freud's somewhat reluctant speculation, especially in the *Three Essays on the Theory of Sexuality*, that sexual pleasure occurs whenever a certain threshold of intensity is reached, when the organization of the self is momentarily disturbed by sensations or affective processes somehow "beyond" those connected with psychic organization. Reluctant because, as I have argued elsewhere, this definition removes the sexual from the intersubjective, thereby depriving the teleological argument of the *Three Essays* of much of its weight. For on the one hand Freud outlines a normative sexual development that finds its natural goal in the post-Oedipal, genitally centered desire for someone of the opposite sex, while on the other hand he suggests not only the irrelevance of the object in sexuality but also, and even more radically, a shattering of the psychic structures themselves that are the precondition for the very establishment of a relation to others. In that curiously insistent, if intermittent, attempt to get at the "essence" of sexual pleasure—an attempt that punctuates and interrupts the more secure narrative outline of the history of desire in the *Three Essays*—Freud keeps returning to a line of speculation in which the opposition between pleasure and pain becomes irrelevant, in which the sexual emerges as the *jouissance* of exploded limits, as the ecstatic suffering into which the human organism momentarily plunges when it is "pressed" beyond a certain threshold of endurance. Sexuality, at least in the mode in which it is constituted, may be a tautology for masochism. In *The Freudian Body*, I proposed that this sexually constitutive masochism could even be thought of as an evolutionary conquest in the sense that it allows the infant to survive, indeed to find pleasure in, the painful and characteristically human period during which infants are shattered with stimuli for which they have not yet developed defensive or integrative ego structures. Masochism would be the psychical strategy that partially defeats a biologically dysfunctional process of maturation. From this Freudian perspective, we might say that Bataille reformulates this self-shattering into the sexual as a kind of nonanecdotal self-debasement, as a masochism to which the melancholy of the post-Oedipal superego's moral masochism is wholly alien, and in which, so to speak, the self is exuberantly discarded.

The relevance of these speculations to the present discussion should be clear: the self which the sexual shatters provides the basis on which sexuality is associated with power. It is possible to think of the sexual as, precisely, moving between a hyperbolic sense of self and a loss of all consciousness of self. But sex as self-hyperbole is perhaps a repression of sex as self-abolition. It inaccurately replicates self-shattering as self-swelling, as psychic tumescence. If, as these words suggest, men are especially apt to "choose" this version of sexual pleasure, because their sexual equipment appears to invite by analogy, or at least to facilitate, the phallicizing of the ego, neither sex has exclusive rights to the practice of sex as self-hyperbole. For it is perhaps primarily *the degeneration of the sexual into a relationship that condemns sexuality to becoming a struggle for power*. As soon as persons are posited, the war begins. It is the self that swells with excitement at the idea of being on top, the self that makes of the inevitable play of thrusts and relinquishments in sex an argument for the natural authority of one sex over the other.

Far from apologizing for their promiscuity as a failure to maintain a loving relationship, far from welcoming the return to monogamy as a beneficent consequence of the horror of AIDS, gay men should ceaselessly lament the practical necessity, now, of such relationships, should resist being drawn into mimicking the unrelenting warfare between men and women, which nothing has ever changed. Even among the most critical historians of sexuality and the most angry activists, there has been a good deal of defensiveness about what it means to be gay. Thus for Jeffrey Weeks the most distinctive aspect of gay life is its "radical pluralism." Gayle Rubin echoes and extends this idea by arguing for a "theoretical as well as a sexual pluralism." Watney repeats this theme with, it is true, some important nuances. He sees that the "new gay identity was constructed through multiple encounters, shifts of sexual identification, actings out, cultural reinforcements, and a plurality of opportunity (at least in large urban areas) for desublimating the inherited sexual guilt of a grotesquely homophobic society," and therefore laments the "wholesale de-sexualisation of gay culture and experience" encouraged by the AIDS crisis. He nonetheless dilutes what I take to be the specific menace of gay sex for that "grotesquely homophobic society" by insisting on the assertion of "the diversity of human sexuality in *all* its variant forms" as "perhaps the most radical aspect of gay culture." *Diversity* is the key word in his discussions of homosexuality, which he defines as "a fluctuating field of sexual desires and behaviour;" it maximizes "the mutual erotic possibilities of the body, and that is why it is taboo."

Much of this derives of course from the rhetoric of sexual liberation in the 1960s and 1970s, a rhetoric that received its most prestigious intellectual justification from Foucault's call—especially in the first volume of his *History of Sexuality*—for a reinventing of the body as a surface of multiple sources of pleasure. Such calls, for all their redemptive appeal, are, however, unnecessarily and even dangerously tame. The argument for diversity has the strategic advantage of making gays seem like passionate defenders of one of the primary values of mainstream liberal culture, but to make that argument is, it seems to me, to be disingenuous about the relation between homosexual behavior and the revulsion it inspires. The revulsion, it turns out, is all a big mistake: what we're really up to is pluralism and diversity, and getting buggered is just one moment in the practice of those laudable humanistic virtues. Foucault could be especially perverse about all this: challenging, provoking, and yet, in spite of his radical intentions, somewhat appeasing in his emphases. Thus in the *Salmagundi* interview to which I have already referred, after announcing that he will not "make use of a position of authority while [he is] being interviewed to traffic in opinions," he delivers himself of the highly idiosyncratic opinions, first of all, that "for a homosexual, the best moment of love is likely to be when the lover leaves in the taxi" ("the homosexual imagination is for the most part concerned with reminiscing about the act rather than anticipating [or, presumably, enjoying] it") and, secondly, that the rituals of gay S & M are "the counterpart of the medieval courts where strict rules of proprietary courtship were defined." The first opinion is somewhat embarrassing; the second has a certain campy appeal. Both turn our attention away from the body—from the acts in which it engages, from the pain it inflicts and begs for—and directs our attention to the romances of memory and the idealizations of the presexual, the courting imagination. That turning away from sex is then projected onto heterosexuals as an explanation for their hostility. "I think that what most bothers those who are not gay about gayness is the gay life-style, not sex acts themselves," and, "It is the prospect that gays will create as yet unforeseen kinds of relationships that many people cannot tolerate." But what is "*the* gay life-style"? Is there one? Was Foucault's lifestyle the same as Rock Hudson's? More importantly, can a nonrepresentable form of relationship really be more threatening than the representation of a particular sexual act—especially when the sexual act is associated with women but performed by men and, as I have suggested, has the terrifying appeal of a loss of the ego, of a self-debasement?

We have been studying examples of what might be called a frenzied epic of displacements in the discourse on sexuality and on AIDS. The government talks more about testing than it does about research and treatment;

it is more interested in those who may eventually be threatened by AIDS than in those already stricken with it. There are hospitals in which concern for the safety of those patients who have not been exposed to HIV takes precedence over caring for those suffering from an AIDS-related disease. Attention is turned away from the kinds of sex people practice to a moralistic discourse about promiscuity. The impulse to kill gays comes out as a rage against gay killers deliberately spreading a deadly virus among the "general public." The temptation of incest has become a national obsession with child abuse by day-care workers and teachers. Among intellectuals, the penis has been sanitized and sublimated into the phallus as the originary signifier; the body is to be read as a language. (Such distancing techniques, for which intellectuals have a natural aptitude, are of course not only sexual: the national disgrace of economic discrimination against blacks is buried in the self-righteous call for sanctions against Pretoria.) The wild excitement of fascistic S & M becomes a parody of fascism; gay males' idolatry of the cock is "raised" to the political dignity of "semiotic guerrilla warfare." The phallocentrism of gay cruising becomes diversity and pluralism; representation is displaced from the concrete practice of fellatio and sodomy to the melancholy charms of erotic memories and the cerebral tensions of courtship. There has even been the displacement of displacement itself. While it is undeniably right to speak—as, among others, Foucault, Weeks, and MacKinnon have spoken—of the ideologically organizing force of sexuality, it is quite another thing to suggest—as these writers also suggest—that sexual inequalities are predominantly, perhaps exclusively, displaced social inequalities. Weeks, for example, speaks of erotic tensions as a displacement of politically enforced positions of power and subordination, as if the sexual—involving as it does the source and locus of every individual's original experience of power (and of powerlessness) in the world: the human body—could somehow be conceived of apart from all relations of power, were, so to speak, belatedly contaminated by power from elsewhere.

Displacement is endemic to sexuality. I have written, especially in *Baudelaire and Freud*, about the mobility of desire, arguing that sexual desire initiates, indeed can be recognized by, an agitated fantasmatic activity in which original (but, from the start, unlocatable) objects of desire get lost in the images they generate. Desire, by its very nature, turns us away from its objects. If I refer critically to what I take to be a certain refusal to speak frankly about gay sex, it is not because I believe either that gay sex is reducible to one form of sexual activity or that the sexual itself is a stable, easily observable, or easily definable function. Rather, I have been trying to account for the murderous representations of homosexuals unleashed and "legitimized" by AIDS, and in so doing I have been struck by what might be called the aversion-displacements characteristic of both those representations and the gay responses to them. Watney is acutely aware of the displacements operative in "cases of extreme verbal or physical violence towards lesbians and gay men and, by extension, the whole topic of AIDS"; he speaks, for example, of "displaced misogyny," of "a hatred of what is projected as 'passive' and therefore female, sanctioned by the subject's heterosexual drives." But, as I argued earlier, implicit in both the violence toward gay men (and toward women, both gay and straight) *and* the rethinking among gays (and among women) of what being gay (and what being a woman) means is a certain agreement about what sex should be. The pastoralizing project could be thought of as informing even the most oppressive demonstrations of power. If, for example, we assume that the oppression of women disguises a fearful male response to the seductiveness of an image of sexual powerlessness, then the most brutal machismo is really part of a domesticating, even sanitizing project. The ambition of performing sex as *only* power is a salvational project, one designed to preserve us from a nightmare of ontological obscenity, from the prospect of a breakdown of the human itself in sexual intensities, from a kind of selfless communication with "lower" orders of being. The panic about child abuse is the most transparent case of this compulsion to rewrite sex. Adult sexuality is split in two: at once redeemed by its retroactive metamorphosis into the purity of an asexual childhood, and yet preserved in its most sinister forms by being projected onto the image of the criminal seducer of children. "Purity" is crucial here: behind the brutalities against gays, against women, and, in the denial of their very nature and autonomy, against children lies the pastoralizing, the idealizing, the redemptive project I have been speaking of. More exactly, the brutality is identical to the idealization.

The participation of the powerless themselves in this project is particularly disheartening. Gays and women must of course fight the violence directed against them, and I am certainly not arguing for a complicity with misogynist and homophobic fantasies. I am, however, arguing against that form of complicity that consists in accepting, even finding new ways to defend, our culture's lies about sexuality. As if in secret agreement with the values that support misogynist images of female sexuality, women call for a permanent closing of the thighs in the name of chimerically nonviolent ideals of tenderness and nurturing; gays suddenly rediscover their lost bathhouses as laboratories of ethical liberalism, places where a culture's ill-practiced ideals of community and diversity are authentically put into practice. But what if we said, for example, not that it is wrong to think of so-called passive sex as "demeaning," but rather that *the value of sexuality itself is to demean the seriousness of efforts to redeem it?* "AIDS," Watney writes, "offers a new sign for the symbolic machinery of repression, making the rectum a grave." But if the rectum is the grave in which the masculine ideal (an ideal shared—differently—by men *and* women) of proud subjectivity is buried, then it should be celebrated for its very potential for death. Tragically, AIDS has literalized that potential as the certainty of biological death, and has therefore reinforced the heterosexual association of anal sex with a self-annihilation originally and primarily identified with the fantasmatic mystery of an insatiable, unstoppable female sexuality. It may, finally, be in the gay man's rectum that he demolishes his own perhaps otherwise uncontrollable identification with a murderous judgment against him.

That judgment, as I have been suggesting, is grounded in the sacrosanct value of selfhood, a value that accounts for human beings' extraordinary willingness to kill in order to protect the seriousness of their statements. The self is a practical convenience; promoted to the status of an ethical ideal, it is a sanction for violence. If sexuality is socially dysfunctional in that it brings people together only to plunge them into a self-shattering and solipsistic *jouissance* that drives them apart, it could also be thought of as our primary hygienic practice of nonviolence. Gay men's "obsession" with sex, far from being denied, should be celebrated—not because of its communal virtues, not because of its subversive potential for parodies of machismo, not because it offers a model of genuine pluralism to a society that at once celebrates and punishes pluralism, but rather because it never stops re-presenting the internalized phallic male as an infinitely loved object of sacrifice. Male homosexuality advertises the risk of the sexual itself as the risk of self-dismissal, of *losing sight* of the self, and in so doing it proposes and dangerously represents *jouissance* as a mode of ascesis.

THE IMPACT OF AIDS ON THE ARTISTIC COMMUNITY

FRAN LEBOWITZ

from The New York Times

| **September 13, 1987** |

1. The Impact of AIDS on the Artistic Community is that when a 36-year-old writer is asked on a network news show about the Impact of AIDS on the Artistic Community particularly in regard to the Well-Known Preponderance of Homosexuals in the Arts she replies that if you removed all of the homosexuals and homosexual influence from what is generally regarded as American culture you would be pretty much left with "Let's Make a Deal."

The interviewer's lack of response compels her to conclude that he has no idea what she is talking about and she realizes that soon many of those who do know what she is talking about will be what is generally regarded as dead.

2. The Impact of AIDS on the Artistic Community is that on New Year's Eve Day a 36-year-old writer takes a 31-year-old photographer to get a chest X-ray and listens to him say with what can only be described as a certain guarded hope, "Maybe I just have lung cancer."

3. The Impact of AIDS on the Artistic Community is that a 36-year-old writer has a telephone conversation with a dying 41-year-old book editor whom even the most practiced verbal assassin has called the last of the Southern gentlemen and hears him say in a hoarse whisper, "I'm sorry but I just hate old people. I look at them and think, 'Why don't *you* die?' "

4. The Impact of AIDS on the Artistic Community is that an aspiring little avant-garde movie director approaches a fairly famous actor in a restaurant and attempts to make social hay out of the fact that they met at Antonio's and will undoubtedly see each other at Charles's and Antonio's and Charles's are not parties and Antonio's and Charles's are not bars and Antonio's and Charles's are not summer houses in chic Tuscan towns—Antonio's and Charles's are funerals.

5. The Impact of AIDS on the Artistic Community is that a 36-year-old writer is on the telephone with a 38-year-old art director making arrangements to go together the following morning to the funeral of a 27-year-old architect and the art director says to the writer, "If you get there first sit near the front where we usually sit and save me the seat on the aisle."

6. The Impact of AIDS on the Artistic Community is that a 24-year-old ballet dancer is in the hospital for 10 days following an emergency appendectomy and nobody goes to visit him because everyone is really busy and after all he's not dying or anything.

7. The Impact of AIDS on the Artistic Community is that a 36-year-old writer takes time out at a memorial service for the world's preeminent makeup artist and a man worth any number of interesting new painters to get angry because the makeup artist's best friend and eulogist uses a story that she has for years been hoarding for her book which she can't write anymore anyway unless she writes it as a historical novel because it's about a world that in the last few years has disappeared almost entirely.

8. The Impact of AIDS on the Artistic Community is that a 36-year-old writer runs into a 34-year-old painter at a party and the painter says to the writer that he is just back from Los Angeles and he says with some surprise that he had a really good time there and he asks why does she think that happened and says it's because New York is so boring now that Los Angeles is fun in comparison and that's true and it's one reason but the real reason is that they don't know the people who are dying there.

9. The Impact of AIDS on the Artistic Community is that a 36-year-old writer has dinner every night for 11 nights in a row with the same 32-year-old musician while he waits for his biopsy to come back because luckily for her she is the only one he trusts enough to tell.

10. The Impact of AIDS on the Artistic Community is that a 36-year-old writer trying to make plans to go out of town flips through her appointment book and hears herself say, "Well, I have a funeral on Tuesday, lunch with my editor on Wednesday, a memorial service on Thursday, so I guess I could come on Friday, unless, of course, Robert dies."

11. The Impact of AIDS on the Artistic Community is that when the world's most famous artist dies of complications following surgery at the age of 61 it doesn't seem like he really died at all—it seems like he got off easy.

12. The Impact of AIDS on the Artistic Community is that at a rather grand dinner held at a venerable New York cultural institution and catered by a company famous for the beauty of its waiters a 39-year-old painter remarks to a 36-year-old writer that the company in question doesn't seem to employ as many really handsome boys as it used to and the writer replies, "Well, it doesn't always pay to be popular."

WHITE NIGHTS

RANDY SHILTS

from And the Band Played On

| 1988 |

June 11, 1988
Stockholm, Sweden

So close to midsummer's eve and so near the Arctic Circle, the skies darkened only briefly in the deepest hours of the night. After a fleeting interlude of blackness around midnight, the sky faded to ghastly gray, an eerie shade not characterized by light so much as by the absence of darkness. In the northern latitudes, these long hours of twilight pallor before sunrise are called the white nights.

The white nights wreaked havoc on the sleep patterns of those not acclimated to the land of the midnight sun, and like many Americans, Jim Curran lay awake in his hotel room. Each year since the first international AIDS conference was held in Atlanta, Curran had delivered an opening address to the gatherings, detailing the current epidemiology of acquired immune deficiency syndrome in the United States. Tomorrow would be no different, and like every night before this talk, Curran was having a hard time sleeping.

He had come to view his speech each year as something of an annual report on AIDS in America, a time to review and a time to project. It was hard not to personalize the increasingly depressing statistics he was called upon to recite each June. An American was diagnosed with AIDS on the average of once every fourteen minutes, this year's speech read. The nation's

AIDS caseload, which had hit 50,000 with the New Year, now exceeded 65,000—though, Curran knew, what with reporting delays and undiagnosed cases, the nation's real AIDS caseload was more like 75,000, maybe 80,000. Official numbers, of course, would hit these levels soon enough, probably by the end of the summer. As many as 1,000 Americans were being diagnosed with AIDS every week.

The larger bombshell of Curran's presentation the next day would come with the new official projections of AIDS incidence over the coming four years. The U.S. Public Health Service had struck on the idea of AIDS projections in 1986 at the Coolfant conference in hopes of garnering media attention to the proportions that the AIDS problem would soon assume. Those projections, predicting 270,000 AIDS cases by 1991, were proving startlingly accurate, albeit somewhat conservative. In fact, the true numbers of AIDS cases reported in 1986 and 1987 amounted to 109 percent of the numbers forecast at Coolfant. Days before the Stockholm conference convened, the CDC had come up with its new divinations. By the end of 1992, 365,000 Americans would be suffering from AIDS, the statisticians figured; in that year alone, 80,000 would be diagnosed with the disease—many more people than had been diagnosed in the entire first seven years of the epidemic.

The extent to which so many old-timers had remained in AIDS work continued to surprise Curran. From the CDC, a number of old hands had come to Stockholm, the ones who had been with AIDS since those first frustrating days when the entire federal effort consisted of a dozen researchers fielding calls in an obscure corner of Building 6—Harold Jaffe, Dale Lawrence, and Bill Darrow. From California, Don Francis, now done with his African assignment, had also come to Stockholm. In a few weeks, San Francisco's newly elected mayor, Art Agnos, was slated to announce that Francis was going to serve as San Francisco's AIDS coordinator.

When Curran ran into Donna Mildvan in Stockholm, she reminded him of the talk he had given at the New York Physicians for Human Rights in 1982. By anyone's memory, Mildvan was the first person to speak words of warning about the new epidemic when, after treating several mysteriously ill gay men, she called Dr. Dan William eight years ago to insist that "there is a new disease going around." Like most of the doctors in the 1982 physicians' meeting, she hadn't believed Curran when he said they would spend the rest of their careers as AIDS doctors. Now Mildvan, who still worked at Beth Israel Medical Center on Manhattan's East Side, treated hundreds of AIDS patients. In New York City, where the AIDS toll was nearing fifteen thousand, she could barely conceive of the scope the problem would have in a few years when there were 50,000 cases in that one city alone. She suspected it would take a miracle to save New York City a few years down the road. For her part, all she could do was keep managing.

Such determination awed Curran, for he knew that ultimately, AIDS work, whether in the clinic or in government, was a thankless task. AIDS experts spent their days issuing warnings that were rarely heeded and seeking opportunities that, if taken at all, seemed always to arrive too late. This was part of the epidemic that hadn't changed much at all since those first frustrating years of AIDS.

In fact, it occurred to many of the veterans lying sleepless on that white night, little in the fundamental plot of the AIDS story had changed in all these years. To be sure, AIDS had assumed a much grander scale: Cases were counted in the hundreds of thousands, not the hundreds, and the dollars now directed against it numbered in the billions. Outbursts of concern at the failure of the federal government to fight the problem aggressively were coming from ever more prestigious sources, but the ability of the American government to ignore such warnings even more resolutely had grown proportionately, too. As it always had been, the scale of the response was not even remotely commensurate with the scale of the problem.

It was a prescription for terminal frustration to any but the most committed Cassandras, and yet they hung in there. Burnout claimed few victims, though AIDS took its share. Jim Curran had worked with many gay physicians and AIDS activists over the years, whom he would see at these conferences; at one conference he would see that they had lost weight, and then at the next conference they wouldn't be there.

These were the faces behind all the numbers that he would read the next morning. The only thing that Curran hated more than reading the predictions of future AIDS cases was seeing those predictions come true, year after year. After seven years, he had the feeling that he was being swept along in a storm and there was nothing else to do than to hold on.

The first days of June each year seemed to usher in a rush of AIDS news that in turn tended to shape the context of the annual AIDS meeting. In 1987, the first AIDS speeches by President Reagan and Vice President Bush had provided a thoroughly political framework for the Washington conference. This year the challenges confronting the AIDS battle were defined by a pair of reports issued in the days preceding the conference.

The first blow to the federal AIDS bureaucracy came from the prestigious Institute of Medicine of the National Academy of Sciences. The report, an update of its 1986 critique, "Confronting AIDS," bluntly blamed "the absence of strong federal leadership" for the dimensions the AIDS problem had assumed. Lack of federal leadership had failed to provide "overarching direction" to bring together "all components of the government and private sector" in a coordinated fight against the epidemic.

The day after the academy report, the Reagan administration got an even sharper condemnation from its own Presidential Commission on the HIV Epidemic. Decrying a "distinct lack of leadership" from the federal government regarding the AIDS crisis, commission chairman James Watkins summarily issued his recommendations for the commission's final report, due a few weeks later. It was a stunning repudiation of just about every aspect of the Reagan administration's handling of AIDS, as well as a sweeping battle plan for how the nation might cope with the epidemic in coming years. Among Watkins's 579 specific recommendations was a call for spending $1.5 billion a year on rehabilitation programs for intravenous drug users, for only such a response could put a meaningful dent in intravenous drug-related transmission and its corollary problems of the spread of heterosexual AIDS and pediatric AIDS. And with the medical systems of major cities across the country facing collapse from the growing burden of AIDS cases, Watkins also called for the establishment of a public health nursing corps and new scholarships to attract the medical personnel who would be needed to treat AIDS in the years to come.

Like nearly everybody else involved in the AIDS war, both Watkins and the National Academy of Sciences concurred that widespread voluntary testing was a valuable weapon in the fight against the epidemic. Testing would alert HIV-positive people of their infectivity, prod drug users into rehabilitation programs, and help prevent births of AIDS-infected babies, they reasoned. Also like just about everybody involved in the AIDS fight, Watkins understood that people would not take the AIDS antibody test if they had to worry about losing their jobs and homes because they tested positive. There were enough horror stories of discrimination against HIV carriers to discourage many people at risk for AIDS from testing; calls from rabid conservatives such as U.S. Senator Jesse Helms for possible quarantine of the HIV-infected weren't doing much to promote such programs either. Watkins, therefore, proposed sweeping federal legislation to ban discrimination against AIDS or ARC sufferers or the HIV-infected, calling such discrimination the "greatest single barrier" to overcome in the battle against AIDS.

If this wasn't enough to give conservatives apoplexy, Watkins added a skillfully crafted final chapter to his recommendations, calling for a new public health emergency response system. Under the proposed system, once the president declared a health emergency, all powers for guiding administration policy would go to the surgeon general, who would have broad powers to cut through red tape in all federal agencies and expedite a swift response. Considering the problems AIDS research faced in the perplexing federal funding system, Watkins felt the proposal was reasonable enough. As a military man used to *getting things done*, Admiral Watkins couldn't believe that research on AIDS treatments was being hung up by officials at the Office of Management and Budget refusing to allow the National Institutes of Health to build new labs or hire more staffers. He was incredulous at the mixed signals on AIDS policy emanating from the administration. The experts at the Centers for Disease Control counseled against AIDS discrimination in the workplace, for example, but the conservative Justice Department issued a legal opinion saying such discrimination was just fine. AIDS was war, Watkins reasoned, and in a war *somebody must be in charge*; that's how you *get things done*. In interviews shortly after the release of his statements, Watkins said he hoped Congress would enact his proposal and that the surgeon general would get his emergency powers by the end of the year.

For all its logic, the political implications of Watkins's recommendations set congressional aides chortling to each other all over Washington. Few had any reasonable expectation that such a public health response system would be enacted. Even Watkins privately doubted that his proposal would get past his own commission. It was really something of a rhetorical statement to the cognizant from a man who wanted to impart an important message while still appearing loyal to the president. But insiders realized that by choosing the surgeon general as the man who should wield broad emergency powers, Watkins was offering a scornful assessment of the ability of the HHS secretary and the assistant secretary for health to handle AIDS, even in 1988. Moreover, as some congressional aides noted, the surgeon general is one of the few high-ranking administration officials who does not serve at the pleasure of the president, staying in office, instead, for a fixed term. Once in charge of AIDS, therefore, the surgeon general could, in effect, tell even the president to stuff it. Some believed Watkins's plan was a delicate way of suggesting that the president ought not to have too great a say in AIDS policy, given his past record.

Such implications were duly noted by a White House that already had faced a bad year in AIDS policy-making. Indeed, the appointment of the AIDS commission just days after the president's first address on the epidemic a year earlier had touched off the first wave of unhappy days. Coerced by Congress into forming a commission it never wanted, White House domestic policy adviser Gary Bauer, a protégé of ultraconservative Education Secretary William Bennett, stacked the membership largely with conservative ideologues who had little background at all in AIDS but who could be counted on to support a New Right agenda. These appointees included the president of Project Hope, who, by a strange coincidence, was Bennett's uncle; the president of Amway products, who, as a former finance chair of the Republican Party, had raised millions of dollars for conservatives; the wife of the Tennessee finance chair of Vice President Bush's presidential campaign; an Illinois legislator who was a protégé of antifeminist crusader Phyllis Schlafly; and New York City's conservative John Cardinal O'Connor, an outspoken foe of gay civil rights. Bauer argued vociferously against including a gay member on the commission. Homosexual geneticist Dr. Frank Lilly was appointed only after a reported personal intervention by First Lady Nancy Reagan, who was becoming increasingly concerned with how history would judge the Reagan AIDS record.

The commission promptly dissolved into fierce ideological squabbling as conservatives pushed their various causes. Within four months, the commission chair was so distressed at the infighting that he resigned; the vice chair, disgusted at the politicking, quickly followed suit, as did the commission staff. Reagan then put Watkins in charge, secure that the retired admiral would prove a pliable presence. A committed Roman Catholic, the fifty-nine-year-old Watkins was a former chief of naval operations and member of the Joint Chiefs of Staff, a conservative who had staunchly defended the military's blanket exclusions of gays. However, Watkins also possessed a quality that was altogether inimical to what the Reagan administration wanted from the leader of its AIDS commission—he was fair-minded, with little interest in pursuing an ideological agenda on the epidemic.

While the commission industriously held its hearings throughout late 1987 and early 1988, various altercations within the administration on other fronts prevented anything resembling a cohesive response to the various challenges of the epidemic. The White House had long ago decided that Surgeon General C. Everett Koop had been brainwashed by militant homosexuals, and presidential aides roundly ignored his suggestions. In fact, Reagan had never so much as had a meeting with Koop to discuss the epidemic. Carrying more weight was Education Secretary Bennett, who had gone ga-ga over the potential offered by massive AIDS testing. In one proposal privately circulated at the White House, Bennett set forth an aggressive plan to test fifty-seven million Americans at a cost of $306 million. Testing mania was so rabid on Pennsylvania Avenue that the White House pressured the Veterans' Administration to test every patient coming into its massive complex of facilities. VA administrators resisted the suggestion by pointing out that such testing was probably illegal.

The administration steadfastly opposed laws that would protect the confidentiality of AIDS test results and protect HIV-infected people from discrimination. That, the administration privately reasoned, would be coddling those people who were infected, and amounted to little more than backdoor approval of gay rights. CDC officials argued that the goal of AIDS testing was not to punish the infected but to stop the spread of the disease, but they too were viewed as captives of homosexual interest groups.

Nor were White House conservatives keen on the idea of AIDS-prevention programs that told people how not to contract the AIDS virus in the first place. Convinced that AIDS-education programs were cleverly designed covers to promote sodomy and sexual promiscuity, Bennett issued an official Department of Education handbook, approved by the White House, that urged teachers to stress "appropriate moral and social conduct" as the first line of defense against AIDS. Meanwhile, the CDC's proposal for a national mailing from Koop's office, like comparable mailings completed more than three years earlier in all of western Europe, was repeatedly stalled by administration officials for this or that bureaucratic reason. The mailing only went out in the days before the Stockholm conference—after it was specifically ordered by two acts of Congress.

With the failure of the executive branch of the American government, Congress once again assumed leadership in both uncovering administration lassitude and giving some coherence to the nation's response to the epidemic. Solons from both parties showed an amazing willingness to forge a bipartisan consensus on issues of research and education. The year's largest AIDS spending package, a $655 million bill for treatment and prevention, was shepherded through the U.S. Senate under the cosponsorship of Senator Edward Kennedy, one of the body's most liberal senators, and Senator Orrin Hatch, one of its most conservative. The bipartisan consensus tended to fall apart on politically touchy issues like nondiscrimination, and ultraconservative Senator Jesse Helms was usually on hand to offer this or that amendment decrying homosexuality. What direction did exist to federal AIDS policy, however, continued to come from the legislative branch.

June 12
Stockholmsmassans Convention Center

The full orchestra played a dignified anthem while all seven thousand delegates to the Fourth International Conference on AIDS stood politely, craning their necks to watch His Royal Majesty King Carl XVI Gustaf enter the sprawling hall. The Swedish prime minister welcomed the conferees and, with more stately overtures from the orchestra, the conference's first session was convened.

The opening ceremony of the AIDS conference demonstrated the extent to which the epidemic had become not only respectable, but wholly institutionalized. Between the elegant music and the solemn first speeches, the evening was more like a PBS special than a scientific conference. The senior statesmen of AIDS research, Drs. Robert Gallo and Luc Montagnier, delivered the opening scientific addresses. Neither researcher had much new to offer, but their speeches were now part of AIDS conference ritual. For Gallo, who had made it through another controversial year, it was still something to continue to dominate center stage as the so-called co-discoverer of the AIDS virus.

With participants from 140 countries, the meeting also had the atmosphere of a scientific United Nations. Over the past year, the international mobilization against the epidemic was the most significant single development in the AIDS story. The epidemic had become the first disease ever singled out for discussion on the floor of the U.N. General Assembly. In January, delegations from 142 nations, including 120 health ministers, had assembled in London for an international AIDS summit. And under the leadership of a charismatic CDC epidemiologist, Dr. Jonathan Mann, the World Health Organization's Global Programme on AIDS had emerged as the world's fastest-growing health bureaucracy. The WHO budget for AIDS now approached $100 million a year, donated largely by the developed nations of North America and Europe, spawning a global network of AIDS control plans in 75 nations. The unprecedented international cooperation in the fight against AIDS fuelled visionaries' hopes that one day health issues would be confronted by a united humankind who, at least in this arena, could lay aside differences of race and of political ideologies. In his speech at the opening ceremony, Mann outlined the dimensions of the problem: at least 200,000 people had AIDS internationally, between 5 and 10 million were infected worldwide, and there would be 1 million AIDS cases by the early 1990s. Gravely, he concluded, "There has never been anything like this before, and the world will change forever as its result."

With the growing international AIDS network, the catchword of the 1988 conference became the "institutionalization" of AIDS. The Stockholm conference launched an international AIDS society with San Francisco General Hospital's Dr. Paul Volberding as its president-elect. The society would sponsor future conferences and publish its own journal of AIDS research. Nobel Prize–winning virologist Dr. David Baltimore marvelled at the existence of a conference that could bring epidemiologists from Katmandu, Nepal, and Lima, Peru, to rub shoulders with Soviet molecular biologists and Danish immunologists. "As a virologist, I can't describe what it's like to see seven thousand people get together to talk about just one virus," enthused Baltimore. "The international Congress of Virology meets once every three years and gets only half this number of people to talk about all the viruses in the world."

Dr. Marcus Conant listened to Jim Curran's presentation with impatience and growing anger. What Curran seemed to be saying, Conant thought, was that the government was doing a great job of counting bodies and an even better job of predicting how many bodies they would be counting in the future. What Conant was more interested in hearing about was what the government was going to do to stop those bodies from piling up. Conant had come to the conference to get information that could help patients; instead, he was just getting mad.

The dearth of good news from the conference was by now the talk of AIDS clinicians in the hallways of the modernistic Stockholmsmassans Convention Center. Problems with AIDS vaccine development had refueled researchers' fears that they would never find a safe, effective vaccine against the disease. Even worse, there were few reported advances in the search for long-term treatments for AIDS sufferers or those infected with HIV. The lack of advancements in this area particularly galled Conant, because he knew impediments stemmed almost entirely from the sluggish bureaucracy of the National Institutes of Health, the agency in charge of developing AIDS treatments.

This highlighted the central irony of AIDS research in 1988: On one hand, researchers like Conant had grown ever more optimistic about their ability to overcome the biological barriers to finding successful long-term treatments for AIDS. They were convinced that at some point in the not-too-distant future, AIDS could become a manageable, chronic medical condition like diabetes, which, while troubling, would not be lethal. On the other hand, never before was there greater pessimism about overcoming the bureaucratic barriers to reaching that day. The problems were not biological or scientific, but political.

Of course, Conant, like everyone else treating AIDS patients, had heard all the official explanations from the NIH. Government scientists continued to insist that the delays in finding meaningful therapies for AIDS were entirely beyond their control. Yes, the NIH insisted repeatedly, they had the money and manpower they needed to do the job, and they were moving as fast as they *responsibly* could. People who suggested they move faster, NIH doctors would add a bit smugly, were out to undermine *good, responsible science*. "Responsible science" was the favored term in Bethesda AIDSpeak now.

Conant and physicians on the front lines of AIDS research knew better. Bureaucratic delays and endless red tape had so clogged the process of approving clinical trials for AIDS drugs that clinicians complained they would be far better off working without the government than working with it. The NIH was not only not helping things, they said; it was actually getting in the way. Conant himself was conducting drug trials out of his office in conjunction with private pharmaceutical companies who were loath to be mired in the red tape and byzantine scientific politics of the NIH bureaucracy.

This was not the way things were supposed to work. Since 1986, Congress had appropriated hundreds of millions of dollars for an AIDS Treatment and Evaluation Unit system, or ATEU, designed to rapidly put promising AIDS treatments into clinical trials to see if they were effective. After nearly two years in existence, however, the only drug that had received much testing at the ATEUs was AZT, a drug for which the NIH could claim credit. In fact, some 90 percent of the 3,500 people in ATEU trials were in one or another AZT study. The other fifty treatments that were promising enough to be in some phase of FDA approval tended to get lost in the shuffle. Criticism of the ATEU's sluggishness became so pronounced by late 1987 that NIH brass grandly announced that they would bend to public pressure and . . . change the name of the ATEU system.

Several months later, this was followed by the announcement that Dr. Anthony Fauci, director of the National Institute of Allergy and Infectious Diseases, would become the associate NIH director for AIDS. It was not clear what difference the new title would make. Fauci remained NIAID director, a full-time job in itself, considering that the agency was supposed to administer, monitor, and plan for $310 million in AIDS studies alone in the next fiscal year. Fauci also continued to do immunological research at the NIH hospital. The piling up of responsibilities was in keeping with an NIH management mentality that seemed to hold that billion-dollar AIDS programs should be run like a mom-and-pop store, with Dad stocking the shelves, running the cash register, and doing the books at night.

Not surprisingly, NIH management problems persisted, adding horrendous delays to even the simplest AIDS research projects. One planned CDC study of the effect of AZT on healthy people infected with the AIDS virus, for example, was delayed five months while the NIH bitterly fought for control of the research, insisting the NIH, not the CDC, should conduct the study. When the NIH won the turf battle, it refused to use the already prepared CDC protocol, and so the study waited two more months while a near-identical protocol was written by an NIH doctor. It took four months to find placebo tablets that looked like AZT; apparently, nobody had thought of this detail before it could delay the study. And then recruiting actual study subjects was delayed many months more while each hospital participating in the study submitted the protocol to their institutional review boards, some of which met only once every few months. A year and three months after the CDC had been ready to launch the study, fewer than one-half the study subjects had been enrolled in the NIH program. And this study, which might determine whether AZT could halt the almost-certain progression from HIV seropositivity to AIDS, was, everyone agreed, the most important piece of AIDS clinical research in the United States. Even more frightful stories accompanied attempts to move other drugs into clinical trials. When pressed, however, NIH officials, particularly Dr. Fauci, insisted that there were no internal problems. The NIH had all the staff and money it needed, he said, to conduct its research, which must be done in a manner that was *scientifically responsible*.

For Conant, who had several hundred HIV-positive patients waiting apprehensively for some medicine that might keep them from contracting AIDS, the delays in such studies were mortifying. New projections from the San Francisco hepatitis cohort now held that 99 percent of people infected with HIV would develop the lethal disease in time if no treatments were forthcoming. With the federal government saying that between 1 and 1.5 million Americans were infected with HIV, such studies predicted deaths far greater than even Curran's bleak forecasts. And yet, studies on treatments that might prevent this wholesale death languished because of agency turf wars and unnecessary delays.

Because of the torpid pace of NIH research, most advancements in clinical management of AIDS patients were made outside the government by private physicians. Private doctors like Conant, for example, had pioneered the use of an aerosolized version of pentamidine, which seemed to prevent the appearance of *Pneumocystis carinii* pneumonia, still the major killer of AIDS patients. Aerosolized pentamidine was no ultimate answer for AIDS, of course. It did not solve the problem of the underlying immune deficiency, so instead of getting *Pneumocystis*, the patient got some other opportunistic infection. But that usually came much later in the course of the disease. By most counts, there were easily several thousand Americans alive by mid-1988 who would otherwise be dead without the drug.

Among AIDS insiders, however, the aerosolized-pentamidine issue was a paradigm of how the NIH and FDA not only retarded good research, but actually prevented the results of what research was accomplished from helping people. Because the experiences of Conant and other AIDS clinicians represented evidence that was only "anecdotal," the FDA had not yet approved aerosolized pentamidine as a PCP prophylaxis. That meant that people on private insurance could not get reimbursed for pentamidine costs, because most insurance companies only pay for FDA-approved treatments. Moreover, some doctors outright refused to use any treatment lacking FDA approval. Since only the better-connected physicians in the gay community were even aware of its use, the treatment was generally not used outside of gay men, which meant that poor minorities were simply left to die. But before the FDA could solve these problems and approve the treatment, it wanted the results of randomized clinical trials, which were supposed to be conducted by the NIH. Indeed, the NIH had put aerosolized pentamidine on its list of "priority" drugs for rapid testing in early 1987—but no trials had begun.

The issue exploded into a major embarrassment just weeks before the Stockholm conference, when U.S. Representative Ted Weiss called Fauci and other officials from the NIH and FDA to his oversight subcommittee, the site of so many revealing AIDS hearings in the early 1980s. Weiss put Fauci under oath, and only then did the truth about the NIH management problems come out. Under sharp questioning, Fauci admitted that the problems in getting aerosolized pentamidine into testing stemmed "almost exclusively" from the lack of staff at the NIH. In fact, under further interrogation, it turned out that Fauci had requested 127 staff positions to handle AIDS treatment protocols at the NIAID; the administration had granted him only eleven employees. When pressed by U.S. Representative Nancy Pelosi, the freshman legislator who had been elected to the seat of the late Representative Sala Burton of San Francisco, Fauci admitted that if he were ailing he would seek out aerosolized pentamidine himself, even if it meant he had to get it "in the street."

The admission that the administration was still nickel-and-diming the NIH was damning enough. Even worse was the fact that it was Fauci who had spent much of the past year assuring reporters that the only barriers to AIDS treatments were unavoidable delays that were all in the interest of *responsible science*. It was now clear that Fauci had spent much of the past year not telling the truth. What stunned congressmen even more was that the only way to get the NIH's top-ranking AIDS official to admit the staffing shortfalls publicly was to put him under oath and, in effect, threaten him with penalty of perjury. It brought back all the murky memories of the deceitful health officials streaming to congressional committees in 1982 and 1983 to insist that *government scientists have all the funds they need . . . no stone is being left unturned*. Government scientists, it seemed, still were less interested in protecting the public health than in saying what the Reagan administration wanted them to say, even if it meant that thousands would die as a result.

Fauci's testimony fuelled a brief burst of outrage from predictable quarters. As feisty as ever, Larry Kramer took time off from working on two new plays to pen another attack on the federal government in the *Village Voice*, calling Fauci a "murderer" and bluntly asking, "Why did you keep quiet for so long? I don't know (though it wouldn't surprise me) if you kept quiet intentionally. I don't know (though it wouldn't surprise me) if you were ordered to keep quiet by Higher Ups somewhere. You are a good lieutenant, like Adolf Eichmann." In the mainstream press, however, Fauci's startling testimony received only a whisper of comment.

This led to a second area of anger for Conant, one that was only piqued further as he watched reporters respectfully scurrying after NIH scientists at the conference. "Where are the journalistic watchdogs?" he railed to one San Francisco newsman. "Where are the reporters who are supposed to protect the public's interest?"

Media nonreaction to stories of deceit at the highest levels of Washington's AIDS bureaucracy highlighted the fact that the press still had not grasped what was important in the ongoing AIDS drama. Inarguably, AIDS reporting now featured some of the best medical and science writing in the history of journalism. A lot of this writing, however excellent, continued to miss the point. Breakthroughs in complicated issues of molecular virology or the elegant genetics of the AIDS virus would be of little real significance if federal agencies had neither the personnel nor the management expertise to put them to good use. Moreover, it was never clear what good were long, in-depth analyses on the state of AIDS vaccine and treatment development if the NIH officials who were quoted—and NIH officials were often the *only* people quoted—had the propensity not to tell the truth.

Media recalcitrance to devote serious investigative journalism to federal AIDS policy was, by 1988, downright astounding. Some reporters covering AIDS had allowed themselves to be reduced to mere NIH sycophants; more commonly, others feared that an adversarial tone might cost them all-important access to government researchers. At the Stockholm conference, Dr. Gallo was already holding press conferences by-invitation-only, excluding all but the most respectful reporters. Network television coverage, meanwhile, was little more than a diary of the obvious. No television network had assigned a reporter full-time to cover the unfolding story, and none of the networks' already overworked science correspondents had demonstrated either the background or the disposition to challenge the administration's official press releases.

The media's lack of interest in the serious politics of AIDS created a presidential primary season in which the A-word was rarely uttered aloud. Though polls in every region of the country showed the epidemic was near the top of the list of voters' domestic policy concerns, reporters rarely asked candidates about their AIDS platforms, sometimes groaning aloud if another reporter, usually one from San Francisco, insisted on raising the issue during a press conference. Presidential hopefuls, who rarely volunteered stands on any controversial subjects unless asked, spoke only in the broadest platitudes about AIDS, when they spoke at all. Democratic candidate Reverend Jesse Jackson and Republican aspirant Senator Robert Dole had well-developed AIDS policies, but their rhetoric failed to nudge the ultimate nominees, Vice President George Bush and Governor Michael Dukakis, to be similarly forthcoming. In fact, by the end of the primary campaign, neither Bush nor Dukakis had set forth a detailed plan on exactly what he would do about the disease that was projected to claim 365,000 American casualties during the next presidential term. Interviews with both candidates' staffs made it clear that neither had chosen a specific course of action. No matter who won the presidential election, it did not appear likely that a new president would hit the ground running, clean house in the federal AIDS bureaucracy, and get things done.

Conant was crestfallen as the Stockholm conference progressed. "I've got to go back to the office next Monday and tell dying men that there's nothing new to help them," he sighed. "And why? Because the government's not doing its job, and the press isn't doing its job either. So little has changed."

The assessment was shared by many doctors at the Stockholmsmassans that week. On the surface, it looked as if the history of AIDS had entered a new era: The disease had become infinitely more respectable as a cause and subject of discussion. As a cultural topic, in fact, AIDS was nearly ubiquitous now. Moreover, it was clear that most Americans wanted to respond compassionately to the problem and do whatever it took to get the mess solved. This, however, did not mean that the nation's most powerful institutions were actually doing things much differently than they had in the past. What remained most noteworthy about AIDS in America during 1987 and 1988 was how, in Congress, in the White House, at the National Institutes of Health, and in the media, very little had fundamentally changed. The band still played on.

Throughout the conference, whenever the lights in the grand hall dimmed, two spotlights cut through the darkness and illuminated two huge tapestries on either side of the dais. On each hanging were stitched the names of people who had died. As Cleve Jones watched the faces in the crowd study the names, he recalled the cold, drizzly night in San Francisco when the idea had first occurred to him. He had led the traditional candlelight march that night to commemorate the assassinations of Supervisor Harvey Milk and Mayor George Moscone. He also had asked marchers to bring a hand-lettered sign with the name of someone they knew who had died in the epidemic. At the end of the march, after they had left their candles on the statue of Abraham Lincoln, Cleve directed the demonstrators to the side of the nearby Federal Building. Each participant taped a name on the grey concrete walls of the building and within a few minutes, there were hundreds of names. Everyone stood spellbound, staring at the wall with all the names of the dead. Put together, the squares looked like those of a patchwork quilt, Cleve thought.

The idea of a quilt stuck with Cleve—a quilt with all the names of the dead. It wasn't much more than a year ago, after one of his closest friends had died, that he had made a tapestry for the man, Marvin Feldman. He began to talk up the idea and promoted the concept aggressively at the 1987

Gay Freedom Day Parade in San Francisco. He wanted a massive quilt to unfold at the foot of the U.S. Capitol when hundreds of thousands gathered for the March on Washington for Lesbian and Gay Rights in October 1987. By September, only three hundred panels had arrived in the office Cleve opened on the last site of Harvey Milk's old camera store near Castro Street, but the idea took hold as various newspapers began reporting on the poignant project to memorialize the dead. Within weeks, Cleve's office was flooded with quilt panels, and nearly two thousand had been stitched together for the march on Washington, covering two acres of the Capitol Mall.

Each quilt panel was six by three feet, the size of a human grave. Friends and family who sewed the panels usually added some personal touches for the departed. The one for civil-rights lawyer Felix Velarde-Munoz featured the scales of justice; Bill Kraus's had the palm trees of Hawaii, his favorite vacation spot; on Rock Hudson's was the Hollywood sign; Liberace's was sewn with sequins from his favorite cape. There were panels for the people who had played roles great and small in the history of the epidemic: Paul Popham and Elizabeth Prophet, Olympic decathlete Tom Waddell and U.S. Rep. Stewart McKinney, the first congressman to die of AIDS. Each panel represented individual loss; stitched together and stretching farther and farther, they were for many people a glimmer of how much had been lost to the disease. Few could wander for more than several minutes among the names and not be moved to tears.

Cleve was enthralled, not only with what the quilt did to people, but also with what it meant. Quilts resounded with good old-fashioned American virtue, of Conestoga wagons, working together at barn raisings and quilting bees, and everybody helping one another out on the night of the terrible flood. The quilt also encouraged people to respond compassionately to the plight posed by AIDS, while advancing no overt political message. With all the color and drama of the quilt, Cleve also knew it would be irresistible to the media.

The Names Project, as Cleve called it, proved a sensation. At the national march, which fell on Cleve's thirty-third birthday, publicity on the quilt far overshadowed even the news of 300,000 lesbians and gay men marching on the Capitol. Local Names Project chapters sprang up in thirty cities. In early 1988, the quilt had launched an American tour, garnering a band of quilt groupies—the "Thread Heads"—who followed the project from city to city. A full-color book on the project was published in 1988, with a documentary film in the making. Pope John Paul II viewed the quilt on his trip to the San Francisco basilica, where he told one hundred sufferers of AIDS and ARC that "God loves people with AIDS, without distinction, without limit."

By the time Cleve brought the huge panels to the Stockholm conference at the invitation of the Swedish government, the outpouring of attention and support for the quilt had easily made him the most prominent gay leader in the United States. Both the World Health Organization and the Centers for Disease Control were negotiating with Cleve to sponsor events built around the quilt. Cleve was surprised at how simple his message, the message of the tapestry, had become—Americans needed to take care of one another and accept one another, no matter what seemed to separate them. When stripped of political rhetoric, Cleve realized this had always been the message of his embattled community. Cleve never was more convinced that this message would be heard as when he sat in the back bleachers of the Stockholm convention center and saw the spotlights brightening the panels of his quilt.

Cleve knew that many more of his friends would die, far more than those among the five thousand cases now counted in San Francisco. But Cleve remained healthy. His vitality defied those people who, knowing of his well-publicized status as an HIV-positive gay leader, met him and indecorously exclaimed, "Cleve—I'm surprised you're still alive." Cleve's overriding interest had always been the gay community, this dream moving through time. Today, he looked wryly at the angst he and other gay leaders had spent in the early years, worrying about an AIDS-bred, antigay backlash. It hadn't happened. The Reagan years were almost over; nothing, Cleve hoped, could be worse. For all the new rhetoric AIDS gave to the old foes of homosexuals, it was clear that the disease was making the gay community few new enemies; rather, people were coming to understand the value of a gay person's life and the great injustice that had been committed against gay people in the course of the epidemic. The future Cleve envisioned was not so much one of bright triumph, as one with an absence of darkness, with the potential of a new dawn ahead, someday. It had been a long hard journey from the glory days of gay liberation, but Cleve now truly believed that some good might ultimately come from all this suffering, even if he were not around to see it.

There was a romantic tenor to Cleve's analysis which was widely shared in the gay community, though it was at odds with another emerging appraisal of what AIDS would mean to America and the world. The second, antithetical trend of thought was generally held by people who were working on AIDS among intravenous drug users in the American inner cities, or among the impoverished masses of the Third World. These people, riding a later wave of the epidemic, saw the disease as a naturalistic drama with little that could be considered heartening. There was, after all, scant evidence that AIDS would wash away the barriers of racism and economic inequities that separated the Bronx from the affluent Upper East Side of New York. The tales of pediatric AIDS were not of mother-and-child reunions but of abandonment or orphanhood. In worn-out hospitals of São Paulo, clinicians treating the burgeoning numbers of teenagers showing their first ARC symptoms did not have the luxury of contemplating the spiritual growth an AIDS diagnosis might bring the patient. Nor did the doctors in Kampala or Kinshasa find any happy ending even vaguely implicit in the staggering prevalence of HIV in their teeming urban slums.

It was on the shoulders of such physicians in the Third World and in American inner cities that the true weight of the future AIDS epidemic would fall. You could read the story of AIDS in the measured desperation in their eyes, even while they gleaned every medical report from the Stockholm conference for some hint of hope, something that might stop the avalanche of death that lay ahead.

The Stockholm conference marked a time when the story of AIDS in the gay community at last diverged from the broader story of AIDS in America and in the world. The fact that educational programs had all but eliminated new HIV infections from gay men meant that the turbulent changes that marked gays' adjustment to the epidemic in the early 1980s were completed. That work was largely done, and as the disease spread rapidly in the underclass, gay men made up an increasingly smaller proportion of its cases. The fact that AIDS had been perceived as a gay disease had everything to do with how it was dealt with by various institutions in the early years, but that phase was now effectively over as well. To be sure, the epidemic would define the future of the gay movement and hold vast political and cultural implications for homosexuals worldwide for many decades to come. But while AIDS would play a central role in gay history, it was clear that gays would not play the most central role in the future history of AIDS. They were separate stories now, the story of AIDS among gays and the story of AIDS elsewhere, and they were stories that shared very little except their common historical roots and the physical suffering wrought by a horribly cruel and insidious virus.

Rakai, Uganda

From the shadows of his mud hut, the gaunt and weary young man stares outside to the pigs playing in the dust under the banana palms. His chest is covered with open sores; skin rashes have left his ebony arms looking as if they are covered in chalk; his army fatigues hang loosely around his waist.

Outside, Charles Lwanga glances toward his ailing second son and lowers his voice. Last year, when the Ugandan army gave him his medical furlough, his son was sick, but at least he could walk, says Lwanga. Now he cannot walk, and his son's young wife has returned to her village, where she recently gave birth to the couple's child. The baby too is very ill now; it may not survive. A few huts away, down a one-lane dirt path, another couple suffers from "slim," Lwanga says, and he hears that many are dying in his father's village.

Lwanga's brows are furrowed; he has the face of a man who is watching his son die. His eyes sharpen when he hears that an American journalist knows many of the Western doctors working on the disease. The aging man has no intelligence of byzantine scientific intrigues and timorous reporters, or of esoteric distinctions between American political factions. He knows only that the United States is a country of immense wealth, and that the medicine that will save his country and his son will probably come from there. Tears gather in his brown eyes, and he asks, "When will it come? When will there be the cure?"

THE ABSENCE OF ANGER

ANDREW HOLLERAN

from Ground Zero

| 1988 |

"Youre not angry yet. You don't feel the gun at your head," says the man who has taken the podium after a series of speakers have addressed the crowd at the community center on Thirteenth Street. He looks out at them and says this in the calm, slightly amazed voice of someone who has seen the symptoms of apathy so many times he can perceive them even through wild applause—in this case, the wild applause of a room filled with people seated on every available chair, bench, ledge, and shelf and standing in the back corners on tiptoe to see and hear the speakers who have gone before. "You just don't feel the gun at your head," he repeats, almost to himself, in amazement, in a sort of dream voice, marveling. He surveys them for a moment with a smile on his lips, a smile of wonder and, perhaps, condescension and amusement—from the height of his own anger, his own suffering, his own knowledge of what it does feel like to have the gun barrel on his temple, that is, to have AIDS. "What will it take? What will it take to make you angry?"

In truth, of course, nobody knows. He does not know. Nor, even worse, does the audience—the people who have just been asked the question. They were, at the outset of the first speech, asked to stand if they had or knew someone who has AIDS. Most did. They were asked again to stand up—in every other row of folding chairs, starting from the first—and told, once they were on their feet: "That's how many of you will not be here in five years." And later: "By 1992, half of the people in this room will be dead." Why then, aren't they angry? Why *don't* they feel the gun is at their heads?

I have come here wondering exactly that—I feel I should be angry, and I'm not—though the fact that I'm late getting here for the meeting, and the reason I'm late getting here for the meeting, provides me already with a partial answer. The reason I'm late is that I was having dinner with a friend who is sick with AIDS and did not want to rush off after coffee because I do not know when I'll see him again (I am leaving New York tomorrow), and because I did not want to tell him I was going to a meeting he is probably too weak to attend, since he must conserve his strength for the six flights of stairs he must climb to and from his loft every time he goes out. That is one reason I am not angry, I guess—anger is subsumed, lost, in sadness. It did not even seem a matter of choice—being with E. was far more important than arriving on time for a political meeting. Sorrow, moreover, is a sort of immobilizing emotion. It requires stillness, removal, withdrawal from the world. We sat in the dark loft while the Four Last Songs of Strauss played (*How can he bear this?* I wondered) and talked about books, friends, fate, as we watched the city sky darken and the lighted towers of Wall Street become sharp as diamonds. (It is exactly this the activists protest against: our turning philosophical when we should be angry. And it is exactly the opposite the gay men organizing home care for people with AIDS accuse the activists of: playing politics when they should be sitting at bedsides.) Eventually I left—slowly; as if I had nothing to do afterward, as if I were not leaving him by himself—and ran uptown to this meeting already in progress, the friend (whose speech I'd come to hear) already speaking. And, like a concertgoer who arrives after the start of a symphony, I wait in the hall. Beside me the black lesbian security guard is talking to two men in yarmulkes about a woman in Brooklyn with AIDS. On the bulletin board are the notices and advertisements endemic to universities everywhere that are still associated with the sixties—that changeless universe of yoga classes, guitar lessons, marches on Washington, shares in an apartment, requests for a room—including one that reads, "Two leather men, one from Argentina, one from Amsterdam, need place to stay in Chelsea. Close to bars, with room for weight-lifting equipment." Such a duo would have set hearts thumping in the seventies; now they remind me of that Polish ship that arrived ten days too late for the Bicentennial celebration. Times have changed, fellas. One no longer wants to be close to bars. One comes instead to places like the community center, the old Firehouse born out of its ashes, the sixties coming back relentlessly to life, like some mummy in a horror film. There is nothing quite so depressing as the doctrine of eternal recurrence. One wants to go up to people on Saint Marks Place with long hair and headbands, take them by the shoulders, and say, "Don't you know all this has been *done?*" Which is why even this—the call for demonstrations—seems like one more dreary consequence of AIDS, and why it may have fallen on indifferent ears; like the ads for yoga class, the clutter of this bulletin board, the anger of the speakers inside, it merely seems something out of the past that has just been wound up again, like an old Victrola.

The trouble is, of course, that there may be reasonable cause, now, for anger—just how reasonable is what I've come to this place to find out. A certain bitterness comes easily already. It is easy to be angry with God, or the virus, or the general arrangement of the universe in which a microbe takes man from the summit, the apex, of mammalian life to the nadir of bacterial existence, which changes him from a paragon a little lower than the angels to the doormat of every germ that comes through the door; nature's punching bag. It is easy to be disgusted by the fact that the same phenomenon that caused Rice-A-Roni to drop its jingle ("The San Francisco Treat") apparently kept President Reagan from even saying the word AIDS till only recently: AIDS does not sell political programs or noodles. Even the most apathetic citizen cannot help but compare the government's response to AIDS with its reaction—speedy, alarmed, passionate—to a disease contracted by Legionnaires having a convention at a hotel in Philadelphia during the seventies. But one is also cynical enough to realize the ramifications of the fact that AIDS is *not* spread by an air conditioner at a hotel occupied by a convention of Legionnaires. AIDS is spread by sex; in America, sex among homosexuals. And needles; needles used by drug addicts. That queer quartet that introduced the subject of AIDS to North America—Haitians, homosexuals, hemophiliacs, and heroin addicts—has never really left the minds of most Americans, no matter how many people not in those categories have died since then. Forget the babies, receivers of blood transfusions, African heterosexuals—it is still a gay disease, and as it moves into the black and Hispanic ghettos of the northern cities (those apparent pools of excess humanity mainstream America can see no role for besides breakdancing and rap music), AIDS solidifies itself as divine eugenics—that forbidden science Hitler was the last to try, that lurking fantasy people still harbor ("If only the human race, the population of this corrupt world, could be *edited*"). And so there is no national pressure to solve the problem, so long as it remains within these communities. The resources of the entire nation have not been marshaled because the entire nation has not been threatened; AIDS remains the problem of a special-interest group, in the eyes of conservatives, who, like Robert Novak on the television program *Crossfire*, suggest gays *hope* straight people will contract AIDS, so they can get more funding.

This is indeed politics at its most cynical, but no doubt in their heart of hearts, Hispanic drug addicts who abandon their babies with AIDS and homosexual activists are not exactly people America *wants* within its borders. A few years ago William Safire suggested that homosexuals simply remain invisible, and that is probably the consensus still. By now homosexuals have become accustomed to the idea that there are people who would like to see them simply subtracted from society. Including the religious. The early Christians were shocked by the custom of exposing unwanted babies in the marketplace or on the roadside in ancient Rome—to die of exposure, unless someone picked them up, and took them home—but one cannot help but see a different instinct in some of their descendants. The house-burning in Arcadia, Florida, the treatment of schoolchildren like Ryan White, is just part of the urge to keep the victims of AIDS outside the community, the home, the school, the marketplace, to wither away alone. Homosexuals rebelled against nature, and now nature is taking its revenge, wrote Pat Buchanan—before he was hired by the White House as its communications director. It is a view that allows those willing to brand homosexuals lepers the instant they had an excuse for doing so, to write off a portion of the human race in a vast collective hiss of "I told you so." Why? Because AIDS is not caused by an air conditioner in Philadelphia; AIDS is transmitted through sex. Famine gets rock stars to hold benefits, but no one packs stadiums because Africans are dying in even greater numbers of AIDS.

But even this malice isn't enough to make most homosexuals angry—this hysteria and hatred are things most of them are long familiar with. When the brother of a conservative activist takes an ad out in the *Washington Post* to say the deceased activist was not homosexual and, while dying, reconciled himself with the church by repenting his past (like the lawyer who defends his client by saying not only was his client not in the hotel that night, but if so, he did not assault the waiter), they shake their heads and smile a bitter smile. What lengths, what depths, people will go to in their aversion! Ditto the obituaries that refuse to list AIDS as the cause of death—as if there were only one thing worse than being dead and that is being homosexual. The high-pitched giggle Pat Buchanan broke into whenever interviewing a homosexual on *Crossfire*—the blush, the expression of a nine-year-old boy telling a dirty joke that inevitably suffused his face, the near falsetto of his voice when homosexuality was the subject of the program—only typifies the way legions of people like him view homosexuals: as an off-color joke. Homosexuals, I suspect, *expected* the length of time it took the president to even say the word *AIDS* in public, considered it part of the way things are, something they had and would always have to live with. And there was something else—

AIDS had also induced a kind of shock—a numbness—those first few years; the sense of unreality that occurs to us when our car begins to spin on a patch of ice or collide with another vehicle. *What is going on?* That is the chief question. One is not angry. One is dumbfounded.

Of course *all* these questions that come under the heading of "Why aren't you angry?"—Why do homosexuals not have elected leaders? Why do they not support a national organization? Why do they not employ a lobby in Washington to further their interests? Why do they not donate to gay candidates?—had been around long before AIDS. They were one of the perplexing enigmas that followed the Stonewall rebellion. Why had liberation largely expressed itself as promiscuity?

Well, for one thing, homosexuality is about sex. Most animals wish to be alone when they lay their eggs. It's hard to base a political platform on what one does behind closed doors—or in the toilets of subways. For another, homosexuality is for the most part invisible. If blacks have no choice in the matter, homosexuals could pass; and did so. The perfectly natural desire to conduct one's private life in private—an instinct common to everyone—in this case contravenes the need to stand up and be counted; and show the rest of society how average, random, and like everyone else most homosexuals are. Who wanted to be a target? Who wanted to be a lightning rod for the hatred of people from Pat Buchanan to the thug on the street who, in the company of six other adolescents, went looking for gays to bash? Life was too short to waste precious time on goons. The easiest way to be homosexual was to be homosexual in private—that's where one's homosexuality occurred, anyway. And so the attempts, long before AIDS arrived, to gather the tribe together, to consolidate money, support, political clout, collided with the universal desire to keep one's sexual life as private as everyone else's. As Freud said years ago, "Homosexuality is no vice, Madame, but assuredly no advantage."

And let us not forget that homosexuals *are* like most people, and like most people, indifferent to politics and loath to burn tires in the streets. The percentage of politically militant homosexuals is probably the same in every generation and probably the same in the general population—a fervent few. Political agitation is simply a vocation few people have in life; and those who have it are always asking, How can we get everyone else off their butts? Complicating the picture is no doubt another fact: Some homosexuals disapprove of their homosexual self. That self-repudiation is something that has never been addressed fully in gay life; it may lie beneath so many layers of apparently well-adapted behavior that the problem of people who have counted themselves out on some deep level, lowered their ambitions, stayed away from arenas in which they felt they could not succeed, is similar perhaps to that of blacks. No one even sees the self-hatred. They take William Safire's advice to simply keep quiet. And finally, even the homosexual population has its common selfishness; Scott Fitzgerald's description of the man who cares not if the whole world crashes down so long as it spares his own house applies here. *Let me just hide till all this is over*, people think, *smear blood upon the door, and let the Angel of Death pass over this house*. And so anger has been lost in a general withdrawal—an attempt to escape the general fate.

That is, the virus was just the latest in a series of diseases that no amount of money or research seems able to cure; as horrible and implacable as muscular dystrophy, multiple sclerosis, Parkinson's, Alzheimer's, Lou Gehrig's disease. In short, not all the anger or all the money in the world could eliminate these blights on human health—we had to wait for some accident, some breakthrough, some genius in a laboratory that might or might not be one of those funded by the government. We had to wait for an apple to fall on Newton's head; for Archimedes to shout "Eureka!"

And so, despite the charge by Larry Kramer that the incompetence, stupidity, and bureaucratic paralysis of the government-medical establishment amounted to genocide—that homosexuals are this generation's Jews being led off to the showers—there was little anger against the government. The government was considered just the government, not helpful to gay men but not conspiring to murder them either, coldly and consciously, that is. Most people are simply not conspiracy-minded; most people do not believe this is genocide. If San Francisco surpassed New York immeasurably in the care and treatment of AIDS patients, San Francisco had always surpassed New York in everything having to do with issues of gay life. But most homosexuals did not think Mayor Koch was Hitler. Most homosexuals, in fact, turned away from the public arena altogether and made this a personal matter. Sickness usually is. As in: Why did I let this happen to me? The anger was just a "God damn it," directed under one's breath, on walks late at night, against fate; this fate that has no favorites, intercedes never on our behalf, merely unfolds. If one was angry, one was angry at the virus—this dumb, lifeless, blind, greedy microbe that was so stupid it killed the very thing it fed on, reproducing itself to no purpose. And, no doubt, one was angry with oneself. Because in searching for the answer to that question, "Why aren't you angry?" it would be wrong to overlook one of the most bizarre things about accidents (like AIDS)—that people to whom they happen blame themselves, as if bad luck were a moral failing. Nothing is so difficult for the human mind to accept as the fact that much suffering in life is random, meaningless, and in a sense completely trivial: the wrong place at the wrong time. Once the plague established itself, gay men in doctors' offices all over Manhattan were weeping over their pasts. AIDS had simply tapped into the remorse, the conviction ("I have been unlucky in life") harbored by homosexuals who may not even suspect they have these feelings. Echoing Pat Buchanan, they say, "If only I had not been homosexual, this never would have happened." Strictly true, perhaps. But their being homosexual did not cause the illness; the virus simply exploited their homosexuality. But like someone whose child is injured on a hike they took them on, they blame themselves for ever having gone walking.

And so, as with victims of rape or any misfortune, gay men have been silenced by a peculiar guilt induced by the misfortune—which makes the minority who have formed organizations, raised money, prodded the government, gone on television to educate others, defended themselves against the Pat Buchanans and Robert Novaks and Jerry Falwells, all the more admirable. The fact that gay men did not throw rocks, set cars on fire, or besiege the White House was chiefly because they did other things that seemed more constructive at the time. They did march on Washington, they did print newspapers, they did criticize elected politicians. They did picket the airlines when Northwest refused to fly a sick man back from the Orient because he had AIDS. It is a long battle ahead, after all, and it will be necessary, of course, to confront this sort of unacceptable behavior each time it occurs. The fact is that in some curious way, though the people in this room have been told flat out that half of them will be dead in five years, none of them knows what else he can do about it—except for what he has already done. And because, most curious of all, most odd, most marvelous, the truth is none of them is really chilled by the assertion—each of them thinks he will escape, I suspect. As Freud also said, "No one really believes in his own death."

FROM BORROWED TIME

PAUL MONETTE

| 1988 |

I don't know if I will live to finish this. Doubtless there's a streak of self-importance in such an assertion, but who's counting? Maybe it's just that I've watched too many sicken in a month and die by Christmas, so that a fatal sort of realism comforts me more than magic. All I know is this: The virus ticks in me. And it doesn't care a whit about our categories—when is full-blown, what's AIDS-related, what is just sick and tired? No one has solved the puzzle of its timing. I take my drug from Tijuana twice a day. The very friends who tell me how vigorous I look, how well I seem, are the first to assure me of the imminent medical breakthrough. What they don't seem to understand is, I used up all my optimism keeping my friend alive. Now that he's gone, the cup of my own health is neither half full nor half empty. Just half.

Equally difficult, of course, is knowing where to start. The world around me is defined now by its endings and its closures—the date on the grave that follows the hyphen. Roger Horwitz, my beloved friend, died of complications of AIDS on October 22, 1986, nineteen months and ten days after his diagnosis. That is the only real date anymore, casting its ice shadow over all the secular holidays lovers mark their calendars by. Until that long night in October, it didn't seem possible that any day could supplant the brute equinox of March 12—the day of Roger's diagnosis in 1985, the day we began to live on the moon.

The fact is, no one knows where to start with AIDS. Now, in the seventh year of the calamity, my friends in L.A. can hardly recall what it felt like any longer, the time before the sickness. Yet we all watched the toll mount in New York, then in San Francisco, for years before it ever touched us here. It comes like a slowly dawning horror. At first you are equipped with a hundred different amulets to keep it far away. Then someone you know goes into the hospital, and suddenly you are at high noon in full battle gear. They have neglected to tell you that you will be issued no weapons of any sort. So you cobble together a weapon out of anything that lies at hand like a prisoner honing a spoon handle into a stiletto. You fight tough, you fight dirty, but you cannot fight dirtier than it.

I remember a Saturday in February 1982, driving Route 10 to Palm Springs with Roger to visit his parents for the weekend. While Roger drove, I read aloud an article from *The Advocate*: "Is Sex Making Us Sick?" There was the slightest edge of irony in the query, an urban cool that seems almost bucolic now in its innocence. But the article didn't mince words. It was the first in-depth reporting I'd read that laid out the shadowy nonfacts of what till then had been the most fragmented of rumors. The first cases were reported to the Centers for Disease Control (CDC) only six months before, but they weren't in the newspapers, not in L.A. I note in my diary in December '81 ambiguous reports of a "gay cancer," but I know I didn't have the slightest picture of the thing. Cancer of the *what*? I would have asked, if anyone had known anything.

I remember exactly what was going through my mind while I was reading, though I can't now recall the details of the piece. I was thinking: How is this not me? Trying to find a pattern I was exempt from. It was a brand of denial I would watch grow exponentially during the next few years, but at the time I was simply relieved. Because the article appeared to be saying that there was a grim progression toward this undefined catastrophe, a set of preconditions—chronic hepatitis, repeated bouts of syphilis, exotic parasites. No wonder my first baseline response was to feel safe. It was *them*—by which I meant the fast-lane Fire Island crowd, the Sutro Baths, the world of High Eros.

Not us.

I grabbed for that relief because we'd been through a rough patch the previous autumn. Till then Roger had always enjoyed a sort of no-nonsense good health: not an abuser of anything, with a constitutional aversion to hypochondria, and not wed to his mirror save for a minor alarm as to the growing dimensions of his bald spot. In the seven years we'd been together

I scarcely remember him having a cold or taking an aspirin. Yet in October '81 he had struggled with a peculiar bout of intestinal flu. Nothing special showed up in any of the blood tests, but over a period of weeks he experienced persistent symptoms that didn't neatly connect: pains in his legs, diarrhea, general malaise. I hadn't been feeling notably bad myself, but on the other hand I was a textbook hypochondriac, and I figured if Rog was harboring some kind of bug, so was I.

The two of us finally went to a gay doctor in the Valley for a further set of blood tests. It's a curious phenomenon among gay middle-class men that anything faintly venereal had better be taken to a doctor who's "on the bus." Is it a sense of fellow feeling perhaps, or a way of avoiding embarrassment? Do we really believe that only a doctor who's *our* kind can heal us of the afflictions that attach somehow to our secret hearts? There is so much magic to medicine. Of course we didn't know then that those few physicians with a large gay clientele were about to be swamped beyond all capacity to cope.

The tests came back positive for amoebiasis. Roger and I began the highly toxic treatment to kill the amoeba, involving two separate drugs and what seems in memory thirty pills a day for six weeks, till the middle of January. It was the first time I'd ever experienced the phenomenon of the cure making you sicker. By the end of treatment we were both weak and had lost weight, and for a couple of months afterward were susceptible to colds and minor infections.

It was only after the treatment was over that a friend of ours, diagnosed with amoebas by the same doctor, took his slide to the lab at UCLA for a second opinion. And that was my first encounter with lab error. The doctor at UCLA explained that the slide had been misread; the squiggles that looked like amoebas were in fact benign. The doctor shook his head and grumbled about "these guys who do their own lab work." Roger then retrieved his slide, took it over to UCLA, and was told the same: no amoebas. We had just spent six weeks methodically ingesting poison for no reason at all.

So it wasn't the *Advocate* story that sent up the red flag for us. We'd been shaken by the amoeba business, and from that point on we operated at a new level of sexual caution. What is now called safe sex did not use to be so clearly defined. The concept didn't exist. But it was quickly becoming apparent, even then, that we couldn't wait for somebody else to define the parameters. Thus every gay man I know has had to come to a point of personal definition by way of avoiding the chaos of sexually transmitted diseases, or STD as we call them in the trade. There was obviously no one moment of conscious decision, a bolt of clarity on the shimmering freeway west of San Bernardino, but I think of that day when I think of the sea change. The party was going to have to stop. The evidence was too ominous: *We were making ourselves sick.*

AIDS IN BLACKFACE

HARLON L. DALTON

from Daedalus

| **Summer 1989** |

My ambition in the pages that follow is to account for why we African-Americans have been reluctant to "own" the AIDS epidemic, to acknowledge the devastating toll it is taking on our communities, and to take responsibility for altering its course. By the end, I hope to convince you that what may appear to the uninitiated to be a crazy, self-defeating refusal to stand up and be counted is in fact sane, sensible, and determinedly self-protective. The black community's impulse to distance itself from the epidemic is less a response to AIDS, the medical phenomenon, than a reaction to the myriad social issues that surround the disease and give it its meaning. More fundamentally, it is the predictable outgrowth of the problematic relationship between the black community and the larger society, a relationship characterized by domination and subordination, mutual fear and mutual disrespect, a sense of otherness, and a pervasive neglect that rarely feels benign.

If I am right, then there is a profound need to reorient the public health enterprise so that it can succeed in a multicultural society. Public health officials cannot simply wander uptown (or wherever the local black ghetto is situated), their expertise in one hand, their goodwill in the other, and expect to slay the disease dragon. They must first discern just who this particular public is and how it sees itself in relation to them. How does the black community see its own health needs, and how do they stack up against its other concerns? And, not least, just what has been the black community's prior experience in dealing with government do-gooders?

Answering these questions is not an impossible task, even in the midst of an epidemic. Consider, for example, the extent to which the relationship between the white gay community and the public health establishment changed in the mid-1980s. Much has been written about the latter's failure to intervene in a timely and sensitive way early on, when the AIDS epidemic might have been successfully contained. I do not quarrel with the explanations usually proffered for this failure—the health establishment's inability to identify with or care about the gay men who were viewed as the disease's principal targets, bureaucratic ineptitude and infighting, and an administration in Washington mindlessly committed to reducing social spending no matter what. I do, however, want to highlight an additional factor, the fact that initially most public health officials approached AIDS as solely a biomedical phenomenon and exhibited little comprehension of the many ways in which culture, politics, and disease intersect. Thus they failed to realize how much freight would attach to their well-intentioned attempts to safeguard the public's health and did not anticipate that both the gay community and the larger society would react in ways reflective of the social distance between the two.

The moment of truth arrived shortly after the Food and Drug Administration approved the first HIV antibody test for the screening of the nation's blood supply. Many health officials advocated that the test be used diagnostically as well, to determine whether persons in so-called high-risk groups had been exposed to the virus. The officials were surprised to discover that most gay organizations and AIDS support organizations took the opposite view and strongly recommended that gay men, including those who had engaged in high-risk activity, *not* take the test.

At first, the public health establishment saw this resistance as misguided, irresponsible, and self-destructive. In fairly short order, however (thanks largely to the efforts of "bridge" people who served, in effect, as bicultural interpreters), key officials began to see past the bare fact that their recommendations were being opposed, to the concerns underlying the gay community's opposition: that the test was not sufficiently accurate to be used for diagnostic purposes; that testing would produce needless mental anguish for many; that persons seeking the test might thereby open themselves to criminal liability by admitting to having engaged in sodomy or the use of illicit drugs; that testing would facilitate the quarantining of persons who tested positive; that absent strict confidentiality, testing would lead (at least for seropositives) to the loss of insurance, employment, and housing, and to social isolation and vilification as well. These concerns, the officials realized, were as much the lived reality of AIDS as helper-T cells and transmission routes.

It became apparent that to reach the gay community, public health officials had to learn to view the epidemic from the perspective of the gay community. Consequently, today even the most control-minded health officials take care to involve the gay community in decision-making and emphasize the need for a high degree of test accuracy, for strict confidentiality, and for enhanced laws against discrimination. The moral of this story is plain. The public health establishment *can* take account of community differences if it has to. It *can* take account of the sociopolitical contexts in which it operates. It *can*, if pressed, recognize that its targets are, in an important sense, its teachers. My hope is that the failure of New York's needle-exchange program, together with other failures to reach the black community, will, like the white gay opposition to testing in the mid-1980s, provoke thoughtful reconsideration of how the public health enterprise should operate in a society deeply divided along racial lines.

I have arrived at the conclusions in this essay in much the same way a reporter, or perhaps a biographer, would. Rather than engage in rigorous empirical research, I have relied on my store of impressions formed over several years of communicating about AIDS with the black community and, more important, listening to concerns voiced outside that community. The comparison to reporting and biography is less than perfect inasmuch as I do not claim to be neutral. I do not pretend to be solely a channel for the experiences and expressions of others. On the contrary, as a member of the black community I have personally experienced most of the sentiments and dynamics about which I report, and like human beings in general, tend to view others' experience through the prism of my own. My hope is that the texture and depth of the result will more than offset any distortions.

My approach rests on two assumptions—that an African-American subculture exists (marked by shared sentiments, sensibilities, experiences, and history) and that I am sufficiently linked to it (by virtue of upbringing, kinship ties, and spirit) to be qualified to interpret it.

The first proposition is, I should think, relatively unproblematic so long as we remain near the subculture's core and resist the temptation to specify its precise contours. As for the second proposition, you are, I am afraid, going to have to trust me, at least provisionally. The true test of my entitlement to speak about (not for) the black community will be whether my words resonate for the majority of its members (and for the small set of others who know it well).

On occasion I will take the liberty of treating you, dear reader, as a stand-in for white America. That is to say, I will speak directly to *it* through *you*. My goal in so doing is not to artificially divide (though that is certainly a risk I take), but rather to speak in a way that captures the timbre as well as the pitch of the community sentiments I seek to convey.

THE IMPACT OF AIDS

Unquestionably, AIDS has hit the black community hard. We are losing our sons and daughters at an alarming rate. Twenty-five percent of all persons with AIDS in the United States are African-American. Among the newly diagnosed, the figure exceeds 36 percent. In many eastern cities, blacks and Latinos constitute a majority of the AIDS cases. In New York City, where AIDS is the number-one killer of women between the ages of twenty-five and thirty-four, black women, with their Latina sisters, account for 84 percent of the adult female AIDS cases. Nine out of ten children with AIDS in New York City are black or Latino. In the Bronx one baby in forty-three is born infected. Across the board, black people are disproportionately represented. Thus, even among gay and bisexual men and intravenous drug users, blacks are more likely to be infected than are their white counterparts. On average, black persons with AIDS (PWAs) are sicker at time of diagnosis than white PWAs and die nearly five times as rapidly.

Notwithstanding this bleak picture, public health officials and AIDS organizations around the country have been frustrated in their efforts to organize the black community to deal with AIDS. While the vast majority of such people and organizations are predominantly white, even black and Latino officials and activists have run into more than their fair share of walls. Resistance within the community ranges from the simple refusal to acknowledge that AIDS is a problem for black people (an increasingly difficult position to maintain in the face of the overwhelming numbers) to the rejection of programs designed to stem the transmission of HIV. In between these extremes, our leaders, however defined, seem to run away from the issue of AIDS. They talk about it as little as possible and even more rarely involve themselves in efforts to develop constructive solutions.

Perhaps the most dramatic example of the black community's resistance to AIDS intervention involves New York City's pilot needle-exchange program. The goal of the program is to test whether addicts will, if given a chance, exchange used needles for clean ones, and if so, whether that step will appreciably lower the incidence of HIV infection in the addict population. Originally designed to operate in neighborhoods where drug abuse is prevalent, the program was located instead, thanks to pressure from black and Latino community leaders, in a downtown government office building, far away (geographically and otherwise) from its target population. This concession of city officials (a move that, in the view of most observers, severely compromised the program's prospects for success) did not, however, dampen community opposition. On the contrary, word of the program's grand opening "ignited," in the words of one reporter.

Typical of the reaction was Harlem city council member Hilton B. Clark, who characterized the program as a "genocidal campaign." A key opponent was New York's police commissioner, Benjamin Ward, who explained that as a black person, he had "a particular sensitivity to doctors conducting experiments, and they too frequently seem to be conducted against blacks." One month after needle exchange began, the New York City Council, led by its black and Hispanic caucus, urged the health commissioner to cancel the program. In commenting on the nonbinding resolution, which passed on a vote of 31–0, caucus chair Enoch Williams explained that "the city is sending the wrong message when it distributes free needles to drug addicts while we are trying to convince our children to say no to drugs."

City officials were not the only ones to join the chorus. For example, the Reverend Reginald Williams of the Addicts Rehabilitation Center in East Harlem promised that "there will never be a needle-exchange program here. I think the communities and neighborhoods would rise up in opposition. They tell me this is what we must try. . . . Why must we again be the guinea pigs in this genocidal mentality?" To the surprise of many, the needle-exchange program was even opposed by the likes of Dr. Beny J. Primm, a highly respected leader in the field of substance abuse and a belated addition to former President Reagan's AIDS Commission. Primm took issue with the claim that needle exchange would lower the incidence of HIV transmission and, as an alternative, pushed for a more rational system of assigning addicts to available treatment program openings. There were, of course, some blacks and Latinos who lined up in favor of the program, most notably the Brooklyn-based Association for Drug Abuse Prevention and Treatment (ADAPT), led by Yolanda Serrano. For the most part, however, the community response was exceedingly negative.

THE RELUCTANCE TO "OWN" AIDS

Already, a set of stock explanations for this reluctance has emerged. We are told that for too long the media have inaccurately portrayed AIDS as a disease that almost exclusively afflicts white gay men, that for too long public health officials have failed to use media appropriate to the black community, and that the black church has stood in the way of effective AIDS education because of its opposition on moral grounds to homosexuality and drug use. While valid to a point, these explanations have, in my opinion, been very much overblown. First, the mass media are scarcely the only avenues of communication in the black community (a point made by some of the same people who seek to pin the misrepresentation tail on the media). Moreover, we have long since learned to view the media with suspicion and to discount their distortions when our own experiences contradict them. Second, even though the public health establishment has relied on media not well suited to reaching the black population (too many pamphlets and not enough radio spots, for example), by and large health officials have used the same media that arguably have succeeded at presenting a distorted picture of who has AIDS.

As for the third stock explanation, it does a disservice, in my view, to the black church. It is, of course, true that much of the church is doctrinally fundamentalist and socially conservative. These characteristics, however, are constraints not so much on what can be done in the realm of social action as on how to do it. In practice, the church has proved adaptable, pragmatic, and even crafty when need be. To paraphrase former President Nixon, if you want to understand the black church, watch what it does, not what it says. Time and again, the church has demonstrated its awareness of the variability of human existence and the fragility of the soul under siege. Time and again, the church has been responsive to the needs, spiritual and nonspiritual, of the community. The civil rights movement of the 1950s and 1960s is simply the most dramatic example in recent memory.

What else, then, accounts for the black community's reluctance to grapple with AIDS? I have isolated five overlapping factors that I think explain a great deal. The first is that many African-Americans are reluctant to acknowledge our association with AIDS so long as the larger society seems bent on blaming us as a race for its origin and initial spread. Second, the deep-seated suspicion and mistrust many of us feel whenever whites express a sudden interest in our well-being hampers our progress in dealing with AIDS. Third, the pathology of our own homophobia hobbles us. Fourth, the uniquely problematic relationship we as a community have to the phenomenon of drug abuse complicates our dealings with AIDS. And fifth, many in the black community have difficulty transcending the deep resentment we feel at being dictated to once again.

Blame

Early on in the AIDS epidemic, and continuing for some time, scientists, the press, and the public seemed curiously fixated on the origins of the virus associated with AIDS. From the perspective of the black community, interest in HIV's possible African roots seemed insatiable. Article after article appeared, recirculating identical hypotheses. The discovery of a similar virus in the African green monkey stirred the pot and prompted endless speculation about how it might have traveled from an "animal reservoir" into the human species. When pressed to explain why so much time and energy were being devoted to so marginal a concern, white people usually responded that determining where the virus originated might lead to the discovery of ways to slow it down or eliminate it altogether. Perhaps. Black folks, however, offer a different explanation. We understood in our bones that with origin comes blame. The singling out of Haitians as a so-called risk group simply confirmed our worst fears.

Although the society's fixation with the origin of AIDS has faded and Haitians are no longer officially viewed as synonymous with AIDS, for us the memory dies hard. Our exasperation and sometimes rage lingers just below the surface. Were I to go out tomorrow and speak about AIDS to a black audience anywhere in this country, I guarantee you that once the discussion gets going, someone would ask about the disease's origins. The question "Is it true that it started in Africa?" would quickly become "Why do they keep trying to pin it on Africa?" "Why do they keep trying to pin it on us?" and eventually I would be asked the clincher: "What are they trying to say we *did* with that monkey?"

More than insult and affront are at issue here. So long as we African-Americans continue to worry that any hint of connection with AIDS will be turned against us, we will remain leery of accepting responsibility for its impact on our community.

Suspicion and Mistrust

It is difficult to overemphasize the extent to which the black community, qua community, reflexively responds with suspicion and mistrust to what are perceived as "white" initiatives. Just as Jews admonish each other to "never forget," we do not wish to forget the bitter lessons we have been taught since being brought to these shores. Slavery, a subject one does not bring up in polite company, exists within our extended memory; my father used to sit around the dinner table with his grandmother, a former slave. Segregation was upon us only yesterday. Today we must deal with Ed Koch, David Duke, and political campaigns that showcase people like Willie Horton. Push just a little bit and you will tap into wellsprings of mistrust even in those of us who live much of our lives within the ambit of the larger society and negotiate it with apparent ease (though not without cost).

Frequently, our acute mistrust manifests itself as resistance, as sparring, as buying time until we are sure we are safe. The early "negotiations" with the black community regarding AIDS seem largely to have followed this pattern. Given enough time, we can together work our way out of the pattern by building up trust, but time is at a premium where AIDS is concerned. A second way out is for black people to reconceptualize AIDS as not something white America is insisting we deal with but rather as a set of issues we ourselves want to take on. In other words, in order to "own" AIDS even in part, we may need to own it outright.

Homophobia

A third reason the black community has been slow in responding to AIDS is that many of us do not want to be associated with what is widely perceived as a gay disease. More than once I have heard of black parents readily volunteering, so as to forestall even more embarrassing speculation, that their HIV-infected children are addicts. Homophobia is not, of course, unique to the black community, but it takes on a particular character within the context of African-American history and culture. Precious little has been written on the subject. Straight black authors tend to ignore the subject altogether. A notable exception is Bell Hooks, who deftly captures the complexity of black attitudes toward homosexuality and the imperfect connection between those attitudes and actual behavior. Gay black writers seem to find it easier to train their fire on racism within the white gay community than on homophobia within the straight black community. Recently a small but hardy band of academics has begun extensive research on the life experiences of black gay men and lesbians. In time, this work will provide a rich base from which a fuller picture of the character and consequences of black homophobia can be drawn.

If we in the black community are to make progress coping with AIDS, we must deal simultaneously with our homophobia. As a first step, we must name the problem, map its contours, and develop an understanding of how it is detrimental to us as a community. I will not attempt to advance this enterprise very far here, in part because I am not sure that this essay is the best vehicle for doing so. I feel obliged, however, having flagged the issue, to at least say a bit more.

First, let me distinguish between homophobia that is directed at whites and homophobia that is internal to the black community. As we seek to understand the former, it will be difficult, I suspect, to disentangle it from an animus based on race. That is to say, gay whites who encounter hostility from blacks may be the target of antigay sentiment, antiwhite sentiment, or both. Even the originators of the hostility may not know where one motivation ends and the other begins. Moreover, racial prejudice and homophobia may well activate or reinforce each other. It stands to reason that someone who is viewed as an "other" along one dimension will more easily be viewed as an "other" along a second and third. Internal homophobia does not suffer this complication, but it scarcely lacks complexity. Like most aspects of the African-American subculture, its roots are dual. The black community has doubtless been influenced by the larger society's attitudes toward sexual minorities even as its historical experience has produced a distinctive set of attitudes and practices. I would like to focus briefly on the latter.

In the manner in which homosexuality is spoken about, the black community differs markedly from the larger society. In our denunciation of homosexuality and of persons thought to be gay, blacks (including closeted gays) tend to be much more open and pointed than whites. Our verbal attacks seem tinged with cruelty and are usually delivered with an offhandedness that many white observers find unnerving. At the same time, there is, within the black community, an enormous gulf between talk and action, or for that matter, between talk and belief. What we say and what we think, or do, need not be congruent. In fact, a cruel tongue is often used to hide a tender heart. Bell Hooks tells of a "straight black male in a California community who acknowledged that though he often made jokes poking fun at gays or expressing contempt as a means of bonding in group settings, in his private life he was a central support person for a gay sister." "Such contradictory behavior," she adds, "seems pervasive in black communities."

On reflection, none of this is surprising. We, as a people, are given to verbal excesses, to hyperbole, to put-downs meant for sport rather than wounding. People of my generation and older grew up "playing the dozens," verbal horseplay that involved the most scandalous imaginable accusations about the families and acquaintances of the other participants. So long as you stayed within certain well-understood (albeit unwritten and unspoken) bounds of propriety, you could say vicious things without anybody thinking you really meant it. A similar dynamic attends verbal gay bashing. There is a common understanding of which nasty things are acceptable to say, and as long as one stays within the canon, one can claim an absence of malice.

There is, however, a key difference. In the dozens, the participants stand on equal footing; typically they alternate between the role of the slanderer and the role of the slanderized. In addition, there is no necessary relationship between the calumnies heaped on an individual and those heaped on her or his real-life position. In fact, one of the unwritten rules is that you tread lightly around areas of true vulnerability.

In practice, black communities across the country have knowingly and sometimes fully embraced their gay members. But the price has been high. In exchange for inclusion, gay men and lesbians have agreed to remain under wraps, to downplay, if not hide, their sexual orientation, to provide their families and friends with "deniability." So long as they do not put the community to the test, they are welcome. It is all right if everybody knows as long as nobody tells. That is more easily accomplished than you might imagine. For the most part, even the pillars of the black community are content to let its gay members be, and to live alongside them in mutual complicity. This is true even within the church. Indeed, it is a well-kept secret, or more precisely, it is well-denied knowledge, that gays are disproportionately represented within the ministry, including (and perhaps especially) the ministry of many of the more fundamental denominations.

This complex relationship works most successfully when gay men and lesbians are willing to carry on appearances, to live, in effect, straight lives. Many gay black men seek the ultimate cover and become ostentatiously involved with women. One noteworthy consequence of this phenomenon is that their female sexual partners may unknowingly be exposed to an increased risk of HIV infection.

What accounts for the way in which the black community has approached homosexuality—boisterous homophobic talk, tacit acceptance in practice, and a broad-based conspiracy of silence? I have a theory (and it is no more than that) that within the black community, internal homophobia has less to do with regulating sexual desire and affectional ties than with policing relations between the sexes. In this view, gay black men and lesbians are made to suffer because they are out of sync with a powerful cultural impulse to weaken black women and strengthen black men. They are, in a sense, caught in a sociocultural cross fire over which they have little control.

Among the many horrors of slavery is the havoc it wreaked on relations between black men and women. Slave couples were not allowed to form stable bonds, and those relationships that did develop were burdened in ways painful to recount. Men were torn away from their families, women were subjected to the slavemasters' bidding, and both were, on occasion, bred like animals. As a result, men were unable to provide for, much less protect, "their" women and women were unable to rely on their men. This emasculation of black men (when measured against traditional gender role expectations and concepts of male prerogative) boded ill for male-female relations in the postslavery era in the absence of a fundamental redefinition of gender. The near century of Jim Crow that followed—legalized discrimination backed up and surrounded by powerfully disintegrative social forces—simply added to the strain. Black people in general, and black men in particular, were "kept in their place," routinely excluded from places that would bring them honor and respect or that would allow them to serve as family providers. While women could usually find employment as domestics, black men frequently drifted and did not, could not, come close to pulling their own weight.

For me, this reality is best captured by something that happened on the old Art Linkletter show during the 1950s, I believe. The show included a segment entitled "Kids Say the Darnedest Things," in which Linkletter interviewed children about whatever was on their minds. Somehow the word spread that on this particular day Linkletter would have a black kid on the show, a rare occurrence. Like hundreds of thousands of other black folk, I eagerly tuned in and watched with fascination and horror as this little kid, who looked a lot like me, answered the question "What do you want to be when you grow up?" "I want to be a white man," he answered quickly and confidently. Linkletter gulped, paused, and then plunged ahead. "Why?" he asked. "Because," answered the kid, "my momma says that black men aren't worth shit!"

The network instantly broke for a commercial, and when the show returned, the little black kid had been whisked off the set, but no commercial break could stanch the psychic wound opened up in an entire community in that moment of childlike innocence. Black people talked about that show for months, amidst much handwringing and headshaking. Yet, despite the countless retellings and postmortems, the message implicit in the little boy's answer—that relations between black men and women had reached a parlous state—was never disputed.

What does this have to do with homophobia? My suspicion is that openly gay men and lesbians evoke hostility in part because they have come to symbolize the strong female and the weak male that slavery and Jim Crow produced. More than even the mother quoted on the Linkletter show, lesbians are seen as standing for the proposition that "black men aren't worth shit." More than even the "no account" men who figure prominently in the repertoire of female blues singers, gay men symbolize the abandonment of black women. Thus, in the black community homosexuality carries more baggage than in the larger society. To address it successfully, we may have to take on such larger issues as the social construction of gender and the nature of male-female relations.

Drug Abuse

A fourth impediment to our efforts to grapple with AIDS is the association of the disease with drug abuse. We as a community have a complex relationship with illicit drugs, a relationship that often paralyzes us. On the one hand, blacks are scared to even admit the dimensions of the problem for fear that we will all be treated as junkies and our culture viewed as pathological. On the other, we desperately want to find solutions. For us, drug abuse is a curse far worse than you can imagine. Addicts prey on our neighborhoods, sell drugs to our children, steal our possessions, and rob us of hope. We despise them. We despise them because they hurt us and because they *are* us. They are a constant reminder of how close we all are to the edge. And "they" are "us" literally as well as figuratively; they are our sons and daughters, our sisters and brothers. Can we possibly cast out the demons without casting out our own kin?

We know that white America cannot comprehend our dilemma. We know that you do not truly share our concerns. Your interest in drug abuse has always been episodic and shallow. During the 1960s, you focused briefly on the problem when you became convinced that most street crime and petty theft are drug related. Although some of you saw this opening as an opportunity to broaden the nation's commitment to drug prevention and treatment, most energy went into keeping white people from being victimized. Meanwhile, the plight of black victims "uptown" didn't even merit lip service. During the 1970s, drug abuse once again briefly took center stage as suburban high school students began to experiment and addicted GIs returned home from Viet Nam. Left in the shadows as usual was the civilian drug problem in our nation's inner cities.

Now, as the 1980s draw to a close, a combination of factors, including the rise of the social Right, the highly visible fall of dozens of professional athletes, the intertwining of drug trafficking and foreign policy, the emergence of crack as the drug of choice among many communities, and, not least, AIDS, has made drug abuse a hotter social issue than at any time in recent history. Yet for all the *Sturm und Drang*, the white community has shown little concern that day by day, drugs are eating away at the heart and soul of the black community. When schoolchildren were gunned down by a maniac in Stockton, California, you furiously debated the wisdom of allowing private citizens to purchase semiautomatic weapons; at the same time, you appeared oblivious to the fact that every day in the inner city *our* children are being gunned down by such armaments in the never-ending struggle over drug turf and profits.

And so we find ourselves paralyzed, caught up in our own conflicting emotions—guilt, anger, shame, horror, fear, sympathy, aversion, affinity—and your uncertain commitment. We know that to deal with AIDS we must deal with drugs. If only we knew how.

Neocolonialism

Although most of my 1960s rhetoric is safely stored away in my mental attic, I was forced to resurrect this trusty old friend, for try as I might, I couldn't come up with a post-postmodern phrase that captures the one-sided relationship now existing between the black community and the larger society, a relationship built on power and control. When we want help, white America is nowhere to be found. When, however, *you* decide that we need help, you are there in a flash, solution in hand. You then seek to impose that solution on us, without seeking our views, hearing our experiences, or taking account of our needs and desires. We tell you that we fear genocide, and you quarrel with our use of the term. Then you try to turn our concerns back on us. "Don't you know," you ask us in an arch tone of voice, "that while you are standing on ceremony, thousands of the very people you say you care about are dying from AIDS?" Struggling to ignore the insulting implication that we are either profoundly retarded or monumentally callous, we respond, "Don't *you* know that they are already dying from drug overdoses,

Uzis and AK-47s, joblessness, despair, and societal indifference?" And, white America, you sigh and say, "What's one thing got to do with the other?" Then we sigh and wonder if you truly do not understand.

In the silence that follows, none of our real concerns gets voiced. Why can't *we* choose which of the many problems facing us to tackle first? Suppose we think that crack is more of a menace than AIDS? Are you willing to help us take on that one? Why do you want *us* to take all the risks? You say that making drug use safer (by giving away bleach or distributing clean needles) won't make it more attractive to our children or our neighbors' children? But what if you are wrong? What if as a result we have even more addicts to contend with? Will you be around to help us then, especially if the link between addiction and AIDS has been severed? Why do you offer addicts free needles but not free health care? Why do you show them how to clean their works but not how to clean up their lives? Why not provide immediate treatment for every addict who wants it? Why not provide us with job training so that our youth will have realistic alternatives to the street? Instead of asking us to accept on faith that we won't be abandoned and possibly worse off once you move on to a new issue, why not demonstrate your commitment by empowering us to carry on the struggle whether you are there or not?

WHERE TO FROM HERE?

Quite simply, we have to learn how to stop talking past each other. We have to figure out a way to communicate across the racial chasm. Our language is the same, but our frames of reference are so different. Admittedly, part of the blame for recent failures to connect rests with the black community. We have been so intent on trying to get your attention that we have occasionally forgotten why. We have been so busy expressing our fears that we have failed to express our hopes. We have been so focused on past fiascos that we have been unwilling to test whether this time we can work together. We have been afraid to say straight out what is on our minds. And too often when we speak, we do so cryptically, metaphorically, or in a code undecipherable by outsiders.

This concern brings me to the term *genocide*. Although I understand its appeal, I regret the use of the term in conversations about AIDS. My regret stems from the fact that *genocide* tends to be a conversation stopper, and I am desperately anxious for genuine conversation to begin. It is so hard to get past the term itself to the sentiments and experiences that animate its use. Yet those sentiments and experiences reveal a good deal about why efforts to organize the black community around AIDS have been disappointing, so let me take a run at it.

What do community leaders (and followers) mean when they accuse seemingly well-intentioned public health officials of engaging in genocide? Admittedly, the term is a useful club, the kind one uses to get a mule's attention. But that is not its sole function. After all, black folks use it meaningfully even when talking among ourselves. It speaks to us. It resonates. It is shorthand for a wide range of fears and expectations, all of which are backed up by shared experience.

In its strong form, the term *genocide* reflects the genuine suspicion of many that the AIDS virus was developed in a government laboratory for the express purpose of killing off the unwanted. This belief is helped along by HIV's curious affinity for those whom the larger society disdains. Lest you judge this a fringe concern, I must tell you that whenever I speak about AIDS to a grassroots audience in a black neighborhood, at some point during the question-and-answer session someone invariably asks me whether I think AIDS was purposefully developed as a means of wiping out black people or, alternatively, whether black people are being used as guinea pigs to test this new form of biological warfare. Others in the room usually murmur their agreement with the statement within the question or wait expectantly for my answer.

Although I answer no, I understand full well where the question comes from and recognize that it must be heard against the backdrop of the larger society's historic disregard for the sanctity of black people's lives. We need not go back to slavery. There are examples aplenty within my lifetime, or that of my parents, of black people's lives being treated casually or worse. Take, for example, the infamous experiment at Tuskegee Institute in which the government purposefully exposed black men to syphilis so as to study the natural course of the disease. Although an effective treatment was developed mid-experiment, the men were never told about it and were never treated, lest the research be compromised. Another well-documented example is the forced sterilization of women on welfare, many of whom were black or brown. In some states, the practice continued unabated into the 1970s. The recent election of former Klansman David Duke to the Louisiana legislature suggests that this unlovely practice, a key element of his platform, has not altogether lost its appeal. A third example, relatively recently come to light, is the FBI's attempt to pressure Dr. Martin Luther

King, Jr., into committing suicide. To these highly visible stories someone in every black audience can add dozens more, stories of people who found themselves the unwitting object of experimentation or the target of government persecution.

Two assumptions underlie the strong claim of genocide. The first is that the hostility of white America toward black America is so powerful, or the disregard so profound, that no depredation is unthinkable. This view is rooted in racial strife and feeds on the storehouse of sins visited upon blacks by whites. The second assumption is that under the right circumstances, the government is not above compromising the lives of innocent citizens. The grist for such a view is considerable. Time and again the government has demonstrated a willingness to jeopardize the lives of even its most favored in order to expand its knowledge or advance its policies. The purposeful exposure of American soldiers to radiation in the Nevada desert comes readily to mind. For black people, the realization that even white skin does not protect one from being expendable is chilling indeed.

Less strongly, the term *genocide* reflects a widespread belief that the federal government willingly let AIDS spread as long as it was confined to populations that straight white America would rather do without. The grist for this view is provided by the government's own spokespersons, among others. At a press conference following her keynote address at the International Conference on AIDS held in Atlanta in 1985, then Health and Human Services Secretary Margaret Heckler caused considerable consternation among people at society's margins when she implored: "We must conquer [AIDS]. . . . before it affects the heterosexual population and threatens the health of our general population." Her parallel statement, that we must also conquer AIDS for the sake of "individuals in every country who fall within the risk categories" was perceived as, at best, a sop. In similar fashion, when called on to explain on a nationally telecast interview show why President Reagan did not speak publicly about AIDS until late 1985, White House chief domestic policy adviser Gary Bauer responded that until then AIDS had not been a problem worth commenting on because "it hadn't spread into the general population yet."

In its weakest form, *genocide* signifies a reckless indifference to, or deliberate disregard of, the black community's vital interests, or at a minimum the subordination of those interests to the distinct concerns of the larger society. Let me illustrate by once again turning to New York City's needle-exchange program. No one, I take it, would quarrel with the proposition that the black community has a legitimate interest in discouraging its young people from using illicit drugs. Yet that very same interest is directly threatened if the fears expressed by the program's many black critics are warranted, that is to say if providing clean needles to addicts creates a substantial risk that the number of young people willing to experiment with intravenous drugs will rise significantly. The fact that the city pressed forward with the program in the face of such concerns contributed to the charge of genocide.

In fairness, it cannot be said that New York City's health commissioner simply disregarded the issue of whether free needles would encourage addiction. Rather, after thoughtfully considering the issue, he concluded that the risk was minimal. The rub is that most black critics of needle exchange rejected that conclusion. Given this disagreement over a matter of fundamental importance to the black community, to proceed anyway looks a lot like indifference or disrespect.

My overriding goal in writing this essay has been to spur conversation about how a country as racially polarized as ours can hope to deal with a virulent disease that, as fate would have it, manifests itself differentially. It is in the pursuit of that goal that I have struggled to give content to a charge that usually produces more heat than light. I have no particular investment in the term *genocide*; I simply want to jump-start the conversation that usually dies out whenever the word is deployed.

My vision is of a conversation that takes place both on the streets and in the academy, by design and by chance. My hope is for conversation characterized by mutual risk taking and mutual candor. In the spirit of candor, I must warn you that not all will be pleasant. For most Americans of African descent, our history, especially our trials and tribulations—slavery, discrimination, malign neglect—is a lived thing, something we experience and feel even when we do not know its particulars. We wear Jim Crow like our skin, with precious little choice in the matter. Because our history is ever with us, we can never consider the slate wiped clean. It is, for example, difficult for us to divorce our dealings with white persons as individuals from our dealings with whites who preceded them. When you extend a hand in friendship, we can't help wondering whether you carry trouble in the other one. When you invite us to dinner, we can't help wondering why. If your manner of speech reflects considerable training and education, we wonder whether you are putting us down. If, instead, you speak in the vernacular, we wonder if you are being condescending. No matter how pure your motives, we will question why you are in our midst. No matter how deep your commitment, we will wonder what you are getting out of it.

My point, then, is that even as I invite you to bridge the chasm, I know it won't be easy. While we insist that you respectfully come calling, we aren't quite ready to put out the welcome mat. When you predictably bridle at our lack of hospitality, we will peer into your soul to determine whether you are simply one more white person who can't stand to see black folks asserting themselves. But even if we decide that your pique is justified (in the sense that you truly have embraced our concerns and are anxious to work with us), we will expect you to be sympathetic to our predicament while we argue that you cannot expect us to be sympathetic to yours.

Perhaps that is a lot to ask. But we as a nation must play the hand that slavery has dealt us. We cannot undo history, except through long, hard struggle. Meanwhile, we must learn to live with AIDS here and now, in the present that we find so bewildering.

In so doing, we must recognize that the face of AIDS is rapidly changing, from mostly white to predominantly black and brown. The implications of this shift for public health policy and practice are profound; we have just begun to explore them. But this much is clear already. As the drama unfolds, we cannot simply ask white actors to put on blackface and favor us with their best rendition of "life in de ghetto." We must increasingly turn to black actors, and to black directors and producers as well, if we are to really capture the social meaning of the darkening epidemic. Nor can we treat as bothersome background noise black America's complex attitudes toward white America, and vice versa. Only by acknowledging such disconcerting realities do we have a prayer of a chance of escaping their constraining force.

FROM AIDS AND ITS METAPHORS

SUSAN SONTAG

| 1989 |

Epidemics of particularly dreaded illnesses always provoke an outcry against leniency or tolerance—now identified as laxity, weakness, disorder, corruption: unhealthiness. Demands are made to subject people to "tests," to isolate the ill and those suspected of being ill or of transmitting illness, and to erect barriers against the real or imaginary contamination of foreigners. Societies already administered as garrisons, like China (with a tiny number of detected cases) and Cuba (with a significant number of the already ill), are responding more rapidly and peremptorily. AIDS is everyone's Trojan horse: six months before the 1988 Olympics the South Korean government announced that it would be distributing free condoms to all foreign participants. "This is a totally foreign disease, and the only way to stop its spread is to stop sexual contacts between Indians and foreigners," declared the director general of the Indian government's Council for Medical Research, thereby avowing the total defenselessness of a population nearing a billion for which there are presently *no* trained hospital staff members or treatment centers anywhere specializing in the disease. His proposal for a sexual ban, to be enforced by fines and prison terms, is no less impractical as a means of curbing sexually transmitted diseases than the more commonly made proposals for quarantine—that is, for detention. The incarceration in detention camps surrounded by barbed wire during World War I of some thirty thousand American women, prostitutes, and women suspected of being prostitutes, for the avowed purpose of controlling syphilis among army recruits, caused no drop in the military's rate of infection—just as incarceration during World War II of tens of thousands of Americans of Japanese ancestry as potential traitors and spies probably did not foil a single act of espionage or sabotage. That does not mean that comparable proposals for AIDS will not be made, or will not find support, and not only by the predictable people. If the medical establishment has been on the whole a bulwark of sanity and rationality so far, refusing even to envisage programs of quarantine and detention, it may be in part because the dimensions of the crisis still seem limited and the evolution of the disease unclear.

Uncertainty about how much the disease will spread—how soon and to whom—remains at the center of public discourse about AIDS. Will it, as it spreads around the world, remain restricted, largely, to marginal populations: to the so-called risk groups and then to large sections of the urban poor? Or will it eventually become the classic pandemic affecting entire regions? Both views are in fact being held simultaneously. A wave of statements and articles affirming that AIDS threatens everybody is followed by another wave of articles asserting that it is a disease of "them," not "us." At the beginning of 1987, the U.S. secretary of Health and Human Services predicted that the worldwide AIDS epidemic would eventually make the Black Death—the greatest epidemic ever recorded, which wiped out between a third and a half of the population of Europe—seem "pale by comparison." At the end of the year he said: "This is not a massive, widely spreading epidemic among heterosexuals as so many people fear." Even more striking than the cyclical character of public discourse about AIDS is the readiness of so many to envisage the most far-reaching of catastrophes.

Reassurances are multiplying in the United States and Western Europe that "the general population" is safe. But "the general population" may be as much a code phrase for whites as it is for heterosexuals. Everyone knows that a disproportionate number of blacks are getting AIDS, as there is a disproportionate number of blacks in the armed forces and a vastly disproportionate number in prisons. "The AIDS virus is an equal-opportunity destroyer" was the slogan of a recent fund-raising campaign by the American Foundation for AIDS Research. Punning on "equal-opportunity employer," the phrase subliminally reaffirms what it means to deny: that AIDS is an illness that in this part of the world afflicts minorities, racial and sexual. And about the staggering prediction made recently by the World Health Organization that, barring improbably rapid progress in the development of a vaccine, there will be ten to twenty times more AIDS cases in the next five years than there were in the last five, it is assumed that most of these millions will be Africans.

AIDS quickly became a global event—discussed not only in New York, Paris, Rio, Kinshasa but also in Helsinki, Buenos Aires, Beijing, and Singapore—when it was far from the leading cause of death in Africa, much less in the world. There are famous diseases, as there are famous countries, and these are not necessarily the ones with the biggest populations. AIDS did not become so famous just because it afflicts whites too, as some Africans bitterly assert. But it is certainly true that were AIDS only an African disease, however many millions were dying, few outside of Africa would be concerned with it. It would be one of those "natural" events, like famines, which periodically ravage poor, overpopulated countries and about which people in rich countries feel quite helpless. Because it is a world event—that is, because it affects the West—it is regarded as not just a natural disaster. It is filled with historical meaning. (Part of the self-definition of Europe and the neo-European countries is that it, the First World, is where major calamities are history-making, transformative, while in poor, African or Asian countries they are part of a cycle, and therefore something like an aspect of nature.) Nor has AIDS become so publicized because, as some have suggested, in rich countries the illness first afflicted a group of people who were all men, almost all white, many of them educated, articulate, and knowledgeable about how to lobby and organize for public attention and resources devoted to the disease. AIDS occupies such a large part in our awareness because of what it has been taken to represent. It seems the very model of all the catastrophes privileged populations feel await them.

What biologists and public health officials predict is something far worse than can be imagined or than society (and the economy) can tolerate. No responsible official holds out the slightest hope that the African economies and health services can cope with the spread of the disease predicted for the near future, while every day one can read the direst estimates of the cost of AIDS to the country that has reported the largest number of cases, the United States. Astonishingly large sums of money are cited as the cost of providing minimum care to people who will be ill in the next few years. (This is assuming that the reassurances to "the general population" are justified, an assumption much disputed within the medical community.) Talk in the United States, and not only in the United States, is of a national emergency, "possibly our nation's survival." An editorialist at the *New York Times* intoned last year: "We all know the truth, every one of us. We live in a time of plague such as has never been visited on our nation. We can pretend it does not exist, or exists for those others, and carry on as if we do not know. . . ." And one French poster shows a giant UFO-like black mass hovering over and darkening with spidery rays most of the familiar hexagon shape of the country lying below. Above the image is written: "It depends on each of us to erase that shadow" (*Il depend de chacun de nous d'effacer cette ombre*). And underneath: "France doesn't want to die of AIDS" (*La France ne veut pas mourir du sida*). Such token appeals for mass mobilization to confront an unprecedented menace appear, at frequent intervals, in every mass society. It is also typical of a modern society that the demand for mobilization be kept very general and the reality of the response fall well short of what seems to be demanded to meet the challenge of the nation-endangering menace. This sort of rhetoric has a life of its own: it serves some purpose if it simply keeps in circulation an ideal of unifying communal practice that is precisely contradicted by the pursuit of accumulation and isolating entertainments enjoined on the citizens of a modern mass society.

The survival of the nation, of civilized society, of the world itself is said to be at stake—claims that are a familiar part of building a case for repression. (An emergency requires "drastic measures," et cetera.) The end-of-the-world rhetoric that AIDS has evoked does inevitably build such a case. But it also does something else. It offers a stoic, finally numbing contemplation of catastrophe. The eminent Harvard historian of science Stephen Jay Gould has declared that the AIDS pandemic may rank with nuclear weaponry "as the greatest danger of our era." But even if it kills as much as a quarter of the human race—a prospect Gould considers possible—"there will still be plenty of us left and we can start again." Scornful of the jeremiads of the moralists, a rational and humane scientist proposes the minimum consolation: an apocalypse that doesn't have any meaning. AIDS is a "natural phenomenon," not an event "with a moral meaning," Gould points out; "there is no message in its spread." Of course, it is monstrous to attribute meaning, in the sense of moral judgment, to the spread of an infectious disease. But perhaps it is only a little less monstrous to be invited to contemplate death on this horrendous scale with equanimity.

Much of the well-intentioned public discourse in our time expresses a desire to be candid about one or another of the various dangers which might be leading to all-out catastrophe. And now there is one more. To the death of oceans and lakes and forests, the unchecked growth of populations in the poor parts of the world, nuclear accidents like Chernobyl, the puncturing and depletion of the ozone layer, the perennial threat of nuclear confrontation between the superpowers or nuclear attack by one of the rogue states not under superpower control—to all these, now add AIDS. In the countdown to a millennium, a rise in apocalyptic thinking may be inevitable. Still, the amplitude of the fantasies of doom that AIDS has inspired can't be explained by the calendar alone, or even by the very real danger the illness represents. There is also the need for an apocalyptic scenario that is specific to "Western" society, and perhaps even more so to the United States. (America, as someone has said, is a nation with the soul of a church—an evangelical church prone to announcing radical endings and brand-new beginnings.) The taste for worst-case scenarios reflects the need to master fear of what is felt to be uncontrollable. It also expresses an imaginative complicity with disaster. The sense of cultural distress or failure gives rise to the desire for a clean sweep, a tabula rasa. No one wants a plague, of course. But, yes, it would be a chance to begin again. And beginning again—that is very modern, very American, too.

AIDS may be extending the propensity for becoming inured to vistas of global annihilation which the stocking and brandishing of nuclear arms has already promoted. With the inflation of apocalyptic rhetoric has come the increasing unreality of the apocalypse. A permanent modern scenario: apocalypse looms . . . and it doesn't occur. And it still looms. We seem to be in the throes of one of the modern kinds of apocalypse. There is the one that's not happening, whose outcome remains in suspense: the missiles circling the earth above our heads, with a nuclear payload that could destroy all life many times over, that haven't (so far) gone off. And there are ones that are happening, and yet seem not to have (so far) the most feared consequences—like the astronomical Third World debt, like overpopulation, like ecological blight; or that happen and then (we are told) didn't happen—like the October 1987 stock market collapse, which was a "crash," like the one in October 1929, and was not. Apocalypse is now a long-running serial: not "Apocalypse Now" but "Apocalypse From Now On." Apocalypse has become an event that is happening and not happening. It may be that some of the most feared events, like those involving the irreparable ruin of the environment, have already happened. But we don't know it yet, because the standards have changed. Or because we do not have the right indices for measuring the catastrophe. Or simply because this is a catastrophe in slow motion. (Or *feels* as if it is in slow motion, because we know about it, can anticipate it; and now have to wait for it to happen, to catch up with what we think we know.)

Modern life accustoms us to live with the intermittent awareness of monstrous, unthinkable—but, we are told, quite probable—disasters. Every major event is haunted, and not only by its representation as an image (an old doubling of reality now, which began in 1839, with the invention of the camera). Beside the photographic or electronic simulation of events, there is also the calculation of their eventual outcome. Reality has bifurcated, into the real thing and an alternative version of it, twice over. There is the event and its image. And there is the event and its projection. But as real events often seem to have no more reality for people than images, and to need the confirmation of their images, so our reaction to events in the present seeks confirmation in a mental outline, with appropriate computations, of the event in its projected, ultimate form.

Future-mindedness is as much the distinctive mental habit, and intellectual corruption, of this century as the history-mindedness that, as Nietzsche pointed out, transformed thinking in the nineteenth century. Being able to estimate how matters will evolve into the future is an inevitable by-product of a more sophisticated (quantifiable, testable) understanding of process, social as well as scientific. The ability to project events with some accuracy into the future enlarged what power consisted of, because it was a vast new source of instructions about how to deal with the present. But in fact the look into the future, which was once tied to a vision of linear progress, has, with more knowledge at our disposal than anyone could have dreamed, turned into a vision of disaster. Every process is a prospect, and invites a prediction bolstered by statistics. Say: the number now . . . in three years, in five years, in ten years; and, of course, at the end of the century. Anything in history or nature that can be described as changing steadily can be seen as heading toward catastrophe. (Either the too little and becoming less: waning, decline, entropy. Or the too much, ever more than we can handle or absorb: uncontrollable growth.) Most of what experts pronounce about the future contributes to this new double sense of reality—beyond the doubleness to which we are already accustomed by the comprehensive duplication of everything in images. There is what is happening now. And there is what it portends: the imminent, but not yet actual, and not really graspable, disaster.

Two kinds of disaster, actually. And a gap between them, in which the imagination flounders. The difference between the epidemic we have and the pandemic that we are promised (by current statistical extrapolations) feels like the difference between the wars we have, so-called limited wars, and the unimaginably more terrible ones we could have, the latter (with all the appurtenances of science fiction) being the sort of activity people are addicted to staging for fun, as electronic games. For beyond the real epidemic with its inexorably mounting death toll (statistics are issued by national and international health organizations every week, every month) is a qualitatively different, much greater disaster which we think both will and will not take place. Nothing is changed when the most appalling estimates are revised downward, temporarily, which is an occasional feature of the display of speculative statistics disseminated by health bureaucrats and journalists. Like the demographic predictions, which are probably just as accurate, the big news is usually bad.

A proliferation of reports or projections of unreal (that is, ungraspable) doomsday eventualities tends to produce a variety of reality-denying responses. Thus, in most discussions of nuclear warfare, being rational (the self-description of experts) means not acknowledging the human reality, while taking in emotionally even a small part of what is at stake for human beings (the province of those who regard themselves as the menaced) means insisting on unrealistic demands for the rapid dismantling of the peril. This split of public attitude, into the inhuman and the all-too-human, is much less stark with AIDS. Experts denounce the stereotypes attached to people with AIDS and to the continent where it is presumed to have originated, emphasizing that the disease belongs to much wider populations than the groups initially at risk, and to the whole world, not just to Africa. For while AIDS has turned out, not surprisingly, to be one of the most meaning-laden of diseases, along with leprosy and syphilis, clearly there are checks on the impulse to stigmatize people with the disease. The way in which the illness is such a perfect repository for people's most general fears about the future to some extent renders irrelevant the predictable efforts to pin the disease on a deviant group or a dark continent.

Like the effects of industrial pollution and the new system of global financial markets, the AIDS crisis is evidence of a world in which nothing important is regional, local, limited; in which everything that can circulate does, and every problem is, or is destined to become, worldwide. Goods circulate (including images and sounds and documents, which circulate fastest of all, electronically). Garbage circulates: the poisonous industrial wastes of St. Etienne, Hannover, Mestre, and Bristol are being dumped in the coastal towns of West Africa. People circulate, in greater numbers than ever. And diseases. From the untrammeled intercontinental air travel for pleasure and business of the privileged to the unprecedented migrations of the underprivileged from villages to cities and, legally and illegally, from country to country—all this physical mobility and interconnectedness (with its consequent dissolving of old taboos, social and sexual) is as vital to the maximum functioning of the advanced, or world, capitalist economy as is the easy transmissibility of goods and images and financial instruments. But now that heightened, modern interconnectedness in space, which is not only personal but social, structural, is the bearer of a health menace sometimes described as a threat to the species itself; and the fear of AIDS is of a piece with attention to other unfolding disasters that are the by-product of advanced society, particularly those illustrating the degradation of the environment on a world scale. AIDS is one of the dystopian harbingers of the global village, that future which is already here and always before us, which no one knows how to refuse.

That even an apocalypse can be made to seem part of the ordinary horizon of expectation constitutes an unparalleled violence that is being done to our sense of reality, to our humanity. But it is highly desirable for a specific dreaded illness to come to seem ordinary. Even the disease most fraught with meaning can become just an illness. It has happened with leprosy, though some ten million people in the world, easy to ignore since almost all live in Africa and the Indian subcontinent, have what is now called, as part of its wholesome dedramatization, Hansen's disease (after the Norwegian physician who, over a century ago, discovered the bacillus). It is bound to happen with AIDS, when the illness is much better understood and, above all, treatable. For the time being, much in the way of individual experience and social policy depends on the struggle for rhetorical ownership of the illness: how it is possessed, assimilated in argument and in cliché. The age-old, seemingly inexorable process whereby diseases acquire meanings (by coming to stand for the deepest fears) and inflict stigma is always worth challenging, and it does seem to have more limited credibility in the modern world, among people willing to be modern—the process is under surveillance now. With this illness, one that elicits so much guilt and shame, the effort to detach it from these meanings, these metaphors, seems particularly liberating, even consoling. But the metaphors cannot be distanced just by abstaining from them. They have to be exposed, criticized, belabored, used up.

Not all metaphors applied to illnesses and their treatment are equally unsavory and distorting. The one I am most eager to see retired—more than ever since the emergence of AIDS—is the military metaphor. Its converse, the medical model of the public weal, is probably more dangerous and far-reaching in its consequences, since it not only provides a persuasive justification for authoritarian rule but implicitly suggests the necessity of state-sponsored repression and violence (the equivalent of surgical removal or chemical control of the offending or "unhealthy" parts of the body politic). But the effect of the military imagery on thinking about sickness and health is far from inconsequential. It overmobilizes, it overdescribes, and it powerfully contributes to the excommunicating and stigmatizing of the ill.

No, it is not desirable for medicine, any more than for war, to be "total." Neither is the crisis created by AIDS a "total" anything. We are not being invaded. The body is not a battlefield. The ill are neither unavoidable casualties nor the enemy. We—medicine, society—are not authorized to fight back by any means whatever. . . . About that metaphor, the military one, I would say, if I may paraphrase Lucretius: Give it back to the war-makers.

FROM BURNING DESIRES

STEVEN CHAPPLE AND DAVID TALBOT

1989

AIDS

"I think that people will look back and say, 'He was a lone voice crying in the wilderness. He rose to a position of notoriety because in an era when there weren't many heroes around, he appeared to be one.'" There is absolutely nothing modest about the U.S. surgeon general. His office at the Department of Health and Human Services is a shrine. Gold plaques, framed awards, and flattering photos cover the walls. Though his term as the nation's top physician is not yet finished, Dr. C. Everett Koop has already located his proper place in history. "I'm the only sane voice on AIDS that is nationally heard," he tells us.

Over six feet tall and barrel-chested, with a chin beard like his Dutch ancestors and a "Rock of Ages" voice that sounds as though it should be delivering sermons in the desert, Koop certainly fits the part of someone chosen to make history. It is the look of an Old Testament prophet, of Abraham Lincoln, of someone touched with glory. "I think he feels that all his efforts now are God-directed," says one of Koop's best friends, pediatric surgeon John W. Duckett.

Five years after being appointed, at the age of sixty-four, to the surgeon general's post by President Reagan, following a distinguished surgical career at Philadelphia's Children's Hospital, "Chick" Koop found his final calling. He was to fight the plague that was desolating parts of the country, by shedding light where there was darkness, saying forbidden words like "condom" and "penis" and "anus," and by preaching good will toward those rendered "untouchable" by the disease.

It was hard to imagine a less likely savior of gays, drug addicts, and the "sexually active." Here was an evangelical Christian who had crusaded throughout his life against legalized abortion and other manifestations of the new sexual morality. He had made scornful speeches about homosexuality and feminism, which he accused of undermining the family. He had loosed his fearsome anger against the disciples of hedonism, those who pursued lives "of convenience, of pleasure, of permissiveness, of undisciplined morality."

Senator Jesse Helms enthusiastically endorsed President Reagan's choice for surgeon general. But congressional liberals like Edward Kennedy held up Koop's nomination for nearly a year. They were unnerved by his moral fervor; he even *looked* like the wrath of God. His opponents labeled him "Dr. Kook." "He frightens me," said Henry Waxman, the Democratic congressman from West Hollywood who turned his House subcommittee on health into a gauntlet for Koop.

There were times during the long confirmation battle when Koop would return dispiritedly to the little Georgetown apartment he and his wife had rented on the assumption that they would soon be moving to the more comfortable quarters reserved for the surgeon general and would suggest that they give up and go home to Philadelphia. It was a galling experience, "the most difficult period of my life," he would later recall. He was one of the founding fathers of pediatric surgery, a man who had separated three sets of Siamese twins, a miracle worker who had performed heroic operations on horribly deformed infants no other surgeons would go near. And yet the *New York Times* was calling him "Dr. Unqualified."

Weathering all this abuse to win a job that had become in recent years nothing more than a figurehead position . . . well, it hardly seemed worth it. Washington mud-wrestling just seemed too demeaning to the proud Dr. Koop, a man long used to a respect that bordered on adoration. But Betty Koop, the woman he had married when he was still a Dartmouth undergraduate, who had raised their four children almost single-handedly while he maintained his frenetic schedule at the hospital, who knew him better than anybody, refused to let him give in. She thought he would always regret it.

Even after he was finally confirmed, it was not apparent he had done the right thing. By 1983, the Reagan administration had declared AIDS to be the nation's "number-one health priority." But Dr. Edward Brandt, the assistant secretary for health, the man to whom Koop reported in the federal bureaucracy, was making sure that the surgeon general got nowhere near the AIDS issue. Brandt, a conscientious but politically careful administrator, was working in his low-key manner to turn down the panic and moral uproar around the disease. The soft-spoken, jug-eared physician from Texas faced the daunting task of keeping White House ideologues and fire-breathing conservative activists at bay, while maintaining lines of communication with suspicious gay groups and carefully building pressure for bigger AIDS budgets. At one point, Brandt was forced to jump in and derail an alarming plan for a quarantine and mass firing of homosexuals that was being cooked up within administration councils. The last thing he needed under these circumstances was a Bible-quoting surgeon general getting in his way.

The rational types at the upper levels of the federal health bureaucracy strongly distrusted Dr. C. Everett Koop. It wasn't just the reputation he brought with him. Maybe it was the way he strutted around the halls at the Humphrey Building in his starched white uniform with the gold epaulets—a getup abandoned long before by his predecessors in the surgeon general's office. He seemed like a pompous martinet; his Washington critics prayed he would stick to smoking, about which, unsurprisingly for a surgeon general, he had nothing but bad things to say.

Though Koop was largely corralled during his early years in office, he did bolt briefly into the headlines in 1983 when he intervened in what became known as the Baby Jane Doe case, fighting to keep alive a severely impaired infant against the wishes of her parents. Koop had operated on thousands of Baby Does back at Children's Hospital in Philadelphia. Many of those who had grown up and become success stories still stayed in touch with the surgeon. The idea of abandoning infants who were helpless, but not entirely hopeless, filled him with righteous anger. That way lay Mengele, Koop sincerely believed, the medical ethics of the Third Reich.

"We're not fighting for this baby," he thundered at the time. "We're fighting for the principle of this country that every life is individual and uniquely sacred." Baby Jane Doe's doctors did finally take measures to keep her alive. But the Baby Doe regulations that Koop helped write, which would have forced hospitals to treat severely handicapped infants over the objections of their parents, were later declared unconstitutional by the Supreme Court.

With the exception of the Baby Doe controversy and a flare-up over cigarette advertising, the lofty voice of the surgeon general was unheard during Reagan's first term, to the immense relief of liberals on Capitol Hill. In the meantime, AIDS cast a longer and longer shadow across the land, and Ed Brandt struggled, with little success, to mobilize the government against the epidemic. The administration's tightfisted attitude toward domestic spending and its moral rigidity were proving to be insurmountable obstacles. Each year, the White House asked for less money to fight AIDS than was recommended by its own Public Health Service, and each year Congress was forced to tack on a higher figure to the budget. The nation's leading AIDS laboratories were financially strapped and important research went unfunded.

It was a recipe for disaster, as Daniel Greenberg would note in *The Nation*: "The simultaneous arrival in the United States in 1981 of an uncompassionate, overtly homophobic presidency and a mysterious, fatal affliction transmitted mainly through the sex practices of male homosexuals" was a truly "horrific coincidence."

As it became clear that a vaccine or effective antiviral drug was years away, safe-sex research and public education aimed at preventing wider transmission of the virus became of paramount importance. Was deep kissing safe? Cunnilingus? Fellatio? What were the safest condoms? Did spermicidal gel provide another line of protection? These were the kinds of life-and-death questions that the public needed answers to. But the Reagan administration, wedded to the notion that abstinence before marriage and absolute faithfulness in marriage was the only proper design for living, resisted disseminating this information in the belief that it would encourage promiscuity.

In 1984, the Mariposa Education and Research Foundation, a Southern California institute run by gay health expert Bruce Voeller, began exploring the possibility that nonoxynol-9, a common ingredient of spermicide gels, could kill the AIDS virus in sufficiently high concentrations. After a long delay, the federal Centers for Disease Control in Atlanta conducted tests in conjunction with Mariposa that confirmed this hypothesis. Here was an important breakthrough in AIDS prevention. The research suggested that spermicide gel, in conjunction with rubbers, could block transmission of the virus and save lives. Dr. Donald Francis, the lead scientist on the project, wanted to rush the findings into print, but CDC officials stalled publication for more than a year, claiming they were unsure of the research methodology. Francis had another explanation: the federal government did not want to publicize the value of nonoxynol-9 because it might be interpreted as condoning morally unsanctioned sex.

For the same reason, it was not until mid-1987, over six years into the epidemic, that the Food and Drug Administration began to step up its inspection of condoms, in an effort to improve their reliability. Similarly, not one of the hundreds of federally funded scientific papers presented at the Third International AIDS Conference in Washington, D.C., that year dealt with safe-sex techniques. Throughout the Reagan years, practical AIDS-prevention research was left almost entirely to folk practitioners—sexologists, prostitutes, porn stars, amateur scientists—many of whom used their own bodies as laboratories. Safe-sex education, too, would fall to the private sector, with gay organizations and civic-minded celebrities showing citizens how to roll on rubbers. The federal government steadfastly refused to teach the public how to shield itself from the virus. Until, that is, the U.S. surgeon general saw the light.

Near the end of 1984, Ed Brandt, reportedly frustrated with the administration's politicized response to AIDS, announced he was stepping down as assistant secretary of health. For over a year, his post would go unfilled; no reputable physician or public health official wanted to step into the same slippery ditch. The administration's war on AIDS, never a marvel of coordination and dedication, seemed more rudderless than ever. One day the president was buttonholed by a reporter: What exactly was he doing about AIDS? The question stumped Reagan. He mulled it over a long time. Finally, the president declared that he would tell his surgeon general to prepare a report.

White House conservatives were pleased with the idea. The report would help forestall criticism that the administration was asleep at the wheel on AIDS, and anything written by Koop would certainly follow conservative doctrine. But gay groups and the career civil servants who worked on AIDS at Health and Human Services were deeply alarmed. "Dr. Kook," whom sensible Ed Brandt had kept on a short chain for so long, was finally unleashed. They knew what he felt about homosexuality, about modern morality. They dreaded the outcome.

In our interviews with Koop, he would insist that while he was critical of the homosexual lifestyle, he had always been comfortable with gays as individuals: "Some of my closest medical colleagues have been gay. I have always been, I think, a broad-minded person." But HHS staff members who worked with him had seen a less tolerant side of Koop. "He would make remarks about gays, ugly stuff—'homo this' and 'homo that,' " recalled a longtime HHS employee who worked on AIDS-information projects and often conferred with gay groups. "He and his wife would give a Christmas party each year at their house out at the National Institutes for Health. I went with my husband in 1982 or 1983, and as we went down the receiving line, Koop—who was kind of in his cups by then—introduced me to his wife by saying, 'Here's the woman who helps the homos.' My husband and I were offended."

But as he labored over his AIDS report during the first nine months of 1986, meeting with more than two dozen organizations and steeping himself in information about the disease, the surgeon general seemed to undergo a transformation. "That terrible plague had begun to consume me," he would later say. "It changed my life." The wrathful moralist in Koop was giving way to the compassionate physician. The gay leaders with whom he met were impressed with his concern and attentiveness. "He didn't cut [the meeting] short with some excuse like he had to meet with the president or have tea with Nancy," said Richard Dunne of New York's Gay Men's Health Crisis. As for Koop, he "was very pleased to see the problem through homosexual eyes."

HHS staff members who read early versions of the AIDS report, which went through a total of twenty-seven drafts, found a number of judgmental "them versus us" statements on high-risk groups. "He had one line, for instance, like 'Everybody finds homosexuality offensive . . .,'" recalled a former Koop aide. "I told him, 'You can't say that.' He was very gracious in accepting my suggested changes." What began to emerge, as Koop carefully wrote and rewrote the report, spending nights and weekends at the stand-up desk in his basement at home, was a document that was remarkably free of conservative dogma and startlingly blunt in its medical advice.

"As soon as I read the final draft, I knew it was going to be important," remembered the Koop aide, who had long been pushing for a more aggressive educational program on AIDS. Koop, too, realized the report's significance, and he was not about to let it be tampered with before it could be released to the public. "I mean, we had people high up in this department who thought you could get AIDS from shaking hands!" exclaimed Koop's aide. The surgeon general wisely decided to circumvent bureaucratic channels at HHS, brashly telling the new secretary of Health and Human Services, Otis Bowen, "I don't want one word changed." Koop was also shrewd enough to print five thousand copies of his report before taking it to the White House domestic policy council, realizing, in the words of his former assistant, that "a published document looks inviolable; a draft just invites revisions."

Koop's timing was fortuitous. His report was presented to the domestic policy council at a moment when there was no conservative hard-liner taking a leadership role on AIDS within the administration. After giving it a quick once-over, the White House council quickly approved the report. The council's haste was due in part to the fact that "there was a little bit of discomfort in talking about [the report] because it mentioned condoms, and Elizabeth Dole [then secretary of transportation and the only female Cabinet member] was there," a council member would tell the *Washington Post*.

The thirty-six-page *Surgeon General's Report on AIDS*, released at a packed Washington press conference on October 22, 1986, was an immediate bombshell. It used explicit language to describe how the AIDS virus was sexually transmitted ("Small tears in the surface lining of the vagina or rectum may occur during insertion of the penis, fingers, or other objects . . ."). While advocating monogamy as the safest practice, it acknowledged the realities of human behavior by counseling those who did not know the antibody status of their partners to wear condoms. It called for AIDS education "at the lowest grade possible," including "information about heterosexual and homosexual relationships." It rejected panicky proposals from the Right, such as compulsory blood testing and quarantine, as medically unwise. And it urged public compassion for those stricken with the disease.

"I was stunned," said Gary MacDonald of the AIDS Action Council. So were Koop's conservative supporters. What in the world had happened to their pillar of righteousness at Health and Human Services? How could the White House let him stray so far from the reservation?

There was nothing in Koop's report that AIDS scientists and doctors had not been saying for a long time. But Koop was a high federal official and his words carried more impact. Up until his report, the government and the media had preferred vague and prissy language when discussing AIDS transmission. (President Reagan could not even bring himself to mention AIDS in public at all.) So America heard only about "the exchange of body fluids," rather than about semen and rips in the sensitive lining of the rectum. For a country whose culture is drenched with sex, the United States remains remarkably prudish. Even in the face of a dread epidemic that demanded straightforward discussion, the country opted for the sanitized version. But Surgeon General Koop was refusing to play this game.

In the months following publication of the report, Koop's former comrades on the Moral Right denounced him in the bitter words reserved for those who have betrayed a cause. While liberals once called him "Dr. Kook," conservative leaders now called him "Dr. Condom." They accused him of corrupting the nation's youth by promoting "safe sodomy" in the schools. They charged that he had turned himself into "the instrument of the homosexual lobby." Under pressure from Phyllis Schlafly, three 1988 Republican presidential hopefuls—Senator Robert Dole, Representative Jack Kemp, and Pete du Pont—withdrew their support from a testimonial dinner on behalf of Koop.

Meanwhile, the administration moved to muzzle him. In the wake of the report, Koop was besieged with interview requests from the media. But his two press aides were ordered not to schedule any more interviews after the initial flurry of press attention, and a speech Koop was to deliver before the National Press Club was suddenly canceled. Soon afterward, his press aides, who had been criticized for the effective way they had launched the AIDS report, were both transferred to dead-end bureaucratic posts. And congressional committees that wanted Koop to testify were told he was unavailable. "The administration has the surgeon general under wraps," complained Tim Westmoreland, an aide to Representative Henry Waxman, in June 1987. "It practically takes a subpoena to get him up to the Hill nowadays."

Koop's enemies were not above the pettiest types of harassment. While Koop was recovering from neck surgery in fall 1986, Dr. Robert Windom, the undistinguished physician who had finally replaced Ed Brandt as assistant secretary of health, had Koop's office moved from an adjoining suite to a more remote corner of the building. "It was just playpen stuff," said one HHS staffer, shaking her head.

Windom, a big, red-faced geriatric doctor from southern Florida who had raised money for the Reagan-Bush campaigns, resented all the publicity Koop was getting as a result of the AIDS report. Eager to eclipse the increasingly well-known surgeon general, Windom began taking diction lessons so he would fare better in radio and TV interviews. But those who worked with him were unimpressed with his grasp of the health crisis confronting the nation. "If his IQ were any lower, you'd have to water him," remarked one congressional aide. Windom was destined to remain in Koop's shadow throughout his Washington stint.

Despite the flak bursting around his head, Surgeon General Koop refused to lapse into a discreet silence. As the attacks from the Right grew more withering, Koop became ever bolder in his public remarks. In February 1987, he slipped his chains and appeared before a House subcommittee chaired by his old nemesis, Henry Waxman, to advocate condom advertising on television. "Well, I'm glad your mother's dead," Betty Koop told her husband that morning before he went off to testify. At a Philadelphia press conference two months later, he declared that sex education should begin in kindergarten. "You have to tell [children] about AIDS and that requires sex education," he said. "If parents don't do it, they've abrogated their responsibility and somebody else has to do it." He also stated that some high schools should begin handing out condoms to students—an even more stunning piece of advice from a Reagan administration official.

But his biggest philosophical shift occurred when Koop announced that a pregnant woman diagnosed with AIDS had the right to be counseled about abortion. He reiterates this position during our interview with him: "I'm not going to judge her on that; a woman with AIDS is a person in crisis. That's not like the woman who says, 'Hey, Harry, we're going to spoil our vacation to Europe this summer if I'm pregnant.'" This shift was too much for his former comrades in the right-to-life camp. March for Life promptly rescinded the annual award it had bestowed upon the surgeon general.

Stung by the criticism from old allies, Koop lashed back at them with equal venom. He, too, preferred a family-oriented society founded on the monogamous bond between man and woman, he said. But conservatives were living in a dream world if they thought that was the dominant American landscape in the 1980s. Unlike Phyllis Schlafly and the rest, Koop roared, he was not prepared to "sacrifice that half of the adolescent population that was sexually active just to keep the other half from knowing there are condoms!" Nor would he join conservatives in flaying the homosexual population. "Some of these people seem more concerned with homosexual genocide, and with things like William Buckley's suggesting that AIDS victims be tattooed, than with the human tragedy," Koop told the *New York Times* in a remarkable display of passion.

He was utterly exasperated with conservatives' sexual squeamishness. There was no more time for priggish posturing. Didn't they realize the AIDS crisis had changed everything? Why, under the circumstances, he had no problem sitting down with his own nine-year-old grandson and discussing sodomy and vaginal intercourse, Koop informed the *Village Voice* in another provocative interview. "None of it is frightening to him . . . and when you say some things to him, he says, 'Oh, gross!' and just walks away."

Through his frequent speeches and interviews, the surgeon general was turning himself into the nation's wise, bearded grandfather, giving us practical advice about sex and health—even if some of us thought it all too gross. To Koop, there was nothing immoral about medical wisdom.

Koop was still the evangelical Christian who believed that science could not fully explain the wonders of life, the devout man who took the word of the Bible literally, starting with God's six-day creation of the universe. But he also understood that faith alone would not rid the land of the plague which had befallen it. Turning his office into a pulpit would only alienate those he most needed to reach, Koop decided. "I'm not the nation's chaplain general," he liked to say. "I'm the surgeon general."

His conservative critics said Koop was a victim of his overweening ego. Traumatized by liberals and the media during his long confirmation ordeal, they charged, he was now basking in the warm glow of Teddy Kennedy, Hollywood and New York gays, and the TV lights. Even his friends would admit there was some truth to this. "He's in hog heaven in the Washington spotlight," said former colleague Dr. Duckett. "He absolutely thrives on it."

But there was more to the surgeon general's dramatic metamorphosis than this. Chick Koop had become imbued with the importance of his office, the importance of his medical mission. History, he told Secretary of Health Bowen one day, would judge them for what they had done to stem the AIDS epidemic.

Koop came to see himself as the heir to Dr. Thomas Parran, President Franklin Roosevelt's great surgeon general, the man who shattered American taboos in the 1930s by openly discussing the country's syphilis problem in nonmoralistic terms and organizing a public health campaign to stamp out the disease. "We both used words we weren't supposed to use in public: 'syphilis' and 'condom,' " Koop told us. "We both decided you couldn't play that game. We saw a health issue and treated it as a health issue."

Parran's pathbreaking work helped convince FDR to become the first president to directly address the problem of venereal disease. Similarly, in the months after his report was released, Surgeon General Koop angled to get President Reagan to break his increasingly bizarre silence and make a public statement about the AIDS crisis. More than 20,000 Americans had died from AIDS, including the president's old Hollywood friend Rock Hudson, and 1.5 million were thought to be infected. But Reagan had yet to publicly acknowledge he was even aware of the scourge. "You know, it's not the most pleasant subject in the world, and the president is an optimistic kind of guy; he likes upbeat things," a White House aide told us at the time. "So who wants to be the one telling him negative stuff?"

When Koop's attempt to brief the president on AIDS failed, he tried unsuccessfully to arrange a meeting with Nancy Reagan, according to one report (later denied by Koop). The surgeon general felt a deep sense of urgency because he knew he was not the only one in administration circles pushing an AIDS battle plan. He worried about the "loose cannons" in the conservative movement who had the ear of White House officials—"the type who push the idea that AIDS can be spread through casual transmission or who are so homophobic that it blinds them to the fact the disease is no longer limited to an exclusive club."

By early 1987, the surgeon general found himself in a critical battle with two other administration officials, Education Secretary William Bennett and White House adviser Gary Bauer, over the future of the government's AIDS policy. After the release of Koop's AIDS report, Bennett and Bauer became his counterpoint within the administration, presenting their ideas as the moral alternative to the surgeon general's nonjudgmental, medical approach. It was Bennett who got the headlines, calling for "value-based education" to teach teenagers sexual restraint and questioning the reliability of condoms. Like Koop, Bennett was an effective manipulator of the media.

But while Bennett was Koop's main public adversary, it was the little-known Bauer who functioned as the surgeon general's most effective opponent within the administration, working quietly at the White House to undermine his AIDS strategy. Bauer was a latecomer to the AIDS debate, brought over from the Department of Education in January 1987 by White House Chief of Staff Donald Regan to shore up his credibility with the far Right. Bauer was known primarily for chairing an administration task force on the American family which concluded that "two liberal decades" had resulted in more crime, illegitimate birth, drug use, teenage pregnancy, divorce, and venereal disease.

Once in place as the president's chief domestic policy adviser, Bauer, whom Senator Lowell Weicker referred to as the administration's "philosophical enforcer," lost no time in bending Reagan's ear about AIDS and other issues high on the Right's social agenda. Not long after joining the White House staff, Bauer succeeded in arranging for the president to finally speak out about AIDS—something Koop had been unable to do.

In his April 1, 1987, speech before the College of Physicians of Philadelphia—Koop's home turf—Reagan said AIDS education in the schools should stress sexual abstinence rather than a "value-neutral" prophylactic approach. Just Say No, his wife's antidrug slogan, was also "a pretty good answer" when it came to premarital sex, he later told reporters. The president's comments marked a defeat for the surgeon general. He had been bested by Bauer, the shrewd political operative who had worked himself up from a dollar-a-week gofer job in the 1980 Reagan-Bush campaign to a top White House position. "I've always been pretty good at infighting," Bauer would later tell us with an impish grin in his unadorned office in the west wing of the White House.

Bauer, who joined the White House staff at the age of forty, was utterly lacking in the surgeon general's commanding physical presence. Short, doughy, with tiny hands, pop eyes, and a pug nose, he looked like he had stepped from a Saturday-morning TV cartoon. Where Koop was boastful and fond of the limelight, Bauer was soft-spoken and shy, and preferred to work behind the scenes. But the presidential aide was fired with conservative idealism and was as determined in his mission as Koop was in his. "The Mouse That Roars," was the title pinned on him by the *New Republic*.

Bauer and Koop came from similar philosophical backgrounds. Like the surgeon general, Bauer was an evangelical Protestant, raised in the bosom of the Southern Baptist Church in Newport, Kentucky. And like Koop, he was sorely troubled by the moral state of the nation. In his youth, Newport was known as "sin city," a honky-tonk town where painted ladies paraded up and down the main street and men of weak flesh spent their last dollar in strip shows and gambling joints. Bauer's entry into politics came in 1961, when, at the age of fifteen, he volunteered in a campaign to clean up the town by electing a reform sheriff.

Later, he would come to see America as a larger version of Newport, a Sodom wallowing in sensuality and desperately in need of moral purging. What clearer indication of the country's degraded condition was there than the AIDS epidemic, he thought. Gays and other sexual revolutionaries had been defying the natural order for years, and now nature was exacting a terrible revenge. "We went through a period where people threw out all the rules and now nature, in the sort of difficult way that only nature does, is telling us how unwise this was," Bauer tells us. "What I think is incredible is that we didn't have some sort of terrible disease come down the pike sooner than this one."

Medicine could not fully explain this viral blight, says Bauer, who is unable to conceal his contempt for "experts" and scientific rationalism during our interview. There is a moral genesis to this epidemic, argues the White House adviser, and there are moral lessons to be learned from it. Bauer even talks of a "silver lining in this tragic situation." AIDS, he says, "may get people, young people in particular, to behave in a way that it has been hard for the community of adults to get them to do until now. There is nothing like the threat of death," adds the diminutive aide with a chilling little smile, "to get the glands under control."

Bauer himself, married at the age of twenty-seven and the father of three children, is a happy family man. But, he confesses, Washington does have its temptations. He has never been the type who turned women's heads. But, as Henry Kissinger had discovered during his years at the political summit, power is an aphrodisiac. "I think it's clearly true that in Washington, there's a certain type of woman who is attracted to individuals they perceive to have power," says Bauer, eager to discuss the subject. "And there have certainly been times when, if I had sent out the right signals, I'm sure I could have worked something out."

How does he manage to ignore the flattery and flirtatiousness, to keep his own "glands under control"? It comes down to his faith and his love for his family. That may not have been enough to protect people like Jim Bakker and Jimmy Swaggart. But Bauer feels his bulwark is made of stronger stuff. "When I think of the worst possible things that could ever happen to me, right at the top of the list would be the breakup of my family."

The battle between Bauer and Koop came to a head in the spring of 1987 over the issue of mandatory AIDS testing. Administration hard-liners, led by Bauer and Bennett, were pushing for widespread, compulsory testing of immigrants, prisoners, hospital patients, those applying for marriage licenses, and other groups. Koop and other public health officials vehemently objected, charging that nationwide testing would produce many false results among low-risk groups and drive high-risk groups underground. Gays and others on the AIDS front lines were already fearful, for valid reason, of breaches in medical confidentiality and discrimination. These fears were fanned when right-wing leaders like Senator Jesse Helms periodically raised the specter of quarantine, with some gay activists charging that compulsory testing was the first step to detention.

Koop, by now deeply sensitized to the human component of the epidemic, realized that if the White House handed down a mandatory-testing order, those in greatest need of help would be even less likely to cooperate with the public health system. Education and gentle persuasion were the best weapons in fighting a disease with such a noxious social stigma, stated Koop.

The confrontation over testing brought Koop's and Bauer's philosophical differences into stark relief. Bauer was determined to take tougher measures to protect God-fearing America—the upright citizens like himself who had resisted the siren calls of the sexual revolution and dutifully raised families—from the legions of sexually (and morally) diseased. The goal of the White House hard-liners, as one told the press, was "to make ourselves the champion of all the people who don't have the disease yet."

But Koop would not put his faith in this Maginot Line between the infected and uninfected. Like Bauer, he was a strong family man, but he had developed a wider conception of the American family. He might still think of gays and other sexual minorities as black sheep, but he refused to abandon them. "When I was a young surgeon in the emergency room and they brought in a wounded policeman and bank robber," he would tell us, "I didn't go over and say, 'I'll take care of the cop first because he's a cop.' I took care of the one that was in worse shape." Koop had come to see infected and uninfected, gay and straight, needle users and drug-free as all part of the same community when it came to critical matters of public health. It was a philosophy that was summed up by Albert Camus when he wrote, "The only means of fighting a plague is common decency."

Reagan was to finally announce the administration's policy on AIDS testing in a May 31 speech before the American Foundation for AIDS Research, a group chaired by his wife's old friend Elizabeth Taylor. Again, both sides fought to put their own words in the president's mouth. Again, it looked like Reagan was about to side with Bauer and the hard-liners and call for mandatory testing. In the days leading up to the foundation dinner, there was intense negotiating over the precise wording of the president's speech. Koop would later call it "the most important week in the history of AIDS as far as government action is concerned."

On Wednesday, May 27, the surgeon general was abruptly called back from Salt Lake City for a White House domestic policy council meeting where the final recommendation to the president was to be decided upon. "I came racing in from the airport, arriving at the southwest gate of the White House on two wheels at exactly 2 P.M., when the meeting was to begin," recalled Koop. Reagan was not present, but Bauer was, and so was his forceful ally, Education Secretary Bennett, who proceeded to argue strongly for the mandatory-testing approach, hammering away at his points like the big collegiate football tackle he once was. "When Bill Bennett talks, he's on the table, chest, shoulders, both elbows, and he's like the turkey in the middle," said Koop.

Otis Bowen, the aging, white-haired secretary of Health and Human Services, was no match for Bennett, realized Koop, so it fell to the big-chested surgeon general in the gleaming white-and-gold uniform to argue for restraint. Koop conceded the necessity of testing certain groups, like inmates of federal prisons, where the disease could be spread through forcible sodomy. But he continued to hang tough against nationwide testing. By the end of the meeting, it was still a stalemate, and the White House staff was ordered to review the opposing arguments and come up with a compromise position.

The wording was to be presented to Reagan at a Cabinet meeting the next day. Koop showed up, prepared to continue battle. "But when I picked up the agenda and looked immediately at item four," he said, "I couldn't believe my eyes. It said, 'The president urges the states to offer routine testing.' Well I know what 'routine' means and I know what 'offer' means and they don't mean mandatory. It was a great victory, not just for me but for the world."

Bauer, too, would claim victory. "I'm glad that Dr. Koop feels good about it," he tells us, "but the bottom line is that we're going to have more testing than we had before—federal prisoners, immigrants, and so on."

But Koop was convinced that he had stifled the administration's worst instincts. Three days later, under a steamy tent filled with Washington socialites, gay activists, and medical celebrities, President Reagan would call for "understanding, not ignorance. . . . This is a battle against disease, not against our fellow Americans." It was a rare display of compassion, but for many of those in attendance, who had suffered much loss and anguish during the epidemic, it was too little, too late. As Reagan read that part of his speech calling for limited AIDS testing, he was met with a growing chorus of boos.

Dr. C. Everett Koop, on the other hand, was greeted with a standing ovation when Elizabeth Taylor presented him with a special award from the AIDS foundation. By then, Koop's former liberal adversaries on Capitol Hill were also hailing him as a hero. Henry Waxman, once "frightened" by Koop, now called him "a man of tremendous integrity. He's done everything a surgeon general should do, and more, to protect the health of the public." Liberals marveled at Koop's transformation. He exemplified, in the judgment of *Washington Post* columnist Colman McCarthy, "the growth-in-office theory of political appointments. The seemingly worst can turn out to be among the certifiably best."

But Chick Koop insisted he was the same man. Just as his deep religious belief in the sacredness of human life had impelled him to become one of the more zealous leaders of the antiabortion movement and had driven him to champion Baby Doe, so it now directed him to stand up for those whose lives were menaced by AIDS. Every life deserved protection, believed Koop, even those he felt had been badly led. No one was to be left behind. He would never give in to the forces of social triage.

In November 1987, Koop, long mute about his religious convictions out of fear of liberal criticism, felt bold enough to reveal the biblical foundations to his AIDS philosophy in a speech before the Union of American Hebrew Congregations in Chicago. Ironically, the physician had found inspiration in the same story from the Book of Genesis that made his fundamentalist critics burn with righteous conviction. "The Lord wants to destroy Sodom," Koop told the gathering of Jewish leaders in his rich Old Testament voice. "But Abraham argues that the Lord might have to save the lives of thousands of not very nice people in order to also save the lives of as few as ten righteous people. . . . [In this] dialogue over the fate of Sodom, I think the Lord was hearing more than just bravado and 'chutzpah' from the newly named Abraham. I think he was hearing a new voice of awareness, of compassion, of human dignity. Call it what you will, but it was clearly a new voice of faith."

The AIDS crisis compelled America to "quickly act upon that powerful Abrahamic tradition of reverence in action." The tendency to blame, to scorn those who "either recklessly engaged in sodomy or swapped dirty needles while shooting dangerous drugs" had to be morally resisted, Koop continued. There were physicians and nurses who violated medical ethics by shunning AIDS patients, he said, and neighbors who had turned against neighbors. But this was unacceptable, he declared. "In this terrible and fearsome period, I maintain—as a physician, as a scientist, but also as a human being—that man *cannot be denied*. AIDS itself would have us do that. People who live in total fear of AIDS would have us do that. And people weakened by the despair of AIDS would have us do that. But we cannot."

Medicine was still no match for the death force of AIDS, Koop told the gathering. "We have no drugs, no vaccines, no magic bullets, nothing that can accomplish that lifesaving job." All we have, he stated, is a commitment to life, a reverence for our fellow human beings. "If mankind is now the victim of a hideous mystery, we cannot give up on him . . . we cannot abandon him for that reason. Rather, as Martin Buber [has] argued, we must affirm his life and his condition. We must 'liberate him from the dread of abandonment'—the *dread* of abandonment—'which is the foretaste of death.'"

Laced with his fundamentalist values, Koop's speech was nonetheless a moving rejoinder to the forces of conservative moralism. "Yes, I thought it was remarkable too," he would tell us with characteristic modesty.

During the final months of the Reagan presidency, it was the judgmental view of the AIDS tragedy advanced by Bauer's hard-line faction that would continue to dominate administration policy. Bauer succeeded in stacking Reagan's national AIDS commission with like-minded conservatives, including a San Diego sex therapist who said AIDS could be caught from a toilet seat and an Illinois state legislator who accused gays of engaging in "blood terrorism" by deliberately donating infected blood. But the commission, under the leadership of retired admiral James Watkins, stunned the White House with its final report, which called among other things for new federal initiatives to prevent discrimination against AIDS patients and coordination of the government's disparate anti-AIDS efforts under the command of the surgeon general. Administration officials decided to accept the report "without fanfare," ignoring its bold recommendations and continuing the policy of benign neglect to the end.

In contrast, Surgeon General Koop continued to use his bully pulpit to promote compassion and condoms, offsetting the doctrinaire tendencies of the administration and fighting against "the dread of abandonment." He spoke out against panicky state initiatives that mandated AIDS testing and that required infected persons to be reported to health authorities. He pushed for more AIDS education aimed at teenagers and drug users. He demanded a halt to the practice of barring students and teachers with AIDS from classrooms.

Koop knew Bauer could not shut him up; his success with the media protected him from White House retribution. The hard-liners continued to win the political battles. But, in a sense, Koop had won the larger war. Through his forthright AIDS report and candid public statements, he had changed the national dialogue on sex. The country's top physician had repeatedly used the taboo word "condom"—a word with disturbingly graphic associations for many Americans—and thereby legitimated its entry into the public arena.

It was an American tale that could only have taken place in these strange days of death and desire. The square-jawed surgeon general with the old-fashioned chin beard and Old Testament zeal had pushed the country one step further along its rocky path toward sexual enlightenment.

AIDS AND POLITICS: Transformation of Our Movement

MAXINE WOLFE

from Women, AIDS, and Activism

| 1990 |

Over most of the thirty years of my political activism, I was somehow always on the "periphery of the periphery." The question, then, is: "How could a nice Jewish girl from Brooklyn, who once described herself as a bisexual, Trotskyist, anarchist, Reichian lesbian-feminist, end up in an organization people continually describe as white, male, bourgeois (worse yet, upper middle class), single issue, not gay identified, arrogant, resource rich, and every other thing that people who describe themselves as 'progressive' don't like?" The second question is: "Why have I stayed in it?"

I came to AIDS activism and to New York ACT UP out of a queer consciousness, a consciousness forced on me by the sexism and homophobia of the male-identified Left in this country and by the homophobia of the women's movement. I came to ACT UP because of the inability of lesbians to organize around or even figure out what their issues were and because of the dead end of the "identity" politics of the early 1980s.

I had joined the reproductive-rights movement in 1978 to organize against the elimination of Medicaid funding for abortion, after I had left the Trotskyist group—whose periphery I had been on for several years. They disparagingly called the reproductive-rights group which I joined "feminist," but I said I would rather argue for my Marxist politics in a feminist group than for my feminist politics in a Marxist group. Five years later, in 1984, I decided I'd rather do neither. And by that time I had decided I didn't want to be in a lesbian-feminist group, and I didn't want to be in a lesbian and gay left group. What had happened?

Some of the things these groups had in common were an outdated concept of organizing, an unwillingness to reach outside their known constituencies, and a rigid set of politics around which everyone had to agree. Then you couldn't question anything or you were suspect.

Identity politics had gotten to the point where, apparently, the only person I was supposed to feel comfortable talking to was another working-class, Jewish, lesbian mother of two children from the Left who was neither vanilla nor chocolate. Everybody was in their own separate box and I didn't have a box to fit into.

By 1984, I was severely depressed. All of the groups I had worked with since 1979 no longer existed. I was forced to reevaluate every political perspective and value I ever had. I started going to every meeting I could find, including lesbian and gay Democrats. I decided I had to clear out my head of previous indoctrination, really listen to what people said, and really look at what they were doing.

I did a range of different things between 1984 and 1987, but three stand out. First, I began my still-weekly treks as a volunteer to the Lesbian Herstory Archives, the only remaining woman-only space in New York, where a truly diverse group of women work together, committed to preserving the full range of lesbian experience. But it was not enough for my activist bones. Second, I went to the first public meeting of the Gay and Lesbian Alliance Against Defamation and saw that at least four hundred gay men and a few lesbians wanted to do activist work around homophobia and AIDS. I didn't join, however, because their operating style was the familiar "progressive" model. In addition, in response to my questions, one of their answers was that they were neither for nor against the closing of the bathhouses. That turned me off. I was against the closing of the bathhouses. The third significant event (or rather, events) were the Hardwick demonstrations after the Supreme Court upheld Georgia's antigay sodomy law—both the spontaneous sit-in of hundreds one night in Sheridan Square and the several thousand who, four days later on July 4, marched into the throngs of tourists at the Statue of Liberty Centennial against the desires of the self-appointed "gay leadership." I realized that the community was ahead of its so-called leadership and willing to put their bodies on the line at the right moment. This gave me hope.

Almost one year later, a week before the Lesbian and Gay Pride March in 1987, a friend of mine told me about an AIDS activist group. As if by fate, at the march I saw this guy selling "Silence = Death" T-shirts. I went over to him and asked, "Are there women in your group?" "Sure," he said. So the next evening I found myself at the Lesbian and Gay Community Center in a group of a couple of hundred men I didn't know and about four women.

Why did I stay when, in terms of political perspective, many things about this group should have told me to leave? For example, I had assumed it was a lesbian- and gay-identified group, but people didn't want to be called lesbian and gay activists; they wanted to be called "AIDS activists." And they seemed to believe in the health-care system, even if it had gone awry. They even respected doctors!

But everything was run democratically, and people got up and said what they thought. I could get up and say what I thought. They wanted to end the AIDS crisis, period, and if you had a good idea they would listen. No one spouted rhetoric; there was no party line. They had great ideas for actions without any pre-set idea of the right way to do things. They thought tabling was a new idea. They had a great sense of the visual and they used the media, but they didn't cater to it. No one quibbled over words on a flyer. If you wanted to do an action, you proposed it. Most likely people would do it. In fact, they did more actions in a week than I'd ever thought possible. And they have made more of an impact, both conceptually and in terms of saving people's lives, than any group I've ever been part of. These were people organizing not from some abstract concept but to save their lives and the lives of people they cared about. And, they were pro-sex at a time when sex was being connected to death.

But I am a realist and not a romantic. I don't think ACT UP is the be-all and end-all. There have been problems. I stayed in ACT UP because it is a place where I can be a lesbian, a woman, and an activist. I stayed in ACT UP because I have seen people *develop* a political perspective, including myself. I have changed and learned or I wouldn't still be there. It is also the first real organizing I feel I've ever done. I have seen men who wanted to hide being gay behind their AIDS activism do a teach-in on lesbian and gay history, become more and more openly gay, and develop a gay-liberation, and not a gay-rights, perspective. I have seen the issues expand—a year ago no one talked about nationalized health care; now we have a national health-care committee and are talking to unions about doing an action together. ACT UP is a true coalition. Everyone puts up with what my mother would call everyone else's *mischigas*—craziness. I have come to appreciate what each person can and will contribute because they share a commitment to the saving of lives.

I no longer feel like I'm on the periphery of the periphery. For the first time, I feel I am acting from my center but not from the mainstream. I feel I'm helping to build a movement that is mine rather than trying to fit into someone else's.

I don't know where ACT UP will go. Your guess is as good as mine. As for our movement, the lesbian and gay and AIDS movement, I believe that in order to take advantage of the momentum for the future, we need to seriously check out our own homophobia and our rigid rules for evaluating political movements. This is especially true for older lesbians and for lesbians and gay men who identify with progressive movements. For example, there are two questions I am always asked by lesbians who look down on AIDS work, and by lesbians and gay men working in other progressive movements. One is: "Would gay men have done the same thing for lesbians if the situation had been reversed?" The first thing I say is, "I am not in this movement for gay men; I am in this movement for myself." And then I ask them: "What have straight women and straight men done for us? What have the antinuclear and anti-intervention movements done for us?" I'm not saying that people shouldn't work in these movements. I am saying, "Check out the homophobia in your question." The second question I am asked is: "If a cure for AIDS happened tomorrow, wouldn't all those gay men go home and not care about access issues?" "Probably a lot would," I answer, "just like all the women who went home after *Roe v. Wade* and only came out again when *Roe* was threatened." The fact is that poor women—and because of institutional racism in this country, black and Latin women are disproportionately among the poor—and young women and rural women have not had access to abortion for many, many years. Where were these women in 1977 when the Hyde Amendment, cutting off federal Medicaid funding for abortion, was passed? Gay men, as a group, are no better and no worse than anyone else. We have to get past this mentality.

In that respect, one of the most important roles that ACT UP plays is that it is a place where many younger gay men and lesbians have come to understand that what we want is the right to exist—not the right to privacy; the right to a life, not to a lifestyle; and a life that is as important as anyone else's, but not any more important than anyone else's. This understanding has formed the basis for work outside of the lesbian and gay community, with other communities affected by the AIDS crisis, and it is why ACT UP has been managing to do some of that work.

Many younger lesbians in ACT UP see themselves as "queer," and both their political and social life is tied to that of gay men. While I have made good gay male and lesbian friends in ACT UP, many of whom will remain my friends for a long time, ACT UP does not satisfy my social needs. But I am not into coupledom or monogamy in my political life any more than in my social life. ACT UP is my political home for now. And, I can honestly say that while in 1979 there were only a handful of gay men in New York I could work with politically, after ACT UP, there will be more. That's not bad.

This is an edited version of a speech presented at the National Gay and Lesbian Task Force Town Meeting, October 6, 1989, in Washington, D.C.

A "MANHATTAN PROJECT" FOR AIDS

LARRY KRAMER

from The New York Times

| July 16, 1990 |

I am so frightened that the war against AIDS has already been lost.

It is beyond comprehension why, in a presumably civilized country, in the modern era, such a continuing, extraordinary destruction of life is being attended to so tentatively, so meekly, and in such a cowardly fashion.

The armies of the infected, their families, loved ones, and friends no longer know how to deliver their pleas for help. Every conceivable method has been attempted, from quietly working from within to noisily demonstrating without.

Millions of people who need not die so young will die so young. As things stand now, everyone who is presently infected can reasonably expect to die. So desperate is the situation that Dr. David Baltimore, president of Rockefeller University, has called for a "Manhattan Project" for AIDS, an equivalent of the scientific effort that produced the atomic bomb. He's right. Only the federal government can manage the project to find, as quickly as possible, the cure that top scientists believe is there and that could stem the ocean of death.

The number of those infected with AIDS is now so terrifyingly large that, even if a satisfactory treatment or cure were found tomorrow, there is no system in existence anywhere in the world that could deliver it in time to save so many people. The numbers of those facing death from AIDS are so large that the eyes should glaze—with tears.

In America, 212 new cases of full-blown AIDS are diagnosed every day; there is one AIDS death every twelve minutes, and a new case of infection every fifty-four seconds. At a minimum, one to one and a half million Americans are infected.

A report by the American Council on Science and Health predicted that one in every twenty-five New York City residents will have AIDS in the next ten years. Last week, another study revealed that AIDS is already the leading cause of death among black women between the ages of fifteen and forty-four.

Worldwide, 386,588 cases have been reported in 151 countries. The World Health Organization estimates that this number is now at least 700,000 and that 6 to 8 million people have the virus that causes fullblown AIDS. By the year 2000, the infected population will approach 20 million.

All of these figures, which are known to be imprecise, are also known to be low. They are mostly based on extrapolations from small samplings from isolated areas or from cases that doctors report to authorities. We know that many doctors and patients do not report their cases, and that large numbers of those infected never see a doctor.

A transmissible virus is loose in the world. It may be one or several. It is completely out of control. Short of a cure, there is no way it can be stopped—not by mandatory or volunteer contact tracing, partner notification, quarantining, incarceration, or legislation. It is out there, everywhere, and it is rampant.

We are living in a time of plague, and two presidents in a row have refused to stem it. Their refusal to act will cost taxpayers a fortune—easily more than the entire cost of the savings and loan bailout.

Six federal studies and more than fifty congressional oversight hearings have all concluded the same thing: The research on AIDS is uncoordinated and the funding cycles are inefficient. No one is in charge.

President Bush has done as little about AIDS as President Reagan. Twenty-four thousand Americans have died from AIDS since he took office. After stumbling on abortion, the secretary of health and human services, Dr. Louis Sullivan, has meekly followed the lead of the White House on AIDS, even though many sense he would like to perform adequately.

It is suspected that the real villain of the piece is John Sununu, the White House chief of staff, whose mission seems to be appeasing the conservative Right. The result is the perpetuation of a federal policy on AIDS that was crafted by Ronald Reagan's AIDS adviser, Gary Bauer, who is now more visibly displaying his rhetoric of hate as head of the Family Research Council.

Ten years into this plague, the federal agencies dealing with AIDS are mired in such bureaucracy that it is next to impossible for them to respond to the crisis. There are so many committees and committees within committees, peer reviews and interagency task forces that few can sort them all out.

Paths of least resistance are the chosen norm. Imagination is not encouraged and exchange of vital information is often nonexistent. The two most important agencies, the National Institutes of Health and the Food and Drug Administration, are both still lacking a permanent director. Rivalries and distrust between them are embarrassingly, visibly rife. International fistfights over who should get the Nobel Prize for AIDS research has destroyed trust universally. Pharmaceutical companies now test their drugs abroad rather than confront the American maze.

The bureaucracy is so byzantine, nobody can or has to make a decision.

Research is delayed not only by a lack of any coherent plan and mature guidance, but also by a lack of first-rate personnel. The chief NIH laboratories have twenty-seven vacancies for AIDS scientists. Vital studies that many assume are being done are not.

Conflict of interest is rampant. Just about every major AIDS researcher with a government grant is also on the payroll of a major pharmaceutical manufacturer as a "consultant." Thus, the only drugs that are being tested are ones controlled by these same manufacturers. Hundreds of promising treatments developed by the less well-connected are simply ignored—and people continue to suffer and die.

President Bush and Dr. Anthony Fauci of the NIH have constantly assured us that more has been learned in record time about AIDS than any disease in history, that everything that can be done is being done. Dr. Fauci, a dedicated and overburdened scientist, is no doubt trying to calm the waters for his boss, the president, who once called him a "hero." But a real hero must tell the truth, even when it is unpopular.

Huge areas of AIDS still aren't understood. Yet government grants that would locate and assign a researcher to a specific AIDS problem are prohibited by some funding regulations.

Dr. Fauci's $500 million program for conducting experimental drug trials at local hospital sites around the country, the AIDS Clinical Trials Group, has fallen tragically short of its goals. Slots for tens of thousands of patients attract only hundreds, mainly because most people with AIDS are excluded from the trials by a battery of illogical and murderous clinical restrictions.

And recent editorials in the *Lancet* and the *Journal of the American Medical Association* seriously questioned the usefulness of AZT, a twenty-five-year-old, exceedingly toxic antiviral treatment on which the NIH spends billions of dollars. AIDS doctors and patients desperately need something more effective, but they won't get it until the AIDS drug pipeline is rerouted and streamlined.

Stopping the tragic delays in research and treatment—delays which are mostly bureaucratic, not scientific—seems impossible. The president is not interested, and while Congress votes money for the war, it abdicates its responsibility to see that these precious funds are spent wisely.

To top it all off, the media have yet to expose most, if not all, of the wrongs enumerated above. They reserve their energies for criticizing the tactics activists have used to compensate for their shameful silence.

Only an all-out effort by the federal government can defeat AIDS. It alone has the resources and authority to win. President Bush must put one person in charge of all aspects of AIDS and grant this person emergency powers to cut through the red tape. And the president must take up Dr. Baltimore's call for a "Manhattan Project" to find that cure.

Anything less will condemn millions to death, and the war against AIDS will indeed be irrevocably lost. And history will record that it was lost because two U.S. presidents and the entire federal government surrendered.

ESTHETICS AND LOSS

EDMUND WHITE

from The Burning Library
Originally appeared in Personal Dispatches

| 1990 |

I had a friend, a painter named Kris Johnson, who died two years ago of AIDS. He was in his early thirties. He'd shown here and there, in bookstores, arty coffee shops, that kind of thing, first in Minnesota, then in Los Angeles. He painted over color photos he'd color-Xeroxed—images of shopping carts in parking lots, of giant palms, their small heads black as warts against the smoggy sun: California images.

He read *Artforum* religiously; he would have been happy to see his name in its pages. The magazine represented for him a lien on his future, a promise of the serious work he was about to embrace as soon as he could get out of the fast lane. Like many people who are both beautiful and gifted, he had to explore his beauty before his gift. It dictated his way of living until two years ago, before his death. His health had already begun to deteriorate and he'd moved to Santa Fe, where he painted seriously his last few months.

By now there have been many articles about how the AIDS virus is contracted and how it manifests itself. The purely medical horrors of the disease have received the attention of the world press. What interests me here is how artists of all sorts—writers, painters, sculptors, people in video and performance art, actors, models—are responding to AIDS in their work and their lives. If I narrow the focus, I do so because of the impact the epidemic has had on esthetics and on the life of the art community, an impact that has not been studied.

The most visible artistic expressions of AIDS have been movies, television dramas, and melodramas on the stage, almost all of which have emphasized that AIDS is a terribly moving human experience (for the lover, the nurse, the family, the patient), which may precipitate the coming out of the doctor (the play *Anti Body*, 1983, by Louise Parker Kelley) or overcome the homophobia of the straight male nurse (*Compromised Immunity*, 1986, by Andy Kirby and the Gay Sweatshop Theatre Company, from England) or resolve long-standing tensions between lovers (William M. Hoffman's play *As Is*, 1985, and Bill Sherwood's beautifully rendered movie *Parting Glances*, 1985). Although Larry Kramer's play *The Normal Heart*, 1985, is almost alone in taking up the political aspects of the disease, it still ends in true melodramatic fashion with a deathbed wedding scene. John Erman's *An Early Frost*, 1985, a made-for-television movie on NBC, is the *Love Story* of the eighties; the best documentary is perhaps *Coming of Age*, 1986, by Marc Huestis, who filmed scenes from the life of a friend of his diagnosed with the virus.

But even on artists working away from the limelight, AIDS has had an effect. Naturally the prospect of ill health and death or its actuality inspires a sense of urgency. What was it I wanted to do in my work after all? Should I make my work simpler, clearer, more accessible? Should I record my fears obliquely or directly, or should I defy them? Is it more heroic to drop whatever I was doing and look disease in the eye or should I continue going in the same direction as before, though with a new consecration? Is it a hateful concession to the disease even to acknowledge its existence? Should I pretend Olympian indifference to it? Or should I admit to myself, "Look, kid, you're scared shitless and that's your material"? If sex and death are the only two topics worthy of adult consideration, then AIDS wins hands down as subject matter.

It seems to me that AIDS is tilting energies away from the popular arts (including disco dancing, the sculpturing of the living body through working out, the design of pleasure machines—bars, clubs, baths, resort houses) and redirecting them toward the solitary "high" arts. Of course I may simply be confusing the effects of aging with the effects of the disease; after all, the Stonewall generation is now middle-aged, and older people naturally seek out different pursuits. But we know how frightened everyone is becoming, even well beyond the "high risk" group that is my paradigm and my subject here.

What seems unquestionable is that ten years ago sex was a main reason for being for many gay men. Not simple, humdrum coupling, but a new principle of adhesiveness. Sex provided a daily brush with the ecstatic, a rehearsal of forgotten pain under the sign of the miraculous—sex was a force binding familiar atoms into new polymers of affinity.

To be sure, as some wit once remarked, life would be supportable without its pleasures, and certainly a sensual career had its melancholy side. Even so, sex was if not fulfilling then at least engrossing—enough at times to make the pursuit of the toughest artistic goals seem too hard, too much work given the mild returns. "Beauty is difficult," as Pound liked to remind us, and the difficulties held little allure for people who could take satisfaction in an everyday life that had, literally, become . . . sensational. Popular expressions of the art of life, or rather those pleasures that intensified the already heady exchange within a newly liberated culture, thrived: the fortune that was lavished on flowers, drugs, sound systems, food, clothes, hair. People who were oppressed by the brutality of the big city or by their own poverty or a humiliating job could create for at least a night, or a weekend, a magical dreamlike environment.

Now all that has changed. I, for one, at least feel repatriated to my lonely adolescence, the time when I was alone with my writing and I felt weird about being a queer. Art was a consolation then—a consolation for a life not much worth living, a site for the staging of fantasies reality couldn't fulfill, a peopling of solitude—and art has become a consolation again. People aren't on the prowl anymore, and a seductive environment is read not as an enticement but as a death trap. Fat is in; it means you're not dying, at least not yet.

And of course we do feel weird again, despised, alien. There's talk of tattooing us or quarantining us. Both the medical and the moralistic models for homosexuality have been dusted off only fifteen years after they were shelved; the smell of the madhouse and the punitive vision of the Rake Chastised have been trotted out once more. In such a social climate, the popular arts, the public arts, are standing still, frozen in time. There's no market, no confidence, no money. The brassy hedonism of a few years back has given way to a protective gray invisibility, which struck me forcibly when I returned to New York recently after being away for several months. As Joe Orton in his diary quotes a friend remarking, all we see are all those dull norms, all norming about.

But if the conditions for a popular culture are deteriorating, those promoting a renewed high culture have returned. Certainly the disease is encouraging homosexuals to question whether they want to go on defining themselves at all by their sexuality. Maybe the French philosopher Michel

Foucault was right in saying there are homosexual acts but not homosexual people. More concretely, when a society based on sex and expression is deeroticized, its very reason for being can vanish.

Yet the disease is a stigma; even the horde of asymptomatic carriers of the antibody is stigmatized. Whether imposed or chosen, gay identity is still very much with us. How does it express itself these days?

The main feeling is one of evanescence. It's just like the Middle Ages; every time you say good-bye to a friend, you fear it may be for the last time. You search your own body for signs of the malady. Every time someone begins a sentence with "Do you remember Bob . . ." you seize up in anticipation of the sequel. A writer or visual artist responds to this fragility as both a theme and as a practical limitation—no more projects that require five years to finish.

The body becomes central, the body that until recently was at once so natural (athletic, young, casually dressed) and so artificial (pumped up, pierced, ornamented). Now it is feeble, yellowing, infected—or boisterously healthy as a denial of precisely this possibility. When I saw a famous gay filmmaker recently, he was radiant, with a hired tan; "I have to look healthy or no one will bankroll me." Most of all the body is unloved. Onanism—singular or in groups—has replaced intercourse. This solitude is precisely a recollection of adolescence. Unloved, the body releases its old sad song, but it also builds fantasies, rerunning idealized movies of past realities, fashioning new images out of thin air.

People think about the machinery of the body—the wheezing bellows of the lungs, the mulcher of the gut—and of the enemy it may be harboring. "In the midst of life we are in death," in the words of the Book of Common Prayer. Death—in its submicroscopic, viral, paranoid aspect, the side worthy of William Burroughs—shadows every pleasure.

The New York painter Frank Moore told me last fall that in developing possible sets and costumes for a new Lar Lubovitch ballet, he worked out an imagery of blood cells and invading organisms, of cells consuming themselves—a vision of cellular holocaust. In his view, the fact of death and the ever-present threat of mortality have added a bite to the sometimes empty rhetoric of East Village expressionalism. "Until now anger has been a look, a pose," he told me. Now it has teeth.

The list of people in the art world who have died of AIDS is long and growing longer. I won't mention names for fear of omitting one—or including one that discretion should conceal (it's not always possible to verify how much a patient told his family).

Maybe it's tactless or irrelevant to critical evaluation to consider an artist, writer, dealer, or curator in the light of his death.

Yet the urge to memorialize the dead, to honor their lives, is a pressing instinct. Ross Bleckner's paintings with titles such as *Hospital Room, Memoriam*, and *8,122+ As of January, 1986* commemorate those who had died of AIDS, and incorporate trophies, banners, flowers, and gates—public images.

There is an equally strong urge to record one's own past—one's own life—before it vanishes. I suppose everyone both believes and chooses to ignore that each detail of our behavior is inscribed in the arbitrariness of history. Which culture, which moment we live in determines how we have sex, go mad, marry, die, and worship, even how we say Ai! instead of Ouch! when we're pinched. Not even the soul that we reform or express is God-given or eternal; as Foucault writes in *Discipline and Punish* (1978), "The soul is the effect and instrument of a political anatomy; the soul is the prison of the body." For gay men this force of history has been made to come clean; it's been stripped of its natural look. The very rapidity of change has laid bare the clanking machinery of history. To have been oppressed in the fifties, freed in the sixties, exalted in the seventies, and wiped out in the eighties is a quick itinerary for a whole culture to follow. For we are witnessing not just the death of individuals but a menace to an entire culture. All the more reason to bear witness to the cultural moment.

Art must compete with (rectify, purge) the media, which has thoroughly politicized AIDS in a process that is the subject of a book to be published shortly in England. It is *Policing Desire: Pornography, AIDS and the Media* by Simon Watney. (Watney, Jeffrey Weeks, Richard Goldstein, and Dennis Altman rank as the leading English-language intellectuals to think about AIDS and homosexuality.)

This winter William Olander at the New Museum in New York has organized "Homo Video—Where We Are Now," an international gay and lesbian program that focuses in part on AIDS and the media. For instance, Gregg Bordowitz's *". . . some aspect of a shared lifestyle"* deals with the contrast between the actual diseases and the "gay plague" image promoted by the media. John Greyson's *Moscow Does Not Believe in Queers*, 1986, inserts lurid Rock Hudson headlines into a taped diary of ten days at a 1985 Moscow youth festival where Greyson functioned as an "out" homosexual in a country that does not acknowledge the rights—or even the legitimate existence—of homosexuals. And Stuart Marshall's *Bright Eyes*, 1986, tracks, among other things, the presentation of AIDS in the English media.

If art is to confront AIDS more honestly than the media has done, it must begin in tact, avoid humor, and end in anger.

Begin in tact, I say, because we must not reduce individuals to their deaths; we must not fall into the trap of replacing the afterlife with the moment of dying. How someone dies says nothing about how he lived. And tact because we must not let the disease stand for other things. AIDS generates complex and harrowing reflections, but it is not caused by moral or intellectual choices. We are witnessing at long last the end of illness as metaphor and metonym.

Avoid humor, because humor seems grotesquely inappropriate to the occasion. Humor puts the public (indifferent when not uneasy) on cozy terms with what is an unspeakable scandal: death. Humor domesticates terror, lays to rest misgivings that should be intensified. Humor suggests that AIDS is just another calamity to befall Mother Camp, whereas in truth AIDS is not one more item in a sequence, but a rupture in meaning itself. Humor, like melodrama, is an assertion of bourgeois values; it falsely suggests that AIDS is all in the family. Baudelaire reminded us that the wise man laughs only with fear and trembling.

End in anger, I say, because it is only sane to rage against the dying of the light, because strategically anger is a political response, because psychologically anger replaces despondency, and because existentially anger lightens the solitude of frightened individuals.

I feel very alone with the disease. My friends are dying. One of them asked me to say a prayer for us all in Venice "in that church they built when the city was spared from the ravages of the plague." Atheist that I am, I murmured my invocation to Longhena's baroque octagon if not to any spirit dwelling in Santa Maria della Salute. The other day I saw stenciled on a Paris wall an erect penis, its dimensions included in centimeters, and the words *Faut Pas Rever* (You mustn't dream). When people's dreams are withdrawn, they get real angry, real fast.

STOP THE CHURCH

DOUGLAS CRIMP WITH ADAM ROLSTON

from AIDS Demo Graphics

| 1990 |

In 1987 the National Conference of Catholic Bishops agreed to allow a limited exception to the ban on contraceptives: because of the extraordinary circumstances of a dangerous epidemic, condom use as a protection against HIV infection would be minimally tolerated by the church. The archconservative Cardinal O'Connor of New York vehemently opposed the ruling and continued to rail against any kind of safe sex teaching other than abstinence within his jurisdiction. O'Connor had been made archbishop of New York in the spring of 1984 and appointed cardinal a year later by Pope John Paul II, whose conservative political and moral positions O'Connor could be counted on to enforce. From the moment he arrived in New York, O'Connor became an outspoken and powerful opponent of progressive politics, taking on the lesbian and gay movement as his particular obsession. The city's Gay Rights Bill was passed in 1986 over his fierce opposition, and he still refuses to abide by the antidiscrimination law in the provision of services contracted by the city. He banned masses held by the gay Catholic organization Dignity from Catholic churches and got an injunction to prevent the group's silent protests in St. Patrick's against the ban. The clear message from O'Connor's pulpit is that gay people are immoral, and fag-bashers have taken heed: violence against lesbians and gays has sharply increased in the past decade.

But O'Connor's most directly murderous pronouncements have been about AIDS. He has consistently opposed safe-sex education and the use of condoms to prevent HIV transmission. This would be lethal enough if it affected only obedient Catholics, but O'Connor's influence extends well beyond the docile minority. As soon as he came to New York he formed a close alliance with his fellow reactionary, Mayor Koch, whose policies were consistently informed by the cardinal's "moral" positions. This means, for one thing, that in the **public** schools, where 85 percent of the students are people of color, AIDS education has been a just-say-no harangue—antigay, antisex, antilife. Statistics show that by the end of high school the vast majority of students are sexually active and many use drugs. Preaching abstinence denies their reality and will ultimately deny many of them their lives.

In early November 1989, the National Conference of Catholic Bishops, under pressure from O'Connor and his conservative cronies in the church hierarchy, rescinded the bishops' earlier stance on condom use to prevent HIV transmission. They now demand total abstinence as the only means of prevention, even if one partner in a sanctioned marriage is HIV-infected. A few weeks later, the Vatican held its first conference on AIDS, where the pope reaffirmed the church's condemnation of homosexuality and ban on all forms of contraception. Monsignor Carlo Caffarra stated the church's attitude about condoms bluntly: their use "is a true and proper anticonceptive act which is never licit under any circumstances or for any reasons." A speech by a theologian from Liechtenstein suggested that AIDS could indeed be seen as God's wrath against homosexuality, leading an American attending the conference to call it "three days of gay-bashing." O'Connor was one of the prime bashers, saying in his speech, "I believe the greatest damage done to persons with AIDS is done by those health-care professionals who refuse to confront the moral dimensions of sexual aberrations or drug abuse." And he went on to claim, "The truth is not in condoms or clean needles. These are lies—lies perpetuated often for political reasons on the part of public health officials." Because such utter disregard for truth and outbursts of hatred toward the suffering are unseemly in a Christian, O'Connor attempted to temper his statements by claiming that he had "sat with, listened to, emptied the bedpans of, and washed the sores of more than 1,100 persons with AIDS." What he meant was that in the hospitals and nursing home facilities the taxpayers pay him to manage through city contracts, he and his minions daily inflict the indignity of their archaic moralism on people dying from a disease he is helping to spread.

ACT UP's plan to STOP THE CHURCH was formulated during the final stages of the fall mayoralty campaign. Because former U.S. prosecutor Rudolph Giuliani, a Catholic, was running on the Republican ticket against Democrat David Dinkins, the church's stranglehold over city politics became an even more pressing issue, as it also concerned a woman's right to choose an abortion. Giuliani waffled on choice, as he waffled on every politically charged subject, but the cardinal didn't. He openly supported Operation Rescue terrorism against family planning clinics and urged the creation of a new order of nuns whose mission would be fighting abortion rights. ACT UP had been active in the struggle to keep abortion legal and accessible for some time by joining counterdemonstrations when Operation Rescue's well-financed intimidation squads attacked New York clinics. ACT UP's support of abortion rights was not solely a matter of individual members' political convictions or of our coalition building with other progressive movements. Apart from the philosophical links between the AIDS activist and pro-choice positions on control of one's own body and health-care rights, there are even more direct connections between AIDS and reproductive-rights issues. Women are routinely excluded from AIDS drug trials because of their "reproductive capacities" (drug companies' concerns about endangering fetuses are, of course, really fears of potential lawsuits). Women are forced to accept sterilization to gain entry into some trials; and often HIV-positive pregnant women are coerced into having abortions against their will. The ACT UP Women's Committee had thoroughly documented these facts and presented them to the entire group within the context of a March 1989 teach-in on women and AIDS. Their *Women and AIDS Handbook* of more than one hundred pages became a primer on the subject, providing essential background information on the present status of women in the United States, the history of women and the medical establishment, and the relationship of the feminist health movement to the AIDS activist movement.

Several busloads of ACT UP members traveled to Washington, D.C., to form a contingent at the huge pro-choice demonstration there on April 9, 1989. We added our militant voices to those of NO MORE NICE GIRLS in an otherwise rather staid march, our chant proclaiming

ACT UP, WE'RE HERE.
WE'RE LOUD AND RUDE, PRO-CHOICE AND QUEER.

Three months later the conservative majority on the Supreme Court struck another severe blow to abortion rights in *Webster v. Reproductive*

Health Services. Although the historic *Roe v. Wade* decision guaranteeing a woman's constitutional right to an abortion was not entirely overturned, the states were now given so much power to restrict access to abortions that in some states many women effectively no longer have the right to choose at all. This is the case in Missouri, where *Webster* was initiated and whose law bans abortion, including counseling and referral, from any institution receiving public funding (poor women have had no meaningful right to choose since the Hyde Amendment denied federal Medicaid payments for abortion).

In response to *Webster*, abortion-rights forces reorganized and became more militant. The New York group WHAM! (Women's Health Action and Mobilization) staged a number of direct actions and teamed up with ACT UP to organize STOP THE CHURCH. Our demo scenario called for a legal picket around St. Patrick's, culminating in a mass "die-in," a tactic of playing dead in the streets often used by ACT UP to symbolize what the protest target was doing to us. At the same time, affinity groups secretly planned civil disobedience inside the cathedral while O'Connor said mass. More than 4,500 people showed up at St. Patrick's Sunday morning to STOP CHURCH INTERFERENCE IN OUR LIVES. Carrying signs saying STOP THIS MAN, CURB YOUR DOGMA, and DANGER, NARROW-MINDED CHURCH AHEAD, we loudly protested THE SEVEN DEADLY SINS OF CARDINAL O'CONNOR AND CHURCH POLITICIANS:

- ASSAULT ON LESBIANS AND GAYS. In the Ratzinger Letter on the pastoral "care of homosexuals," the church declares that people should not be surprised when a "morally offensive lifestyle is physically attacked." This position encourages the escalating violence against lesbians and gays.
- BIAS. Church-governed "morality" and public policy have been militantly opposed to the repeal of antilesbian and antigay discriminatory laws and criminal sodomy statutes. The cardinals and bishops cannot impose their rules on our bodies and our lives.
- IGNORANT DENIAL. In Rome, O'Connor addressed the Vatican Conference on AIDS, stating "good morality is good medicine." No form of church morality can comfort a homeless person with AIDS or get needed medical treatment to people who are sick.
- ENDANGERING WOMEN'S LIVES. O'Connor stated, "I wish I could join Operation Rescue," while urging all "good" Catholics to escalate their attacks on abortion rights and women's health facilities. The National Conference of Catholic Bishops chose O'Connor to spearhead the church's antiabortion political movement. O'Connor's response: "We have to be more aggressive. That's what my bones are telling me." To

be "more aggressive," O'Connor proposes an order of nuns dedicated to full-time legal, medical, and political opposition to abortion.

- NO SAFE-SEX EDUCATION. O'Connor openly opposes education about sex, safer sex, contraception, condoms, and AIDS in both parochial and public schools. The archdiocese has also opposed safe sex education in AIDS health-care facilities, even when these facilities have been donated by the city. By advocating abstinence as the only means of prevention, O'Connor denies reality, denies lifesaving information, and endangers all of our lives.
- NO CONDOMS. Opposition to condom use from the National Conference of Catholic Bishops and O'Connor is a major component in the continued spread of AIDS and is **k i l l i n g** people. HIV infection is now believed to be growing fastest among adolescents. Without immediate information about preventive methods, including condom use, people will continue to die.
- NO CLEAN NEEDLES. Sharing needles is the most frequent mode of transmission for new cases of HIV infection in New York City. The National Conference of Catholic Bishops opposes needle exchange programs, which supply clean needles to IV drug users, as a "quick fix solution." New York's drug treatment programs have a six-month waiting list; sterile syringes can protect a drug user from HIV infection.

During high mass inside the church, angry protestors forced O'Connor to abandon his sermon. Affinity groups lay down in the aisles, threw condoms in the air, chained themselves to pews, or shouted invectives at the cardinal. One former altar boy deliberately dropped a consecrated Communion wafer on the floor. (The media had a field day with that one: by the day after the event, it had become legions of sacrilegious "homosexual activists" desecrating the host.) Forty-three activists were arrested and dragged out of the cathedral; another sixty-eight were arrested in the streets.

Media coverage was extensive, distorted, negative. The immensely powerful Cardinal O'Connor was portrayed as a helpless martyr. "All hatred is terribly disturbing," he was quoted as saying, as if it were not *his* hatred that was at issue. To the press, the politicians, and even to conservative gay "leaders," STOP THE CHURCH went too far: because we went inside the cathedral, we denied Catholic parishioners their freedom of religion. Their rights became the focus; our life-and-death issues were secondary.

Because ACT UP meetings are open to anyone who wants to come to the Lesbian and Gay Community Services Center, the police and others always know of our plans in advance. O'Connor was thus informed and perfectly prepared for our assault. He filled the church not with the usual Sunday faithful, but with Catholic militants and undercover police. Mayor Koch was also there to side with his old buddy. When the sermon was shouted down, O'Connor had photocopies of it ready to hand out. The heavily reported "outrage" of the parishioners at the disruption of the mass was therefore completely orchestrated. If that was to be expected, so too was the brutality of the New York City police, the majority of whom are Irish and Italian Catholics. The barricaded area for the legal picket was so tight as to make us feel like caged animals and incite us to violence, which *we* nevertheless resisted. Outside the barricades, though, one demonstrator was dragged into a doorway and kicked repeatedly in the groin by the good Christian cops. The press noticed none of this. They worried about that wafer.

It had been difficult to build consensus in ACT UP about STOP THE CHURCH. We knew the Catholic church would not change its positions, and we predicted that the media would misrepresent the target of the demonstration as Catholics or Catholicism, rather than the church hierarchy's impact on all of us through the power illegally granted them by the state. But follow-up debate declared STOP THE CHURCH a success on several counts. The demo sent out the message that there aren't any barriers we won't cross—with the exception of our pledge to nonviolence—in order to help save lives. It proved that we can build effective coalitions with other activist movements dedicated to the rights of health care and control over our own bodies. And it made us rededicate ourselves to protecting one another in the face of violence used against us.

Perhaps even more important, STOP THE CHURCH taught us the necessity of applying rigorous political analysis to our choice of targets, with the goal of productive change uppermost in our minds. As soon as STOP THE CHURCH was over, we began strategizing for the second decade of the AIDS epidemic. And in the first weeks of the 1990s, off we went—to Albany to disrupt Governor Mario Cuomo's state-of-the-state address with our demand that he recognize AIDS as a STATE OF EMERGENCY, an emergency in housing and social services, in health care, and in drug treatment. And to Atlanta, Georgia, to demand that the Centers for Disease Control broaden the definition of AIDS to include all HIV-related illnesses, especially those not now counted because they are specific to women.

Less than three weeks into the new decade, though, we learned the hard way just how little we can depend on, how much harder we have to fight. On January 19, 1990, Mayor David Dinkins, the man we'd helped elect, appointed Dr. Woodrow A. Myers, Jr., health commissioner of New York City. Formerly health commissioner of Indiana, Myers was one of that "batch of geeks and unknowns" appointed to Reagan's original Presidential Commission on the HIV Epidemic. In Indiana he supported mandatory name reporting, contact tracing, and quarantine. He failed to disburse grants from the Centers for Disease Control to AIDS organizations, and he opposed PWA representation on the state AIDS advisory council. ACT UP worked tirelessly against the appointment, but we lost. The day the delayed appointment was finally made, the *New York Times* editorialized for Myers and against ACT UP. Deploying a standard deceit, the *Times* called us "a gay activist group" and pitted us against the interests of people of color (Myers is black). The *Times*'s divisive tactic is consistently used against us. It pretends that *we* are all gay—and white, that there's no such thing as a gay person of color, and most insidiously, that opposing punitive AIDS policies that will endanger everyone is a selfish "homosexual" obsession. Castigating Dinkins for the little attention he did pay to ACT UP and our allies, the *Times* editorial ended, "To turn down Dr. Myers because of the hypothetical fears of a vocal minority would be an error."

But in spite of the betrayal represented by Myers's appointment, and in spite of the *New York Times*'s unceasing incomprehension of AIDS activists and the interests we promote, we also won a historic victory. For nearly a week, the New York news media focused on what they termed the first serious political crisis of David Dinkins's mayoralty—his dispute with ACT UP over who should direct city AIDS policy. During the press conference to announce the appointment, Dinkins was conciliatory toward ACT UP, insisting that "we have not come to a parting of the ways." Myers asked for a meeting with ACT UP. In less than three years, our movement has achieved enough recognition, enough respect, enough *power*, that the mayor of New York City cannot ignore us. Now we must teach him, and Woody Myers, that they owe us much more.

SEIZE CONTROL OF THE FDA

DOUGLAS CRIMP WITH ADAM ROLSTON

from AIDS Demo Graphics

| 1990 |

Our takeover of the FDA was unquestionably the most significant demonstration of the AIDS activist movement's first two years. Organized nationally by ACT NOW to take place on the anniversary of the March on Washington for Lesbian and Gay Rights and just following the second Washington showing of the Names Project quilt, the protest began with a Columbus Day rally at the Department of Health and Human Services under the banner HEALTH CARE IS A RIGHT and proceeded the following morning to a siege of FDA headquarters in a Washington suburb.

If "drugs into bodies" had been central to ACT UP from the beginning, the protest at the FDA represented both a culmination of our early efforts and a turning point in both recognition by the government of the seriousness and legitimacy of our demands and national awareness of the AIDS activist movement. This turning point occurred for two interrelated reasons: 1) the demonstrated knowledge by AIDS activists of every detail of the complex FDA drug approval process, and 2) a professionally designed campaign that prepared the media to convey our treatment issues to the public.

The entire body of ACT UP was schooled in advance with knowledge of complicated issues that until then had largely remained the province of Treatment and Data Committee members. The latter, who had been studying treatment issues for over a year and had also profited from knowledge garnered by AIDS activists in other U.S. cities, prepared an *FDA Action*

Handbook of more than forty pages and conducted a series of teach-ins for ACT UP's general membership. This information was then distilled by the Media Committee for presentation to the press. The FDA action was "sold" in advance to the media almost like a Hollywood movie, with a carefully prepared and presented press kit, hundreds of phone calls to members of the press, and activists' appearances scheduled on television and radio talk shows around the country. When the demonstration took place, the media were not only there to get the story, they knew what that story was, and they reported it with a degree of accuracy and sympathy that is, to say the least, unusual.

ACT UP's fundamental contention was that, with a new epidemic disease such as AIDS, testing experimental new therapies is itself a form of health care and that access to health care must be everyone's right. Although Reagan conservatives and pharmaceutical companies attempted to co-opt our agenda, our demands were very different from their profit-driven desire for deregulation. AIDS activists want *consumer* interests protected, not the profits of pharmaceutical companies. We want drugs proven safe and effective, but we want them faster, and we want them equally accessible for everyone who needs them. Our demands to the FDA included the following:

- Shorten the drug approval process. The FDA must ensure immediate free access to drugs proven safe and theoretically effective—that is, as soon as Phase I trials are completed—together with clear information that the drug has not yet been proven effective.
- No more double-blind placebo trials. Because giving a placebo to someone with a life-threatening illness is unethical, the FDA must inform designers of clinical trials that it will not accept data based on placebo trials. Instead, new drugs must be measured against other approved drugs or, where there are none, against other experimental therapies, different doses of the same drug, or against what is already known of the natural progression of AIDS.
- Allowance of concurrent prophylaxis. The FDA must accept no new drug trials that prohibit simultaneously taking another drug to prevent opportunistic infections; it must also allow concurrent prophylaxis in any ongoing trials and insist that researchers inform trial participants of their right to use preventive, lifesaving treatments.
- Include people from all affected populations at all stages of HIV infection in clinical trials. The FDA must mandate that drug trials recruit participants from all groups affected by HIV infection, including

women, people of color, children, poor people, IV drug users, hemophiliacs, and gay men. If a trial requires a homogeneous population, parallel trials must be conducted in other affected populations. Moreover, trials must be opened to people at all stages of HIV infection, not simply those with CDC-defined AIDS.

- The FDA must set clear criteria for proving the safety and efficacy of a drug and coordinate drug trials in order to prevent drug companies from wasting time with new or redundant trials.
- Institutional Review Boards designed to protect trial participants must be broadened to include people with HIV infection or their informed advocates.
- The FDA must release all potentially lifesaving information—for example, follow-up data on already-approved drugs now in use—no matter what information drug companies believe they own. The FDA must also keep a computerized registry of all clinical trials and make it available to people with HIV infection and their doctors. Preliminary results of trials must be made available to participants throughout the trial so that they can make their own health-care decisions.
- The FDA must rewrite the criteria for investigational new drugs (INDs) to include anyone who is HIV-infected, and drug companies must be compelled to release drugs through the IND program. Until the FDA has been given the power to do that, it must release any information concerning new drugs so that AIDS activists can pressure drug companies to apply for an IND designation.
- Medicaid and private health insurance must be made to pay for experimental drug therapies.
- The FDA must support rather than harass community groups working to keep community members alive by conducting community-based research and operating buyers' clubs—in other words, trying to do what the federal bureaucracy has thus far failed to do.

These demands, whose articulateness stemmed from in-depth knowledge of the history and workings of the drug approval bureaucracy, formed the background to ACT NOW's civil disobedience at FDA headquarters. Affinity groups from around the country engaged all day in skirmishes with the Rockville police, who had clearly been ordered to keep the number of arrests low to minimize media drama. When we blocked the departure of buses full of arrestees (176 activists did manage to provoke arrest), they dragged us out of the street and left us sitting in the grass. When we tried to enter the building, they forcibly restrained us, but refused to arrest us. We did, though, manage to stop business as usual, to occupy FDA headquarters at least symbolically. ACT UP graphics and banners covered the building's facade, and demonstrators staged one piece of theater after another as the television cameras rolled on.

Most affinity groups improvised their own costumes and props for the occasion. ACT UP's Majority Actions Committee made a reproducible design for T-shirts and posters, WE DIE—THEY DO NOTHING, spelling out in fine print who WE are [people of color, whether we are Afro-American, Native American, Hispanic Latino, or Asian, women, men, IV drug users, partners of IV drug users, lesbians, gays, straights, the homeless, prisoners, and children affected by the AIDS crisis], who THEY are [Ronald Reagan, George Bush, Michael Dukakis, the NIH, the FDA, the U.S. Congress, the Congressional Black and Hispanic Caucus, our national media, our national minority leaders], and declaring, around the border, WE RECOGNIZE EVERY AIDS DEATH AS AN ACT OF RACIST, SEXIST, AND HOMOPHOBIC VIOLENCE. Gran Fury reworked an earlier image—the bloody hand—for placards, stickers, and T-shirts. The bloodied hand print that had initially appeared to protest New York City health commissioner Stephen Joseph's cut in projected AIDS cases now said THE GOVERNMENT HAS BLOOD ON ITS HANDS. ONE AIDS DEATH EVERY HALF HOUR—a statement that has unfortunately remained true, so the graphic is still in use by AIDS activists.

The success of SEIZE CONTROL OF THE FDA can perhaps best be measured by what ensued in the year following the action. Government agencies dealing with AIDS, particularly the FDA and NIH, began to listen to us, to include us in decision-making, even to ask for our input. Six months prior to SEIZE CONTROL OF THE FDA, members of ACT UP's Treatment and Data Committee had forwarded a detailed critique of the AIDS Clinical Trials Group (ACTG—a reorganized version of the former ATEU system) to the National Institutes of Health. The critique called for a system of parallel trials for experimental AIDS therapies that would allow people excluded from clinical trials to receive the drugs after Phase I studies had been completed. Following the FDA action, ACT UP continued to lobby for parallel trials, meeting with NIH and FDA officials, negotiating with pharmaceutical companies, and testifying before congressional committees. One year after SEIZE CONTROL, ACT UP's idea, now called Parallel Track, was accepted by the NIH and FDA and went into effect for ddI (dideoxyinosine), the first antiviral AIDS drug to become available since AZT.

3

COMING TO TERMS

GOING FOR THE GOLD

MICHAEL CALLEN

from Surviving AIDS

| 1990 |

I believe that a cure for AIDS is within sight. Having finished this book, I intend to concentrate exclusively on saving my own life. I hope to explore the feasibility of the Community Research Initiative of New York testing a multimodal treatment regimen.

I have given up any hope that the federal research effort will ever help me save my life. The outrageously poor quality of science belatedly brought to bear on finding treatments sends the message loud and clear that the lives of those of us affected by AIDS are not deemed worthy of America's best efforts. The country that put a man on the moon first has refused to apply a moon-launch mentality to the formidable task of curing the immune deficiency that we call AIDS.

Federal AIDS treatment research has concentrated almost exclusively on stopping HIV. The plain truth is that the all-eggs-in-one-antiretroviral-basket approach of federal researchers has produced little of value for people with AIDS. Five antiretrovirals have been thrown at AIDS with no success. And yet the government's obsessive focus on antiretrovirals continues, at the expense of serious research into preventing opportunistic infections and correcting non-HIV-related immune defects.

If HIV—a retrovirus—is "the cause" of AIDS, then antiretroviral drugs that prevent HIV replication should make people better. The fact that this doesn't seem to be the case suggests, at a minimum, that we need to broaden our approach to therapies. We need to begin to search for ways to correct other pathological mechanisms.

My own physician, Dr. Sonnabend, has devised a treatment regimen that we both hope will be tested at CRI-New York. The multimodal approach will do what virtually every AIDS researcher says needs to be done—test many drugs and interventions *in combination* in an attempt to correct the many immune defects that characterize AIDS.

The multimodal regimen is based on the multifactorial theory of AIDS first proposed by Dr. Sonnabend. As discussed in an earlier chapter, the multifactoral model for the development of AIDS proposes that AIDS results from a cascade of events. If the multimodal treatment approach can correct any one of the immune system defects, it may be able to stop—or reverse—the vicious cycle of immunosuppression, much as removing several dominos from a line can stop the dominos that come after it from being knocked down.

The multifactorial explanation for AIDS in gay men proposes that the main causes of the profound immunodeficiency in AIDS are a combination of CMV infection, EBV reactivation, and the immunological consequences of these infections, together with immune responses to foreign tissues, i.e., foreign cells in blood and semen. Controlling CMV and EBV activity is the most important goal of the multimodal treatment protocol.

The second major goal is removing immune complexes, interferon, and T-cell autoantibodies. These goals may be achievable using a number of currently available nontoxic drugs and techniques. Each drug or therapeutic procedure is intended to correct a specific defect and much thought has been given to the schedule of events.

The immune system of someone with AIDS has a number of well-established defects, including polyclonal B-cell hyperactivation; sustained levels of interferon and tumor necrosis factor; circulating immune complexes; herpes virus reactions (in particular CMV and EBV). The goal of the multimodal model is to correct each of these defects, in the hope that doing so will break the positive-feedback loop of immune suppression.

Even those who believe that HIV is playing a central role in AIDS admit that controlling intercurrent infections (such as CMV and EBV) and correcting other defects might have beneficial effects.

The first step in the multimodal model is the aggressive diagnosis and treatment of all known active infections. It doesn't make sense to try to cure AIDS itself while the body is battling treatable infections. After treatment for all treatable conditions, prophylaxis must be instituted.

The next goal is to control CMV and EBV. Several approaches will be tried, alone or in combination: high-dose acyclovir; CMV-specific gamma globulin injections; transfer factor; and possibly low-dose oral DHPG.

To control Epstein-Barr virus reactivation (which plays a role in the B-cell hyperactivation characteristic of AIDS), very low doses of a potent cancer chemotherapy drug will be given.

Concurrently, immune complexes will be removed through a combination of regular plasmapheresis with and without staph-A columns.

Low-dose naltrexone will also be prescribed to help lower interferon levels.

During the course of the trial, attention will be paid to proper nutrition and to psychosocial support. The trial may also include holistic components designed to enhance self-healing, including massage and visualization.

Unfortunately, the multimodal treatment protocol will be labor-intensive and expensive. Exclusive of the extensive lab work, the cost of the multimodal model could run as high as $20,000 for six months per person, based on the retail value of each of the components. Even if the multimodal approach doesn't cure AIDS, we should be able to learn a great deal from the trial about immune defects and how they interact.

I keep myself alive by imagining the day when the cure for AIDS is announced. I sometimes feel that my goal is to stay alive long enough to witness the AIDS equivalent of the Nuremberg trials, where the scientists who've squandered so much money and so many lives pursuing dead ends in AIDS treatment research will be held accountable. Mostly, though, I sustain hope by concentrating on alternatives to the failed federal AIDS treatment research effort.

I have a very clear vision of myself free of AIDS. My immediate goal is to see the lesion on my right wrist that I hate so much (because it is a constantly visible reminder that I'm sick) gone by January 1, 1991.

Maybe it's HIV dementia, but I really believe it's possible that I'll live to see the end of AIDS. I intend to fight until all the suffering is over. I, for one, believe that the multimodal model and the community-based research movement are the best hopes we have.

FROM SEX, DRUGS, ROCK-N-ROLL, AND AIDS

IRIS DE LA CRUZ

from Women, AIDS, and Activism

| 1990 |

I remember seeing the prostitutes on Third Avenue. I started getting high with them and before long I was out there turning tricks. I thought it was great. I had enough money to take care of both my heroin habit and my child and to maintain an apartment on East 14th Street. I walked to work at night! By this time I was taking courses at the School of Visual Arts and shooting up before school in the bathroom. My daughter was attending day care (which was affiliated with the Puerto Rican Socialist Party—old habits die hard). And I thought I was doing all right.

When I started hustling, most of the women were white. Nobody turned a trick for less than $25, and if you were picked up for loitering, they let you out in the morning. They even had a squad of cops, known as the "pussy posse," to round up the whores. I thought I had it made. I liked the feeling of power having men honk their horns as I walked the streets. And the idea that these men thought I was pretty enough to pay me for sex was a big ego boost. This went on for years with the drug habit increasing subtly.

During this time I started writing and got a job writing columns on drugs and sex for men's magazines. This was the mid-1970s, and drugs and disco were considered very chic. All the good parties had lines of coke on coffee tables, and sex clubs were making millions. The party continued. Same faces, different drugs. My drug usage escalated. I dropped out of college and sent my daughter to San Francisco to live with her father. I still kept writing.

My editor set up a meeting with a woman who was organizing prostitutes out on the West Coast, and she asked me if I was interested in reviving P.O.N.Y. (Prostitutes of New York). My best friend had just been found nude, under the Brooklyn Bridge, with her throat cut. We used to watch each other's backs out on the stroll. Hookers needed to be protected, since it was obvious the police and government thought we were expendable. I became the spokesperson for P.O.N.Y. and did all kinds of interviews. The media has always been enthralled with articulate "street people." I kept the ratings up. This went on for about a year while I spent more and more time in shooting galleries. Finally, the unions started getting interested in prostitutes, and P.O.N.Y. started becoming enmeshed in politics. I walked away.

A couple of years passed, and my drug habit became the only thing I was interested in. I lost my apartment and was basically living in shooting galleries. I was still hustling, but the wait between tricks became longer and longer. I looked and acted like your basic run-of-the-mill junkie. I had amassed twenty-six arrests, two of them for second-degree assault. I had meant it when I said that no one was ever gonna beat me. I became real good with a knife and felt nothing cutting someone. I felt nothing anyway. If I called my daughter and any feelings of love or regret came up, I would sedate myself. My life consisted of getting high (I was now addicted to heroin, methadone, sleeping pills, and tranquilizers) and turning tricks. Emotions were not something I wanted to deal with. I used to pray to die. I'd overdose almost every month and then raise hell with hospital staff for reviving me. I tried getting into drug treatments, but they were overcrowded and had waiting lists.

This was a very exciting time in my life. Too bad I wasn't there to experience it. I had a boyfriend I really did love (I just wasn't wild about myself). So there was someone to watch my back and get high with. But I was getting tired. There is nothing more pitiful than an old junkie whore.

It was about this time that I started noticing that a lot of my friends were getting sick and dying. When I had to be hospitalized for pelvic inflammatory disease, the rage kicked up again. I returned to the streets with a vengeance and became known as La Blanca Loca (the crazy white woman). I fought with everyone until in a spaced-out rage I stabbed a man that tried to rip me off.

I was given one and one-half to three years. I kicked all the drugs in jail, complete with convulsions, vomiting, and diarrhea. I hated being locked up, and it occurred to me that the main reason people are locked away is because they're a threat either to themselves or to society. On drugs, I was both. I copped to a program after spending eight months dealing with the insanity the New York State Department of Corrections is notorious for. It was time to start over.

I stayed in treatment for about nine months and learned some very important things, like how to channel my rage, and loving support, and encounter groups. I learned how to accept and give love. I also learned why so many of my friends were dying. We started losing people in the program. The enemy finally had a name. It was AIDS.

After I left treatment I took a course and got my license as an emergency medical technician. I had been drug free for some time and was making Narcotics Anonymous meetings. So I worked as an EMT with plans to someday go through medical school. After years of destructive behavior, I really felt I had to pay back for the very fact that I was still alive. I guess it's true what they say about the Lord protecting fools and children. So I worked, and tried to ignore the little things that kept cropping up, such as the white stuff in my mouth and the fatigue.

I used to transport AIDS patients a lot, since I was the only one that didn't give the dispatcher a hard time about it. By this time they were finding out that the disease wasn't airborne, and it was only transmitted by bodily fluids. So I would wear gloves but refused to wear a mask or "suit up" to transport AIDS patients. Emergency Room nurses would run all kinds of guilt trips about what I was bringing home to my family. I once had a big fight with a charge nurse after I suctioned a patient in the E.R. with PCP. He was left for over an hour all congested. Medical staff, on the whole, resented AIDS patients. The feeling was that they were all faggots and dope fiends and deserved what they got. By this time, I knew what the signs and symptoms were. I knew I was positive for the AIDS virus.

I was still working, even though I was tired all the time. Finally I had a patient go into cardiac arrest in the back of an ambulance. The man had a urinary obstruction and was semicomatose. I panicked and started CPR without a mask. I found out later he had active tuberculosis. A few weeks later, after working with soaring fevers, I had to be hospitalized.

My temperature was spiking up to 105.5 degrees, and the nurses were telling my mother to stay with me because I would not make it through the night. I was delirious and spoke with my father and grandmother. They're both dead. But I made it; I guess I'm too much of a bitch to die.

I got out of the hospital ninety days later looking like the national AIDS poster child. I spent the next ten months getting my weight and strength back. Locked in my mom's house, I felt like a germ. Back to feeling ugly and unloved. I didn't want to be touched because I felt unclean. In this society women's bodies are unclean and have to be deodorized before they're acceptable. So now, on top of everything, I was diseased. My mother wouldn't hear it. She kept hugging me despite the fact that I shied away, began attending a mothers' group, and forced me to go out. My first time on a train I sat there looking at lovers and families and thinking that these options are closed to me. I would look at the person next to me and think, "Would they still sit next to me if they knew I had AIDS?"

I started attending a group for women with HIV. I felt like I was the only woman in the world with AIDS. It was all gay white men. This group changed that.

All of a sudden I discovered other women with the virus. There were black women, white women, Latinas, rich women, and poor women. There were addicts and transfusion women. They were mothers and sisters and lovers and daughters and grandmothers. Some were militant lesbians and others were Republicans (imagine that! Even Republicans get AIDS). And we were all connected by the virus. Outside differences became trivial; feelings and survival were everyone's main concern. And I learned that there was still a lot of love left in me. The rage mellowed.

I was diagnosed with AIDS two years ago. I kept attending the women's group until the leader left. Then I took over the facilitator's role along with my best friend, Helen, who has ARC. A few months ago I started a group for bi- and heterosexuals dealing with HIV. I do AIDS outreach and education. I teach safer sex and show addicts how to clean their works. I encourage them to seek treatment. The rage that burned is now a hot anger. I've been to too many funerals with this disease. I'm tired of the newly diagnosed being made to feel dirty. I'm tired of my people being neglected and left dying on the streets. My child is now nineteen and we're very close. The legacy I want to leave her is for her to remember her mama was a survivor. She survived drugs and she survived her own worst enemy, which was herself. And she taught others survival. She may or may not have survived AIDS, but she kicked ass while she was here.

LOVE STORY

How a Father and Son Discovered Each Other in the Shadow of AIDS

JUDITH VALENTE

from The Wall Street Journal

| **March 16, 1992** |

Duncan Henderson grew up on a wheat farm, walked two miles to school every day and always believed he could find answers in the Bible. He lived in a world where sex was private and the most dreaded disease was cancer. Life wasn't easy, but he found comfort in the knowledge that he was making a better life for his only son and his grandchildren-to-be.

On a warm night in April 1973, Mr. Henderson's twenty-six-year-old son, Paul, told him he had a confession to make. "I haven't really been honest with you," Paul said. "I'm gay."

Mr. Henderson, who didn't think he'd ever met a gay person and had been taught homosexuality was a sin, was speechless. Finally, he looked up at his son and said, "Paul, you're our son and we love you." He wrapped his arms around his boy.

Years later, on the evening of May 19, 1989, Mr. Henderson and his wife, Virginia, got a call from their son at their St. Louis home. The parents, their ears cupped to the receiver, knew it was bad news as soon as they heard Paul's voice. "Mom, Dad," he said, "I got some test results back today. I have AIDS."

Over the next months and years, as Duncan Henderson helped his son battle AIDS, he learned things about himself that he had never imagined. He became a stronger and more complex person than even his wife had known. And Duncan and Paul, once intimate strangers, found a deeper love.

"As the years go by, I will always be grateful I went up there and took care of him," says Mr. Henderson.

With so much written, said, and filmed about AIDS, the toll on fathers remains largely an untold story. In many cases, dads who had hoped their sons would follow in their footsteps are forced to deal at once with the shock of their son's sexuality and the ugly specter of AIDS.

R. Duncan Henderson, for one, could never have imagined this. Until he was twenty, he lived on a farm in Canada, then moved in with an aunt in Missouri. His aunt had another boarder, a shy young woman who was a student at Southeast Missouri State College. Mr. Henderson was smitten. "She was just so sincere," he says.

Virginia Weisheyer's provincial new suitor wasn't a college boy and used funny expressions, like "crazy as a jaybird." But she liked the fact that he went to church and didn't drink. On May 3, 1942, the two married. He was twenty-six, she twenty-three. After Mr. Henderson served in the Air Force, they settled in small-town Jennings, Missouri.

The marriage was happy although, in many ways, the Hendersons were opposites. Mrs. Henderson tended to be a perfectionist. "I was a lot more easygoing," Mr. Henderson recalls. "If we had a flat tire or something, I wouldn't start hollering or screaming. We'd get there a little late." Mrs. Henderson played the piano and loved books, theater, and classical music —interests her husband didn't share.

On April 18, 1947, their son was born. Mr. Henderson was mopping floors at his $75-a-week job at Sears when his brother-in-law called to say Mrs. Henderson was in labor. He dropped the mop and ran to catch the bus to the hospital. "I was real pleased to have a son," he recalls. He dreamed of Paul becoming a doctor.

The delivery was difficult, and the Hendersons, worried about future pregnancies, agreed to have no more children. Both had grown up in the Depression. "We thought we'd rather have one child and have him want for nothing than have six children we maybe couldn't afford to send to college," Mr. Henderson says.

"Paul became the focus of their lives," says Mary Graue, a friend for thirty-seven years.

Mrs. Henderson taught kindergarten. Mr. Henderson rose at Missouri Portland Cement Co. to become the company troubleshooter. He was elected an elder of Jennings United Presbyterian Church, but in his own home, he often let his better-educated wife take the lead, especially in raising Paul. He deferred to her on decisions about Paul's education, the kinds of books he read and activities he attended. "I thought her degree in education counted for something," Mr. Henderson says.

Paul and his father joined a Cub Scout troop together. Weekends, they'd sit at the edge of a lagoon and wait for the whitefish to bite. They never talked much on these outings. "I just enjoyed being out with him," Mr. Henderson says.

But as Paul grew into his teens, he came increasingly under his mother's wing. Soon the two were singing together Sundays in the Jennings church choir and attending concerts. "I didn't care for that high-C stuff," Mr. Henderson says. Paul and his mother discussed books and classical music. They shared private jokes. Paul didn't go fishing with his father anymore.

Mrs. Henderson says she only wanted the best for Paul. "I guess I expected perfection of my son," she says. "He was my only child. I wanted so much for him."

Paul saw it another way: "I became aware at an early age that I was my mother's favorite. It was as if I was my mother's ally and my father was some kind of outsider."

"I never did feel badly about it," says Mr. Henderson. "I just accepted that I wasn't qualified in many areas that Paul was interested in. Virginia was."

When Paul was twelve, Mr. Henderson told him he wanted to have an important talk. They got into the family car in the garage. There, Mr. Henderson talked to his son about sex. He explained "the basics," he says, then told his son having sex wasn't a good idea at his age. "He seemed interested, but he didn't ask a whole lot of questions," Mr. Henderson says. And the subject didn't come up again.

That same year, Mr. Henderson did something he thought would bring him closer to his son. He enrolled in college. His wife was working on her master's. Paul was headed for college in a few years. "I just thought Dad should have something," Mr. Henderson says.

In high school, Paul became even more involved in music and theater. He consistently made the honor roll and his classmates voted him Most Active senior. "Whenever Paul went into anything, it was whole-hog," his father says.

Mr. Henderson encouraged Paul to date girls from their church. But when one girl wanted to go steady, "Paul wouldn't have anything to do with her," his father says. Mr. Henderson thought this a bit odd, but never mentioned it.

In 1965, Paul enrolled at Westminster College in Fulton, Missouri. It was his father's suggestion, because the all-male school was affiliated with the Presbyterian Church. Paul had a tough freshman year. "He started coming home on weekends, even when we weren't expecting him,"

Mr. Henderson says. He seemed depressed. "I thought he was lonesome. It was a big transition, going away to school."

In fact, Paul was wrestling with his sexuality. Home for Christmas his sophomore year, he confided to his mother that he loved a boy he was tutoring in French "the way you love Dad." Mrs. Henderson offered to pay for counseling for her son. But the issue was left unresolved. Mrs. Henderson never mentioned the conversation to her husband. She dismissed it, she told him later, as "an adolescent phase."

Paul graduated with honors in June 1969 with a degree in psychology and French. Although he didn't follow his parents' hope that he study medicine, he was thinking about a career as a minister, something that made his father equally happy.

Shortly after Paul's graduation, Mr. Henderson finished his degree in business administration. He enjoys telling people, "My son and I graduated college the same year." It had taken Mr. Henderson ten years of night classes.

THE CONFESSION

Paul got a job teaching French at a private school in Jennings, but the Army drafted him in 1970. He went to Korea—not Vietnam—and spent his tour with the Army Choir. But the separation from her son was more than his mother could bear. "I took Paul down to the recruiting center on a Monday. On Tuesday, Virginia went into the hospital," Mr. Henderson says. The doctors called it a severe ulcer attack, brought about by emotional stress. Mr. Henderson nursed his wife back to health. He even cooked—something his wife had rarely seen him do.

In 1972, Paul returned home, teaching at a local college preparatory school, and the next year the family vacationed together in New Orleans. When they got back, Paul came down with hepatitis. One night, as Paul lay on the living room couch with a fever, his father asked him: "Paul, how do you think you got this? I mean, your mother and I didn't get any hepatitis down there. It's a puzzlement to me." That's when Paul, who may have thought he'd contracted hepatitis from a lover, told his parents that he was gay.

Mr. Henderson's mind went blank. "I hadn't ever come into contact with anyone who was gay," he recalls. Now, face to face with his own son, he says, "I got a real empty feeling in my stomach."

The secrets of twenty-six years tumbled out. How Paul had always been attracted to men. How, as a boy, he'd take his mother's department-store catalogs so he could look at the pictures of male models. How he'd fallen in love with a freshman boy his sophomore year. How, on a trip to New York in his senior year, with the Westminster Men's Chorus, he'd had his first sexual encounter with a man.

Tears filled Mrs. Henderson's eyes. "I was looking forward to grandchildren," she said. Paul simply looked down.

Mr. Henderson put his arms around his son and told him he loved him.

"That's the best you can hope for," Paul said later. "That a parent will see you as the child they loved instead of this monster who came out of nowhere."

That night, the Hendersons stayed up late consoling each other. "We kept saying how sorry we were for him. We knew the obstacles he would face," Mr. Henderson says.

"What did we do wrong?" Mrs. Henderson kept asking.

The Hendersons wondered what to tell their friends. They decided to tell them nothing.

Soon afterward, Paul moved to Chicago to pursue a double master's in divinity and social work from McCormick Seminary and the University of Chicago. Mainly, he felt a gay man could live more freely in Chicago.

In the years that followed, the family talked very little of Paul's homosexuality, Mr. Henderson says, though Paul still came home for birthdays and Christmas. The visits were pleasant, and the Hendersons were eager to hear about his studies. One time, however, Paul brought home a friend he was dating. Though Paul's friend slept in a guest bed, "I wasn't real comfortable with the whole thing," Mr. Henderson says. But he said nothing of his misgivings. "We tried to treat him like any other guest."

Then, as the young man was leaving, he turned to Mr. Henderson and kissed the flabbergasted father right on the lips. Mr. Henderson jumped back. He was furious. But he didn't say anything. "I didn't want to embarrass the fellow." Later, in private, he told his son, "I wasn't expecting anything like that." Paul apologized. He never brought home a date again.

In the summer of 1976, Paul sought ordination as a minister. At the time, a debate was raging over whether the Presbyterian Church should ordain homosexuals. Paul's church supervisors asked about his sexual orientation—and he told them the truth. Despite numerous recommendations and a flawless school record, they rejected him for the ministry.

Paul drove to his grandmother's grave outside St. Louis and spent the afternoon there, crying.

Mr. Henderson was crushed, too—and angry. "We'd always gone to church, we'd always been generous with our money. And here they were being heavy-handed," he says. "Paul never was a problem in school, never went out boozing. Still, they wouldn't have anything to do with him."

But he felt helpless to change things. Leaving the church, he thought, "wasn't the answer." He took to reading books and magazine articles on homosexuality. He tried to figure out if it was something that could be changed, or if "people are just born that way."

A REALIZATION

Paul, meanwhile, embarked on a career in social work. He ran a program for placing troubled youths in foster care. *U.S. News & World Report* wrote about him once. In the interview, Paul said, "It's difficult to accept sometimes that all you can do is just help someone live with the pain."

One morning in 1983, as he walked to the post office, Mr. Henderson, then sixty-six and retired, felt as if "an elephant was sitting on my chest." When the pain didn't subside, his wife called an ambulance. Waiting for it to arrive, Mr. Henderson phoned his son in Chicago. "I wanted him to know what was going on, in case I died. I wanted him to know so it wouldn't come down on him as a big surprise." Paul rushed home.

Mr. Henderson recovered from the heart attack, though he has to take medication for the rest of his life. He and Paul spent a relaxing two weeks together, going for drives, talking about Mr. Henderson's childhood. Those days, Paul said, made him come to a realization: "Dad was always very available. I was the one who shut the door on a closer relationship."

When it came time for Paul to leave, the two stood alone in the family room. For the first time Paul could remember, he put his arms around his father and said, "I love you, Dad." Mr. Henderson burst into tears.

The two walked with their arms around each other to the car. "I watched him back out of the driveway. And then I stood in the middle of the street and watched him until he made his left turn to go on back to Chicago and I couldn't see him anymore," Mr. Henderson says. "I watched him as long as I could see him. I hated to see him leave."

A NEW DISEASE: AIDS

The newspapers were starting to write about acquired immune deficiency syndrome, a new disease predominantly affecting gay men. The Hendersons asked their son about it on his holiday visits home. Paul admitted he was at risk. He had been sexually active in the years before much was known about the disease.

"Take precautions," Mrs. Henderson urged her son.

Back in Chicago, Paul worked tirelessly to open Chicago House, one of the first hospices for AIDS patients. But on New Year's Eve 1988, he ended up in an emergency room with pneumonia. He was treated, but never felt fully well again. His concentration faltered. He tired easily.

Paul's doctor diagnosed his illness as *Pneumocystis carinii* pneumonia, a major killer of AIDS patients. Paul called his parents. The Hendersons heard the dreaded words: "I have AIDS."

Mr. Henderson went numb. "We're just so sorry, Paul" was all he could think to say. His head was swimming. He thought: "You grow old. You think your children are going to take care of you. But we will be burying Paul."

"What can we do to help?" he asked finally. "Do you need us there?"

"Please come, Dad," Paul said weakly.

That night, the Hendersons again stayed up late, talking. "Is there anything we could have done differently?" Mrs. Henderson kept asking.

"The fact that he's gay is just the way things turned out," her husband told her. But that night in bed, Mr. Henderson cried so much his tears soaked both his pajama sleeves.

The Hendersons drove to Chicago from St. Louis whenever Paul needed help. But the six-hour drive was taking its toll. Mr. Henderson was seventy-four, his wife seventy-one.

By November 1990, Paul could no longer climb the stairs to the second floor of his home. Driving back to St. Louis one morning, Mr. Henderson made a decision: They should sell their house in Jennings and move in with Paul. "I just thought that's what parents do," he said later. His wife agreed.

The Hendersons gave away family heirlooms, including the organ his wife inherited from her grandmother. "We had been saving all that for Paul and for our grandchildren. There didn't seem to be much point to it anymore," Mr. Henderson says. Before they left, he put a deposit on an apartment in a retirement home outside St. Louis, for the day they would return without Paul.

When they arrived at Paul's house in Chicago, "I looked around and I saw all the shrubs and hedges running wild, needing trimming. That's when I knew he couldn't do anything," Mr. Henderson says. Paul greeted his parents from the top of the stairs, looking pale and drawn. He apologized for not being able to help them with their suitcases.

When they went inside, the Hendersons saw that Paul had decorated the house for them with fresh flowers. The couple eventually settled into Paul's old rooms on the second floor, and moved Paul downstairs so he wouldn't have to climb steps.

Mrs. Henderson took care of the cooking and cleaning and running the household so Mr. Henderson could tend to his son's medical needs. Though Paul suffered bouts of dizziness and diarrhea, he continued to do volunteer work. Each night he picked up dirty clothes from a men's shelter, then brought them back washed, dried, and folded the next morning. His father often helped him. Paul had never seen his father wash clothes before.

One evening, the family watched a made-for-TV movie about Ryan White, the young Indiana boy who contracted AIDS from a blood transfusion. Paul asked why they'd never told their friends the truth about his illness.

"Do you think we're ashamed of you?" Mr. Henderson asked.

"No," Paul said. "But if people ask what's wrong with me, I think you should answer honestly."

The next morning, Mr. Henderson called all of their friends back in St. Louis. After idle chitchat about Chicago's weather, Mr. Henderson told each one, "I've got some bad news for you. Paul was diagnosed with AIDS." There was "no way of pussyfooting around the thing. They all said, 'We're so sorry to hear that.'"

Paul had always wanted to visit Disney World, so a few months after the Hendersons arrived, they went there with Paul. "As long as I live, I'll be glad we took that trip," Mr. Henderson says. But in July, Paul and his parents traveled to Wisconsin to attend a funeral; the man's death made Paul the last survivor of the original eight members of an AIDS support group.

On the ride home from the funeral, Paul became severely ill with diarrhea. His father constantly had to stop the car by the roadside. "You didn't have to be a genius to know he was going down fast," Mr. Henderson says.

By the time they reached the house, Paul had a 104-degree temperature. Mr. Henderson sent his wife to bed to get some rest, then stayed up all night with Paul, continually placing cold cloths on his head. At times, Paul's eyes rolled back in his head. "There were times I thought he was gone."

Paul's bedroom was only about ten by seven feet, but Mr. Henderson managed to squeeze a cot in beside the bed so he could sleep next to his son. He set the alarm to ring every two hours so he could give Paul his medicine with a glass of orange juice and a teaspoon of sugar. "Many times I said to myself, this can't be happening, this isn't real—it's a nightmare," Mr. Henderson says.

The care his father had given him helped Paul regain his strength. It also gave him new insight into his dad. "For years, I had looked upon him as this sort of bumpkin. I resented the fact that he wasn't more forceful. But I give him credit for a tremendous amount of patience and faithfulness," Paul said then.

Each day, Mr. Henderson took on more of the burden of his son's care. And each day, his son saw new qualities in his dad. "A central theme in my life has always been a need to be perfect," Paul said. "I got that from my mother. In hindsight, I wish I had had more of my father's relaxed attitude, his ability to punt when it was necessary."

THE LIVING WILL

Mr. Henderson was changing too. Now, even when he went out to pick out linoleum for his son's back porch, he told the saleswoman that it was for "my son who has AIDS and isn't expected to live long."

As for Mrs. Henderson, Paul used to joke that she was so conservative that she wore long-sleeve blouses even in the summer. But after Paul became ill, she attended a Christmas concert with him given by the Chicago Gay Men's Chorus and "really enjoyed it," she said. He overheard her one day after church telling a gay man she barely knew, who had lost his companion to AIDS, "I know how you feel."

Another bout with pneumonia took a big toll on Paul. At five-foot-ten, he had never weighed more than 140 pounds. Now he lost 20 pounds in a few weeks. He felt tired all the time. He talked more frequently of death. In mid-July, he gave his father power of attorney over his legal and financial affairs. He wrote a "living will," stating he didn't wish to be kept on life support.

One morning, he handed his father a typewritten page with the heading: Notes on Paul Henderson's Memorial Service. The next day, he asked his father to drive him to the Illinois Cremation Society. Mr. Henderson sat in a wooden armchair in a small, sparsely furnished room as his son handed over the $525 cremation fee.

For Mr. Henderson, the scene was like being in a dream. "You sit there and you can't believe what's going on." He left the office with a splitting headache.

On August 20, Mr. Henderson's seventy-fifth birthday, he awoke at 6 A.M., picked up his Bible and happened upon this passage from James: "We too can bring about healing and other blessings for one another if we are fervent in our prayers." It cheered him. He thought he'd go right downstairs to Paul's room. If Paul was feeling up to it, they could all go out that night and celebrate his birthday with barbecued ribs.

But when Mr. Henderson looked in on Paul, the change in his son was astounding. Dressed only in undershorts, Paul lay in bed in a fetal position, barely coherent. "Please don't let them take me away," he begged Mr. Henderson. He clasped his father's hand and wouldn't let go.

When his mother came downstairs, Paul grabbed her hand, too. When she tried to leave, he held it more tightly and wouldn't let go. He responded to their questions by nodding. No, he didn't want the doctor. No, he didn't want an ambulance.

For the next ten hours, the Hendersons sat on the edge of Paul's bed, holding his hands. Late in the day, Mr. Henderson was able to break away from Paul and get six cookies, the only food he and his wife ate all day. Finally, Mr. Henderson felt he had to do something. "I love my son and I want to do what he wants," he said at the time. "But I can't sit here and watch him commit suicide."

He called Daniel Derman, the internist who had been treating Paul. The doctor came over early the next morning and recommended hospitalization, suspecting the AIDS infection had entered Paul's brain.

THE CONFRONTATION

That night, Paul lay in Chicago's Northwestern Memorial Hospital with one arm strapped down. His hair seemed to have turned completely gray overnight. Pink and white bumps dotted his forehead.

He acted like a deranged man. He would laugh and hum the musical scales one minute. The next, a look of sheer terror would come across his face. He opened his mouth as if to scream, but no sound emerged. Without speaking, he moved his lips and hands as if he were having a conversation with someone.

His parents arrived at his hospital room carrying a vase with red roses. "This is Dad. Do you know me?" Mr. Henderson said. "Got a smooch for me?" he asked, bending over his son to kiss him on the forehead.

Paul simply stared back blankly. That morning, he had told his doctors he heard voices telling him he was already dead. The doctors told the Hendersons that Paul probably would live only a few more days. But they kept performing tests—and Mr. Henderson began to grow angry.

"It's not as if they don't know what's wrong with him," he kept saying to his wife. He was especially upset over the frequent blood draws. One time, it took doctors forty-five minutes to draw enough to fill a sandwich-sized plastic bag. Paul writhed in pain during each new draw.

The next day, a doctor came by again with a plastic vial and needle in hand. This time, Mr. Henderson folded his arms, blocked the doorway, and refused to let the doctor in. He stared her straight in the eye and demanded to know: "Is this going to be another forty-five-minute thing?"

But before the doctor could answer, he started in again. "Because if it is, I'm not sure it's worth Paul going through all the agony again." The doctor, Sandra Swantek, explained that it was necessary to monitor the level of antibiotics in Paul's blood.

With his wife and now one other doctor looking on, Mr. Henderson held his ground. "If it's going to keep him alive for two more days, or two more weeks, is it worth it? What is his quality of life going to be? What he has in there now certainly isn't living."

If they stopped taking blood, they'd have to cut back on Paul's medication, Dr. Swantek said. "You understand, Paul had a very high fever. He was hallucinating. That could be a painful death, too."

"What would you do if you were a parent?" Mr. Henderson asked.

"I'd want to make him as comfortable as possible."

"In that case," Mr. Henderson said, "I want to see about putting Paul in the hospice program."

In a hospice, terminal patients receive medication for pain, but are no longer treated for their illness. Mr. Henderson insisted Paul was ready for such care. The next day, the doctors agreed.

The hospice provided a far different atmosphere. Except for the hospital bed, Paul's private room resembled a parlor. While most of the other AIDS patients on the floor had few or no visitors, Paul's room had a steady stream of friends.

Day after day, when Paul drifted off to sleep, his friends sat outside his room and remembered the man he'd been. From Paul's former boss, Mr. Henderson heard about the time their program for runaways ran out of funds to pay its employees. Paul, a board member, argued that the employees must be paid. To drive home the point, he pulled out his own checkbook and made a donation.

Coworkers told Mr. Henderson that Paul often slept in the office, and bought haircuts and new shoes for youngsters out of his own pocket. Paul had spent hours on his own time counseling a foster mother who had been raped.

Mr. Henderson also learned that Paul once took in a youth whose father, a doctor, had hit him so hard it left the boy deaf in one ear. When the young man died of a brain aneurysm on his school's basketball court, Paul donated a $5,000 scholarship in his memory.

To Mr. Henderson, the stories were remarkable. "We knew generally what Paul was doing. He wrote us all the time, but never put in much details. What we didn't know was how much of himself he put into his job."

Mr. Henderson tried to comfort Paul's friends. He embraced the woman his son had counseled after she was raped, and promised to bake her some bread. He asked if anyone wanted to take in Paul's Siamese cat, Sasha. By focusing on the mundane, the Hendersons kept their own emotions in check.

As the days passed, Mrs. Henderson leaned more heavily on her husband. She let him ask doctors all the questions. He told her when she should try to feed Paul. He decided what Paul should eat.

For the next few days, Paul's breathing seemed forced. He slept with his eyes half-open. "He won't last much longer," a nurse told his friends. Paul himself told his father, "I'm ready to go. Are there any papers to sign?" Mr. Henderson says he "prayed to God that He would take him so he wouldn't suffer anymore."

But each day, Paul somehow pulled through. After he'd been in the hospice nearly a week, a nurse took the Hendersons aside and encouraged Mr. Henderson to tell Paul "it's all right to let go." But Mr. Henderson refused. Instead, he went into Paul's room, kissed him on the cheek and told him he loved him. "No, no way" was he going to encourage his son to die, he said later. "That was up to him—and God."

"YOU FEEL SO HELPLESS"

After seven days, the medical staff at the hospice, which is designed for short-term care, urged the Hendersons to take Paul home. There, the Hendersons nursed their son as they had when he was a baby. Again, Mr. Henderson was the chief caregiver. He sponge-bathed his son and diapered him. He and his wife took turns feeding him. Mr. Henderson learned how to insert a catheter and measure the doses of morphine Paul needed for pain.

Paul slept in a hospital bed Mr. Henderson set up in his living room, next to a window ledge that contained the pair of bronzed baby shoes his coworkers had presented him for his work with troubled children. Mr. Henderson slept alongside Paul on a cot. At night, he awoke every two hours to turn his son.

Paul had withered to eighty-five pounds. His legs and arms looked like a baby's. For the Hendersons, frustration set in. "We watch over him night and day, we wait on him hand and foot. And yet, you feel you haven't done enough. You feel so helpless," Mr. Henderson said then.

The Hendersons went once to a support group for friends and relatives of AIDS sufferers. "It wasn't really for us," Mr. Henderson says. "There was a girl there with a live-in boyfriend who had AIDS and some drug users. We were looking for other parents our own age who were supporting a son with AIDS."

BETWEEN LIFE AND DEATH

Paul continued to decline. He told a friend he could float above his body, held by a string—and the string was getting more fragile. "The line between life and death is thinner than you think," he said.

One day in October, Mr. Henderson noticed his son shivering "like he was freezing to death." He called the hospice and insisted they take Paul in.

The Hendersons vowed to be with their son when he died. On Oct. 10, they spent five and a half hours holding his hand as he gasped for air. By midday, Mr. Henderson says, he couldn't stand to watch any more. "I had to get out of the room." He passed his fingers over Paul's knuckles. They were blue.

Crying, he gave his son a kiss. Then he told his wife they were leaving.

Paul, then forty-four years old, died fifteen minutes later. Mr. Henderson got the news from a nurse over the phone back at Paul's house. "Thank you for calling. I'm glad he's no longer in pain," he said, and hung up the phone. Then, he told his wife, "Paul's passed."

Both stood silent for a minute. Then Mr. Henderson put his arms around his wife, and for the first time since they learned of their son's illness, they cried together.

The Hendersons have moved back to the St. Louis suburbs. They have a two-bedroom apartment in a red-brick retirement home surrounded by spruce trees. Mr. Henderson looks back on his ordeal with a mixture of acceptance and regret. "Sure, I would give anything for grandchildren to spoil," he says. "But I have many things to be thankful for. Paul didn't marry and have three or four children. But in his own way, he did a tremendous amount for society. He touched the lives of hundreds of people."

Of their final months together, he says, "We became closer than we had ever been. I was never interested in music or theater, like his mother was. So I couldn't help him with that. But when he was sick, if he needed turning or needed to be helped to the bathroom, those were things I could do. This was one time I was able to help."

This time it apparently counted the most. Before he died, Paul asked that his ashes be buried with his dad.

ADDRESS ON AIDS
at the Democratic National Convention

BOB HATTOY

| 1992 |

Thank you. I love you. Thank you, California. Thank you, gay and lesbian community. Thank you, Congresswoman Pat Schroeder. Thank you, Aretha Franklin, God.

I am here tonight because of one man's courage and conviction, one man's dedication and daring and yes, one man's true kindness. He's my boss, Bill Clinton. (Applause)

You see, I have AIDS. I could be an African-American woman, a Latino man, a ten-year old boy or girl. AIDS has many faces. And AIDS knows no class or gender, race or religion, or sexual orientation. AIDS does not discriminate, but George Bush's White House does. (Applause)

AIDS is a disease of the Reagan-Bush years. The first case was detected in 1981, but it took forty thousand deaths and seven years for Ronald Reagan to say the word "AIDS." It's five years later, seventy thousand more are dead and George Bush doesn't talk about AIDS, much less do anything about it.

Eight years from now there will be two million cases in America. If George Bush wins, we're all at risk in America. It's that simple. It's that serious. It's that terrible. (Applause)

(Chants of "No second term!")

This is hard. I'm a gay man with AIDS and if there's any honor in having this disease it's because it's an honor being part of the gay and lesbian community in America. (Applause)

We have watched our friends and lovers die, but we have not given up hope. Gay men and lesbians created community health clinics, provided educational materials, opened food kitchens, and held the hands of the dying in hospices. The gay and lesbian community is an American family in the best sense of the word. (Applause)

President Bush, we are a million points of light; you are just too morally blind to see us. Mr. President, you don't see AIDS for what it is—it's a crisis in public health that demands medical experts, not moral judges—and it's time to move beyond your politics of denial, division, and death. It's time to move George Bush out of the White House. (Applause)

We need a president who will take action, a president strong enough to take on the insurance companies that drop people with the HIV virus, a president courageous enough to take on the drug companies who drive AIDS patients into poverty and deny them lifesaving medicine. And we need a president who isn't terrified of the word "condom." (Applause)

Every single person with AIDS is someone worthy of caring for. After all, we are your sons and daughters, fathers and mothers. We are doctors and lawyers, folks in the military, ministers and priests and rabbis. We are Democrats and, yes, Mr. President, Republicans. We are part of the American family and, Mr. President, your family has AIDS and we're dying and you're doing nothing about it. (Applause)

Listen. I don't want to die. I don't want to die. But I don't want to live in an America where the president sees me as the enemy. I can face dying because of a disease, but not because of politics.

So I stand here tonight in support of Bill Clinton, a man who sees the value in each and every member of the American family. And although I am a person with AIDS, I am a person with hope, because I know how different my life and all our lives could be if I could call my boss Mr. President.

Martin Luther King once said that our lives begin to end the day we become silent about things that matter. Fifty thousand people took to the streets in New York today because they will no longer be silent about AIDS. (Applause)

Their actions give me hope. All of you came here tonight; millions more are watching in America. Obviously, we have hope and hope gives me the chance of life. I think it's really important to understand that this year, more than any other year, we must vote as if our life depends upon it. Mine does; yours could—and we all have so much to live for. Thank you.

(Standing ovation)

Act Up. Fight Back. Fight AIDS. Thank you.

ADDRESS ON AIDS
at the Republican National Convention

MARY FISHER

| 1992 |

Less than three months ago, at Platform Hearings in Salt Lake City, I asked the Republican party to lift the shroud of silence which has been draped over the issue of HIV and AIDS. I have come tonight to bring our silence to an end.

I bear a message of challenge, not self-congratulation. I want your attention, not your applause. I would never have asked to be HIV-positive. But I believe that in all things there is a purpose, and I stand before you, and before the nation, gladly.

The reality of AIDS is brutally clear. Two hundred thousand Americans are dead or dying; a million more are infected. Worldwide, forty million, sixty million, or a hundred million infections will be counted in the coming few years. But despite science and research, White House meetings and congressional hearings; despite good intentions and bold initiatives, campaign slogans and hopeful promises—it is, despite it all, the epidemic which is winning tonight.

In the context of an election year, I ask you, here, in this great hall, or listening in the quiet of your home, to recognize that the AIDS virus is not a political creature. It does not care whether you are Democrat or Republican. It does not ask whether you are black or white, male or female, straight or gay, young or old.

Tonight, I represent an AIDS community whose members have been reluctantly drafted from every segment of American society. Though I am white, and a mother, I am one with a black infant struggling with tubes in a Philadelphia hospital. Though I am female, and contracted this disease in marriage, and enjoy the warm support of my family, I am one with the lonely gay man sheltering a flickering candle from the cold wind of his family's rejection.

This is not a distant threat; it is a present danger. The rate of infection is increasing fastest among women and children. Largely unknown a decade ago, AIDS is the third leading killer of young adult Americans today. But it won't be third for long, because, unlike other diseases, this one travels. Adolescents don't give each other cancer or heart disease because they believe they are in love. But HIV is different.

And we have helped it along. We have killed each other—with our ignorance, our prejudice, and our silence. We may take refuge in our stereotypes, but we cannot hide there long. Because HIV asks only one thing of those it attacks: Are you human? And this is the right question: Are you human?

Because people with HIV have not entered some alien state of being. They are human. They have not earned cruelty and they do not deserve meanness. They don't benefit from being isolated or treated as outcasts. Each of them is exactly what God made: a person. Not evil, deserving of our judgment; not victims, longing for our pity. People. Ready for support and worthy of compassion.

My call to you, my party, is to take a public stand no less compassionate than that of the president and Mrs. Bush. They have embraced me and my family in memorable ways. In the place of judgment, they have shown affection. In difficult moments, they have raised our spirits. In the darkest hours, I have seen them reaching not only to me, but also to my parents, armed with that stunning grief and special grace that comes only to parents who have themselves leaned too long over the bedside of a dying child.

With the president's leadership, much good has been done. Much of the good has gone unheralded. As the president has insisted, "Much remains to be done." But we do the president's cause no good if we praise the American family but ignore a virus that destroys it. We must be consistent if we are to be believed. We cannot love justice and ignore prejudice, love our children and fear to teach them. Whatever our role, as parent or policy maker, we must act as eloquently as we speak, else we have no integrity.

My call to the nation is a plea for awareness. If you believe you are safe, you are in danger. Because I was not hemophiliac, I was not at risk. Because

I was not gay, I was not at risk. Because I did not inject drugs, I was not at risk. My father has devoted much of his lifetime to guarding against another holocaust. He is part of the generation who heard Pastor Niemoeller come out of the Nazi death camps to say, "They came after the Jews and I was not a Jew, so I did not protest. Then they came after the Trade Unionists, so I did not protest. Then they came after the Roman Catholics, and I was not a Roman Catholic, so I did not protest. Then they came after me, and there was no one left to protest."

The lesson history teaches is this: If you believe you are safe, you are at risk. If you do not see this killer stalking your children, look again. There is no family or community, no race or religion, no place left in America that is safe. Until we genuinely embrace this message, we are a nation at risk.

Tonight, HIV marches resolutely toward AIDS in more than a million American homes, littering its pathway with the bodies of the young. Young men. Young women. Young parents. And young children. One of the families is mine. If it is true that HIV inevitably turns to AIDS, then my children will inevitably turn orphans.

My family has been a rock of support. My eighty-four-year-old father, who has pursued the healing of the nations, will not accept the premise that he cannot heal his daughter. My mother refuses to be broken. She still calls at midnight to tell wonderful jokes that make me laugh. Sisters and friends, and my brother Phillip (whose birthday is today), all have helped carry me over the hardest places. I am blessed, richly and deeply blessed, to have such a family.

But not all of you have been so blessed. You are HIV-positive but dare not say it. You have lost loved ones, but you dared not whisper the word AIDS. You weep silently. You grieve alone.

I have a message for you. It is not you who should feel shame, it is we. We who tolerate ignorance and practice prejudice, we who have taught you to fear. We must lift our shroud of silence, making it safe for you to reach out for compassion. It is our task to seek safety for our children, not in quiet denial but in effective action. Some day our children will be grown. My son Max, now four, will take the measure of his mother. My son Zachary, now two, will sort through his memories. I may not be here to hear their judgments, but I know already what I hope they are.

I want my children to know that their mother was not a victim. She was a messenger. I do not want them to think, as I once did, that courage is the absence of fear. I want them to know that courage is the strength to act wisely when most we are afraid. I want them to have the courage to step forward when called by their nation, or their party, and give leadership, no matter what the personal cost. I ask no more of you than I ask of myself, or of my children.

To the millions of you who are grieving, who are frightened, who have suffered the ravages of AIDS firsthand: Have courage and you will find support. To the millions who are strong, I issue the plea: Set aside prejudice and politics to make room for compassion and sound policy.

To my children, I make this pledge: I will not give in, Zachary, because I draw my courage from you. Your silly giggle gives me hope. Your gentle prayers give me strength. And you, my child, give me the reason to say to America, "You are at risk." And I will not rest, Max, until I have done all I can to make your world safe. I will seek a place where intimacy is not the prelude to suffering.

I will not hurry to leave you, my children. But when I go, I pray that you will not suffer shame on my account. To all within the sound of my voice, I appeal: Learn with me the lessons of history and of grace, so my children will not be afraid to say the word AIDS when I am gone. Then their children, and yours, may not need to whisper it at all.

God bless the children, God bless us all. Good night.

ROY COHN

PAUL MCCARTHY

from A Promise to Remember: The Names Project Book of Letters

| 1992 |

Roy Cohn was a horrible human being. During the 1950s Cohn served as right-hand man for Senator Joseph McCarthy's Communist and anti-gay witch hunts. Cohn's vicious tactics and innuendo ruined hundreds of lives, and drove who knows how many to desperation and suicide. After the country rightfully saw fit to take away McCarthy's ill-used power, Cohn became legendary as probably the shiftiest lawyer in the country.

Always in the public eye, Cohn was questioned on many occasions about the allegations of his homosexuality. The allegation was always completely refuted. Even after he was hospitalized Cohn denied his homosexuality and claimed his illness to be a liver disease. His medication and hospital records indicated AIDS.

Many people would argue that a shallow grave and a handful of lime would be a fitting tribute to the legacy of Roy Cohn. Many would argue that living a closeted life is one thing, but ruining other lives with a zeal that can only be described as sadistic is unforgivable. And they're right.

But Roy Cohn died of AIDS. And whether you liked him or hated him, the fact remains that Roy Cohn died of AIDS. He was ashamed to be gay, and I'm ashamed that he was one of us. He was a bully, yes. A coward, yes. He was also a victim of this horrible disease.

HOW ILLNESS HAS AFFECTED ME AS A WOMAN AND A WIFE

DAMBUDZO

from Positive Women

| 1993 |

ZIMBABWE

Dambudzo is a young black woman who integrates her traditional customs and beliefs with Christianity. What Dambudzo has to say about living with AIDS and how she says it relates to her own culture.

After dealing with the initial shock of her husband's infidelity, her diagnosis as HIV-positive and the death of a child, Dambudzo has turned her life around. She became involved with the Mashambanzou AIDS Crisis Centre in Harare, Zimbabwe. This centre provides counselling, peer support, and housing. It is supported in part through fund-raising activities such as the sewing workshop which Dambudzo has recently started.

I was sent for more examinations and blood tests. The doctors said we suspect that you have got HIV in your blood.

After that they sent somebody to explain everything about the disease. I was shocked. I found it hard to accept. At first life was bitter and sour, or it was just like a dream. I started to think very hard. Where did I get it from? When? From whom? How am I going to live among others? What is going to happen to me? Is it my husband? Let me say, this husband of mine wasn't satisfied with one woman. Yes, it was very easy for me to point at my husband.

He was an unfaithful husband. Sometimes he left me at home and went for other women. I would even go and pay his girlfriend's accounts. He would go to the racetrack, the Mashonaland Turf Club, with so many different girlfriends at a time, leaving me at home.

I worried myself with so many questions and thinking too much, which led me into a depression which was not good because I thought about suicide. Thinking too much wasn't helping me, but making me feel worse.

Once you have got the virus, the best thing to do is to find comfort. Seek ideas from the counsellors and psychologists. Ask everything you would like to know about the disease. Because you have HIV, an STD, or AIDS does not mean the end of life.

Believe me, for I am telling you out of experience. I have got the virus and I am suffering from it as did my last-born child. She passed away September 10, 1989 when she was two years and two months old. See how innocent people suffer because of one's guilt. Let me not talk about the death of my child because it hurts me very much. I know she really suffered. As her mother, I was always with her until the last minute.

In 1986, I got married to a caretaker. This caretaker of mine was working at the church. I trusted him very much and thought I had made a good choice to marry a Christian. But to my surprise this husband of mine was quite different from what I thought. This man wasn't satisfied with one woman. He used to go to the Borrowdale Racetrack for betting. When I was six months pregnant, my problems started. I told my husband that it was time for me to go to the prenatal clinic. He said, "This month I don't have enough money. You will go next month." When another month was finished, he said the same thing as before.

In this time of discovery I also discovered that this husband of mine had worked for the church for twenty years, but had no savings account, no bed, not even wooden chairs. Nothing that showed this man had worked for so many years. Where was his money going? Girlfriends, the racetrack, and girlfriends' credits.

That's how my problem started. When we stayed together during my pregnancy, he was attacked by VD about six times, but he refused to go to the doctor. When I was seven months pregnant the Lord came to help me. God provided the reverend's wife who came to me and asked me if I was attending the prenatal clinic. I replied that we didn't have money. She said, "Tomorrow, I will take you there." Early in the morning, I got up and got ready. We went to the clinic where she parked the car and remained inside. She sent me to join the others who were standing by the door. The nurse in charge came and asked everybody for their pay slips. I went back to the reverend's wife and said I didn't have a pay slip for my husband. We went together to the nurse. Again she asked how much my husband earned a month. I said I didn't know. Everybody stared at me with surprise. They thought maybe I was trying to be rude. The reverend's wife, without saying a word, took out twenty dollars and paid for me.

After everything was done, I was told that my blood was negative for syphilis. What a big surprise, since I was sleeping with my husband who had all those sores. If I had said no, he would have said, "Pack your things and go right now, at midnight. If you tell anybody that I am sick then don't come back. Stay away forever." Where would I go while I was seven months pregnant?

Indeed, I was in real trouble for sure. I tried to tell the nurse. I explained how he was sick. The nurse said, "Tell him to come here." I told him but he said, "No. I will not go. I will rather go to the *n'anga* (traditional healer), than the doctor." I went and told the nurse again. Then she said, "Now we can't help you because your blood was negative. If it was positive for syphilis, we could force your husband to get treated."

My baby was due June 1, 1987, as the doctor and nurse said. To my surprise June 1 passed without my beginning labour. At first there were no problems, but when the second week passed, the problems started. I was now feeling tired each day. Suddenly on June 11 I went into labour. I was a mother of two already, but the pain of this third pregnancy was quite different from the others. I delivered the baby at 2 A.M., after twelve hours of suffering. By the time I delivered, I was breathing by means of oxygen. The baby was 3,320 grams. A healthy baby everybody said, but nobody knew that the HIV had been passed from father to mother to this otherwise healthy baby.

We came to know this when I was seriously sick after the birth of the baby. I stayed at home for only seven days. On the eighth day, I was admitted to Parirenyatwa Hospital. I had abdominal pain, diarrhea, vomiting, chest pain, swelling and tenderness in every part of my body, and I felt very weak. The abdominal pain was coming in intervals, just as though I was going to deliver another baby. Maybe there was another baby about to come out. I even mentioned it to the doctor and said the pain was just the same as labour pain. This is the most terrible disease I have ever had in my lifetime.

After so many examinations and blood tests, I was told on July 7, 1987 that I was carrying the HIV in my blood. I was shocked, because I didn't understand it as I do now. I thought that it was the end of my life. I even gave all that belonged to me with my relatives. And so many people are still saying there is no AIDS. They are fooling themselves for sure.

Here are some helpful hints on how to live with HIV:

1. Become a believer. Go to church every Sunday. This will help you to find comfort in the word of God. To find comfort from somebody who understands the Bible better than you is a good idea.
2. Follow everything that is said by your doctor, psychologist, and counsellors, and follow your checkup dates correctly. Be careful about the people you take advice from, because this disease is a new thing in Zimbabwe. Some people will frighten you. Take it easy and forgive them because they don't understand it.
3. Keep yourself busy all the time, but not by working too hard. Read books that can help you to forget about the heavy burden you are carrying. Listen to music such as church songs. These will comfort you. Sewing clothes and cross-stitch can make you busy also.
4. Ignore all the world systems of pleasure, for example going to films, bands, beer halls, etc. Don't be a street walker. These will lead you to the temptations of wanting to enjoy the world system. The result of enjoying yourself will be the spread of the HIV virus to other innocent people. Ignoring the world systems and all the sexual practices will also make the virus sleep for a while. I have experienced this.

   Let me tell you, my brother or sister, aunt, uncle, and everybody who knows that they have HIV. God will punish you for spreading it purposely. It's just the same as taking an axe to chop off someone's head. If you know that you have the HIV in you, and you spread it on purpose, then you are a murderer. Be merciful to the other innocent people.
5. Identify the people to whom you can tell your problems. They must be the people you trust, who understand about this new disease. Don't tell everybody. If you do so, some people will run away from you because they don't understand how the disease gets from one person to another.
6. There is another secret in this virus. The virus's actions are just like a tortoise moving in the bush. If it hears a noise or footstep, it stops moving and listens. Then, as the noise comes near, it will hide its head and legs inside the shell. That is the same with the virus. If you avoid or stop sexual practice every day, the virus will sleep for a while. It's only by turning away from the world systems that you will survive for a while.

Is AIDS in Zimbabwe? Not in the country only, but in human beings like me. Brothers, sisters, uncles, aunts, grandfathers and grandmothers, beware of AIDS. Now I am telling you. Believe that there is this disease that they call STD, HIV, AIDS. Believe it now and take the steps to avoid getting it or to stop spreading it.

ELOQUENCE AND EPITAPH:
Black Nationalism and the Homophobic Impulse in Responses to the Death of Max Robinson

PHILLIP BRIAN HARPER

from Writing AIDS

| 1993 |

From June 1981 through February 1991, 167,803 people in the United States were diagnosed as having acquired immune deficiency syndrome. Of that number of total reported cases, 38,361—or roughly 23 percent—occurred in males of African descent, although black males account for less than 6 percent of the total U.S. population. It is common enough knowledge that black men constitute a disproportionate number of people with AIDS in the United States—common in the sense that, whenever the AIDS epidemic achieves a new statistical milestone (as it did in the winter of 1991, when the number of AIDS-related deaths in the United States reached one hundred thousand), the major media generally provide a demographic breakdown of the figures. And yet, somehow the enormity of the morbidity and mortality rates for black men (like that for gay men of whatever racial identity) doesn't seem to register in the national consciousness as a cause for great concern. This is, no doubt, largely due to a general sense that the trajectory of the average African-American man's life must "naturally" be rather short, routinely subject to violent termination. And this sense, in turn, helps account for the fact that there has never been a case of AIDS that riveted public attention on the vulnerability of black men the way, for instance, the death of Rock Hudson shattered the myth of the invincible white male cultural hero. This is not to say that no nationally known black male figure has died of AIDS-related causes, but rather that numerous and complex cultural factors conspire to prevent such deaths from effectively galvanizing AIDS activism in African-American communities. This essay represents an attempt to explicate several such factors that were operative in the case of one particular black man's bout with AIDS, and thus to indicate what further cultural intervention needs to take place if we hope to stem the ravages of AIDS among the African-American population.

THE SOUND OF SILENCE

In December 1988, National Public Radio broadcast a report on the death of Max Robinson, who had been the first black news anchor on U.S. network television, staffing the Chicago desk of *ABC's World News Tonight* from 1978 to 1983. Robinson was one of 4,123 African-American men to die in 1988 of AIDS-related causes (of a nationwide total of 17,119 AIDS-related deaths), but rather than focus on the death itself at this point, I want to examine two passages from the broadcast that, taken together, describe an entire problematic that characterizes the existence of AIDS in many black communities in the United States. The first is a statement by a colleague of Robinson's both at ABC News and at WMAQ-TV in Chicago, where Robinson worked after leaving the network. Producer Bruce Rheins remembers being on assignment with Robinson on the streets of Chicago: "We would go out on the street a lot of times, doing a story . . . on the Southside or something . . . and I remember one time, this mother leaned down to her children, pointed, and said, 'That's Max Robinson. You learn how to speak like him.'" Immediately after this statement from Rheins, the NPR correspondent reporting the piece, Cheryl Duvall, informs us that "Robinson had denied the nature of his illness for months, but after he died . . . his friend Roger Wilkins said Robinson wanted his death to emphasize the need for AIDS awareness among black people." These are the concluding words of the report, and as such they reproduce the epitaphic structure of Robinson's deathbed request, raising the question of just how well any of us is addressing the educational needs of black communities with respect to AIDS.

That these two passages should be juxtaposed in the radio report is striking because they testify to the power of two different phenomena that appear to be in direct contradiction. Bruce Rheins's statement underscores the importance of Robinson's speech as an affirmation of black identity for the benefit of the community from which he sprang. Cheryl Duvall's remarks, on the other hand, implicate Robinson's denial that he had AIDS in a general silence regarding the effects of the epidemic among the African-American population. I would like, in this essay, to examine how speech and silence actually interrelate to produce a discursive matrix that governs the cultural significance of AIDS in black communities. Indeed, Max Robinson, news anchor, inhabited a space defined by the overlapping of at least two distinct types of discourse that, though often in conflict, intersect in a way that makes discussion of Robinson's AIDS diagnosis—and of AIDS among blacks generally—a particularly difficult activity.

As it happens, the apparent conflict between vocal affirmation and the peculiar silence effected through denial is already implicated in the nature of speech itself, in the case of Max Robinson. There is a potential doubleness in the significance of Robinson's "speaking" that the mother cited above urges upon her child as an example to be emulated. It is clear, first of all, that the reference is to Robinson's exemplification of the articulate, authoritative presence that is ideally represented in the television news anchor—an exemplification noteworthy because of the fact that Robinson was black. Bruce Rheins's comments illustrate this particularly well: "Max really was a symbol for a lot of people. . . . Here was a very good-looking, well-dressed, and very obviously intelligent black man giving the news in a straightforward fashion, and not on a black radio station or a black TV station or on the black segment of a news report—he was the anchorman." Rheins's statement indicates the power of Robinson's verbal performance before the camera, for it is through this performance that Robinson's "intelligence," which Rheins emphasizes, is made "obvious." Other accounts of Robinson's tenure as a television news anchor recapitulate this reference. An article in the June 1989 issue of *Vanity Fair* remembers Robinson for "his steely, unadorned delivery, precise diction, and magical presence." A *New York Times* obituary notes the "unforced, authoritative manner" that characterized Robinson's on-air persona, and backs its claim with testimony from current ABC news anchor and Robinson's former colleague, Peter Jennings: "In terms of sheer performance, Max was a penetrating communicator. He had a natural gift to look in the camera and talk to people." A 1980 *New York Times* reference asserts that Robinson was "blessed with a commanding voice and a handsome appearance." A posthumous "appreciation" in the *Boston Globe* describes Robinson as "earnest and telegenic," noting that he "did some brilliant reporting . . . and was a consummate newscaster." James Snyder, news director at WTOP-TV in Washington, D.C., where Robinson began his anchoring career, says that Robinson "had this terrific voice, great enunciation and phrasing. He was just a born speaker." Elsewhere, Snyder succinctly summarizes Robinson's appeal, noting his "great presence on the air."

All of these encomia embody allusions to Robinson's verbal facility that must be understood as praise for his ability to speak articulate Received Standard English, which linguist Geneva Smitherman has identified as the dialect upon which "White America has insisted . . . as the price of admission into its economic and social mainstream." The emphasis that commentators place on Robinson's "precise diction" or on his "great enunciation and phrasing" is an index of the general surprise evoked by his facility with the white bourgeois idiom considered standard in "mainstream" U.S. life, and certainly in television news. The black mother cited above surely recognizes the opportunity for social advancement inherent in this facility with standard English, and this is no doubt the benefit she has in mind for her children when she urges them to "speak like" Max Robinson.

At the same time, however, that the mother's words can be interpreted as an injunction to speak "correctly," they might alternately be understood as a call for speech per se—as encouragement to *speak out* like Max Robinson, to stand up for one's interests as a black person as Robinson did throughout his career. In this case, the import of her command is traceable to a black cultural nationalism that has waxed and waned in the United States since the mid-nineteenth century, but which, in the context of the Black Power movement of the 1960s, underwent a revival that has continued to influence black cultural life in the United States. Geneva Smitherman notes the way in which this cultural nationalism has been manifested in black language and discourse, citing the movement "among writers, artists, and black intellectuals of the 1960s who deliberately wrote and rapped in the Black Idiom and sought to preserve its distinctiveness in the literature of the period. Obviously, Max Robinson did not participate in this nationalistic strategy in the context of his work as a network news anchor. Success in television newscasting, insofar as it depends upon one's conformity to models of behavior deemed acceptable by white bourgeois culture, largely precludes the possibility of one's exercising the "Black Idiom" and thereby manifesting a strong black consciousness in the broadcast context. We might say, then, that black people's successful participation in modes of discourse validated in mainstream culture—their facility with Received Standard English, for instance—actually implicates them in a profound *silence* regarding their African-American identity.

It is arguable, however, that Max Robinson, like all blacks who have achieved a degree of recognition in mainstream U.S. culture, actually played both sides of the behavioral dichotomy that I have described—the dichotomy between articulate verbal performance in the accepted standard dialect of the English language and vocal affirmation of conscious black identity. Although Robinson's performance before the cameras provided an impeccable image of bourgeois respectability that could easily be read as the erasure of consciousness of black identity, he was at the same time known for publicly affirming his interest in the various sociopolitical factors that affect blacks' existence in the United States, thus continually emphasizing his African-American identity. For example, in February 1981, Robinson became the center of controversy when he was reported as telling a college audience that the various network news agencies, including ABC, discriminated against their black journalists, and that the news media in general constitute "a crooked mirror" through which "white America views itself." In this instance, not only does Robinson's statement manifest semantically his consciousness of his own black identity, but the very form of the entire incident can be said to embody an identifiably black cultural behavior. After being summoned to the offices of then ABC News president Roone Arledge subsequent to making his allegations of network discrimination, Robinson said that "he had not meant to single out ABC for criticism," thus performing a type of rhetorical back step by which his criticism, though retracted, was effectively lodged and registered both by the public and by the network. While this mode of protecting one's own interests is by no means unique to African-American culture, it does have a particular resonance within an African-American context. Specifically, Robinson's back-stepping strategy can be understood as a form of what is called "loud-talking" or "louding"—a verbal device, common within many black-English-speaking communities, in which a person "says something of someone just loud enough for that person to hear, but indirectly, so he cannot properly respond," or so that, when the object of the remark *does* respond, "the speaker can reply to the effect, 'Oh, I wasn't talking to you.' " Robinson's insistence that his remarks did not refer specifically to ABC News can be interpreted as a form of the disingenuous reply characteristic of loud-talking, thus locating his rhetorical strategy within the cultural context of black communicative patterns and underscoring his African-American identification.

Roone Arledge, in summoning Robinson to his offices after the incident, made unusually explicit the suppression of African-American identity generally effected by the networks in their news productions; such dramatic measures are not usually necessary because potential manifestations of strong black cultural identification are normally subdued by blacks' very participation in the discursive conventions of the network newscast. Thus, the more audible and insistent Max Robinson's televised performance in Received Standard English and in the white bourgeois idiom of the network newscast, the more secure the silence imposed upon the vocal black consciousness that he always threatened to display. Robinson's articulate speech before the cameras always implied a silencing of the African-American idiom.

Concomitant with the silencing in the network news context of black-affirmative discourse is the suppression of another aspect of black identity alluded to in the above-quoted references to Max Robinson's on-camera performance. The emphasis these commentaries place on Robinson's articulateness is coupled with their simultaneous insistence on his physical attractiveness: Bruce Rheins's remarks on Robinson's "obvious intelligence" are accompanied by a reference to his "good looks"; Tony Schwartz's inventory of Robinson's assets notes both his "commanding voice" and his "handsome appearance"; Joseph Kahn's "appreciation" of Robinson cites his "brilliant reporting" as well as his "telegenic" quality; it seems impossible to comment on Robinson's success as a news anchor without noting simultaneously his verbal ability and his physical appeal.

Such commentary is not at all unusual in discussions of television newscasters, whose personal charms have taken on an increasing degree of importance since the early day of the medium. Indeed, Schwartz's 1980 *New York Times* article entitled "Are TV Anchormen Merely Performers?"—intended as a critique of the degree to which television news is conceived as entertainment—actually underscores the importance of a newscaster's physical attractiveness to a broadcast's success; and by the late 1980s that importance had become a truism of contemporary culture, assimilated into the popular consciousness, through the movie *Broadcast News*, for instance. In the case of a black man, such as Max Robinson, however, discussions of a news anchor's "star quality" become potentially problematic and, consequently, extremely complex, because such a quality is founded upon an implicitly acknowledged "sex appeal," the concept of which has always been highly charged with respect to black men in the United States.

In the classic text on the subject, Calvin C. Hernton has argued that the black man has historically been perceived as the bearer of a bestial sexuality, as the savage "walking phallus" that poses a constant threat to an idealized white womanhood and thus to the whole U.S. social order. To the extent that this is true, then for white patriarchal institutions such as the mainstream media to note the physical attractiveness of any black man is for them potentially to unleash the very beast that threatens their power. Max Robinson's achievement of a professional, public position that mandates the deployment of a certain rhetoric—that of the news anchor's attractive and telegenic persona—thus also raises the problem of taming the threatening black male sexuality that that rhetoric conjures up.

This taming, I think, is once again achieved through Robinson's articulate verbal performance, references to which routinely accompany acknowledgments of his physical attractiveness. In commentary on white newscasters, paired references to both their physical appeal and their rhetorical skill serve merely to defuse accusations that television journalism is superficial and "image-oriented." In Robinson's case, however, the acknowledgment of his articulateness also serves to absorb the threat of his sexuality that is raised in references to his physical attractiveness; in the same way that Robinson's conformity to the "rules" of standard-English-language performance suppresses the possibility of his articulating a radical identification with African-American culture, it also, in attesting to his refinement and civility, actually *domesticates* his threatening physicality that itself *must* be alluded to in conventional liberal accounts of his performance as a news anchor. James Snyder's reference to Robinson's "great presence" is a most stunning example of such an account, for it neatly conflates and thus simultaneously acknowledges both Robinson's *physical* person (in the tradition of commentary on network news personalities) and his virtuosity in standard *verbal* performance in such a way that the latter mitigates the threat posed by the former. Max Robinson's standard-English speech, then, serves not only to suppress black cultural-linguistic forms that might disrupt the white bourgeois aspect of network news, but also to keep in check the black male sexuality that threatens the social order that the news media represent. Ironically, in this latter function, white bourgeois discourse seems to share an objective with forms of black discourse, which themselves work to suppress certain threatening elements of black male sexuality, resulting in a strange reaction to Max Robinson's death in African-American communities.

HOMOPHOBIA IN AFRICAN-AMERICAN DISCOURSE

Whether it is interpreted as a reference to his facility at Received Standard English, whereby he achieved a degree of success in the white-run world of broadcast media, or as a reference to his repeated attempts to vocalize, in the tradition of African-American discourse, the grievances of blacks with respect to their sociopolitical status in the United States, to "speak like Max Robinson" is simultaneously to silence discussion of the various possibilities of black male sexuality. We have seen how an emphasis on Robinson's facility at "white-oriented" discourse serves to defuse the "threat" of rampant black male sexuality that constitutes so much of the sexual-political structure of U.S. society. Indeed, some middle-class blacks have colluded in this defusing of black sexuality, attempting to explode whites' stereotypes of blacks as oversexed by stifling discussion of black sexuality generally. At the same time, the other tradition from which Max Robinson's speech derives meaning also functions to suppress discussion about specific aspects of black male sexuality that are threatening to the black male image.

In her book on "the language of black America," Geneva Smitherman cites, rather unself-consciously, examples of black discourse that illustrate this point. For instance, in a discussion of black musicians' adaptation of themes from the African-American oral tradition, Smitherman mentions the popular early 1960s recording of "Stagger Lee," based on a traditional narrative folk poem. The hero for whom the narrative is named is, as Smitherman puts it, "a fearless, mean dude," so that "it became widely fashionable [in black communities] to refer to oneself as 'Stag,' as in . . . , 'Don't mess wif me, cause I ain't no fag, uhm Stag.' " What is notable here is not merely the homophobia manifested in the "rap" laid down by the black "brother" imagined to be speaking this line, but also that the rap itself, the very verbal performance, as Smitherman points out, serves as the evidence that the speaker is indeed *not* a "fag"; verbal facility becomes proof of one's conventional masculinity and thus silences discussion of one's possible homosexuality. This point touches upon a truism in studies of black discourse. Smitherman herself implies the testament to masculine prowess embodied in the black "rap," explaining that, "While some raps convey social and cultural information, others are used for conquering foes and women;" and she further acknowledges the "power" with which the spoken word is imbued in the African-American tradition (as in others), especially insofar as it is employed in masculine "image-making," through braggadocio and other highly self-assertive strategies. Indeed, a whole array of these verbal strategies for establishing a strong masculine image can be identified in the contemporary phenomenon of "rap" music, a form indigenous to black male culture, though increasingly appropriated and transformed by members of other social groups, notably black women.

If verbal facility is considered as an identifying mark of masculinity in certain African-American contexts, however, this is only when it is demonstrated specifically through use of the vernacular. Indeed, a too-evident facility in the standard white idiom can quickly identify one not as a strong black man, but rather as a white-identified Uncle Tom who must also, therefore, be weak, effeminate, and probably a "fag." To the extent that this process of homophobic identification reflects powerful cross-class hostilities, then it is certainly not unique to African-American culture. Its imbrication with questions of racial identity, however, compounds its potency in the African-American context. Simply put, within some African-American communities the "professional" or "intellectual" black male inevitably endangers his status both as black and as "male" whenever he evidences a facility with Received Standard English—a facility upon which his very identity as a professional or an intellectual in the larger society is founded in the first place. Max Robinson was not the first black man to face this dilemma; a decade or so before he emerged on network television, a particularly influential group of black writers attempted to negotiate the problem by incorporating into their work the semantics of "street" discourse, thereby establishing an intellectual practice that was both "black" enough and virile enough to bear the weight of a stridently nationalist agenda. Thus, a strong Stagger Lee–type identification can be found in the poem "Don't Cry, Scream," by Haki Madhubuti (Don L. Lee):

> swung on a faggot who politely
> scratched his ass in my presence.
> he smiled broken teeth stained from
> his over-used tongue, fisted-face.
> teeth dropped in tune with ray
> charles singing 'yesterday.'

Here the scornful language of the poem itself recapitulates the homophobic violence that it commemorates (or invites us to imagine as having occurred), the two together attesting to the speaker's aversion to homosexuality and, thus, to his own unquestionable masculinity. Although it is striking, the violent hostility evident in this piece is not at all unusual among the revolutionist poems of the Black Arts movement. Much of the work by the Black Arts poets is characterized by a violent language that seems wishfully conceived of as potent and performative—as capable, in itself, of wreaking destruction upon the white establishment to which the Black Power movement is opposed. What is important to note, beyond the rhetoric of violence, is the way in which that rhetoric is conceived as part and parcel of a black nationalism to which all sufficiently proud African-Americans must subscribe. Nikki Giovanni, for instance, urges, "Learn to kill niggers / Learn to be Black men," indicating the necessity of cathartic violence to the transformation of blacks from victims into active subjects, and illustrating the degree to which black masculinity functions as the rhetorical stake in much of the Black Arts poetry by both men *and* women. To the extent that such rhetoric is considered an integral element in the cultural-nationalist strategy of Black Power politics, then a violent homophobia, too, is necessarily implicated in this particular nationalistic position, which since the late 1960s has filtered throughout black communities in the United States as a major influence in African-American culture.

Consequently, Max Robinson was put in a very difficult position with respect to talking about his AIDS diagnosis. Robinson's reputation was based on his articulate outspokenness; however, as we have seen, that very well-spokenness derived its power within two different modes of discourse that, though they are sometimes at odds, both work to suppress issues of sexuality that are implied in any discussion of AIDS. The white bourgeois cultural context in which Robinson derived his status as an authoritative figure in the mainstream news media must always keep a vigilant check on black male sexuality, which is perceived to be threatening generally (and it is assisted in this task by a moralistic black middle class that seeks to explode notions of black hyper-sexuality). At the same time, the African-American cultural context to which Robinson appealed for his status as a paragon of black pride and self-determination embodies an ethic that precludes sympathetic discussion of black male homosexuality. However rapidly the demography of AIDS in this country may be shifting as more and more people who are not gay men become infected with HIV, the historical and cultural conditions surrounding the development of the epidemic ensure its ongoing association with male homosexuality, so it is not surprising that the latter should emerge as a topic of discussion in any consideration of Max Robinson's death. The apparent *inevitability* of that emergence (and the degree to which the association between AIDS and male homosexuality would become threatening to Robinson's reputation and discursively problematic, given the contexts in which his public persona was created) is dramatically illustrated in the 9 January 1989 issue of *Jet* magazine, the black-oriented weekly. That number of *Jet* contains an obituary of Max Robinson that is very similar to those issued by the *New York Times* and other nonblack media, noting Robinson's professional achievements and his controversial tenure at ABC News, alluding to the "tormented" nature of his life as a symbol of black success, and citing his secrecy surrounding his AIDS diagnosis and his wish that his death be used as the occasion to educate blacks about AIDS. The *Jet* obituary also notes that "the main victims [*sic*] of the disease [*sic*] have been intravenous drug users and homosexuals," leaving open the question of Robinson's relation to either of these categories.

Printed right next to Robinson's obituary in the same issue of *Jet* is a notice of another AIDS-related death, that of the popular disco singer Sylvester. Sylvester's obituary, however, offers an interesting contrast to that of Robinson, for it identifies Sylvester, in its very first sentence, as "the flamboyant homosexual singer whose high-pitched voice and dramatic on-stage costumes propelled him to the height of stardom on the disco music scene during the late 1970s." The piece goes on to indicate the openness with which Sylvester lived as a gay man, noting that he "first publicly acknowledged he had AIDS at the San Francisco Gay Pride March last June [1988], which he attended in a wheelchair with the People With AIDS group," and quoting his recollection of his first sexual experience, at age seven, with an adult male evangelist: "You see, I was a queen even back then, so it didn't bother me. I rather liked it."

Obviously, a whole array of issues is raised by Sylvester's obituary and its juxtaposition with that of Max Robinson (not the least of which has to do with the complicated phenomenon of sex between adults and children). What is most pertinent for discussion here, however, is the difference between *Jet*'s treatments of Sylvester's and Max Robinson's sexualities, and the factors that account for that difference. It is clear, I think, that Sylvester's public persona emerges from contexts that are different from those that produced Max Robinson's. If it is true that, as *Jet* puts it, "the church was . . . the setting for Sylvester's first homosexual experience," it is also true that "Sylvester learned to sing in churches in South Los Angeles and went on to perform at gospel conventions around the state." That is to say that the church-choir context in which Sylvester was groomed for a singing career has stereotypically served as a locus in which young black men both discover and sublimate their homosexuality, and also as a conduit to a world of professional entertainment generally conceived as "tolerant," if not downright encouraging, of diverse sexualities. In Sylvester's case, this was particularly true, since he was able to help create a disco culture characterized by a fusion of elements from black and gay communities and in which he and others could thrive as openly gay men. Thus, the black-church context, though ostensibly hostile to homosexuality and gay identity, nevertheless has traditionally provided a means by which black men can achieve a sense of themselves as homosexual and even, in cases such as Sylvester's, expand that sense into a gay-affirmative public persona.

The public figure of Max Robinson, as we have seen, is cut from entirely different cloth, formed in the intersection of discursive contexts that do not allow for the expression of black male homosexuality in any recognizable form. The discursive bind constituted by Robinson's status both as a conventionally successful media personality and as exemplar of black male self-assertion and racial consciousness left him with no alternative to the manner in which he dealt with his diagnosis in the public forum—shrouding the nature of his illness in a secrecy that he was able to break only after his death, with the posthumous acknowledgment that he had AIDS. Consequently, obituarists and commentators on Robinson's death are faced with the "problem" of how to address issues relating to Robinson's sexuality—to his possible *homo*sexuality—the result being a large body of wrong-minded commentary that actually hinders the educational efforts Max Robinson supposedly intended to endorse.

It is a mistake to think that, because most accounts of Robinson's death do not mention the possibility of his homosexuality, it is not conceived of as a problem to be reckoned with. On the contrary, since, as I have attempted to show, the discursive contexts in which Max Robinson derived his power as a public figure function to prevent discussion of black male homosexuality, the silence regarding the topic that characterizes most of the notices of Robinson's death actually marks the degree to which the possibility of black male homosexuality is worried over and considered problematic. The instances in which the possibility of Robinson's homosexuality *does* explicitly figure actually serve as proof of the anxiety that founds the more usual silence on the subject. A look at a few commentaries on Robinson's death will illustrate this well; examining these pieces in the chronological order of their appearance in the media will especially help us to see how, over time, the need to quell anxiety about the possibility of Robinson's homosexuality becomes increasingly desperate, thus increasingly undermining the educational efforts that his death was supposed to occasion.

In the two weeks after Robinson died, there appeared in *Newsweek* magazine an obituary that, once again, includes the obligatory references to

Robinson's "commanding" on-air presence, to his attacks on racism in the media, and to the psychic "conflict" he suffered that led him to drink. In addition to rehearsing this standard litany, however, the *Newsweek* obituary also emphasizes that "even [Robinson's] family . . . don't know how he contracted the disease." The reference to the general ignorance as to how Robinson became infected with HIV—the virus widely believed to cause the suppressed immunity that underlies AIDS—leaves open the possibility that Robinson engaged in "homosexual activity" that put him at risk for infection, just as the *Jet* notice leaves unresolved the possibility that he was a homosexual or an IV drug user. Yet, the invocation in the *Newsweek* piece of Robinson's "family," with all its conventional heterosexist associations, simultaneously indicates the anxiety that the possibility of Robinson's homosexuality generally produces, and constitutes an attempt to redeem Robinson from the unsavory implications of his AIDS diagnosis.

The subtlety of the *Newsweek* strategy for dealing with the possibility of Robinson's homosexuality gives way to a more direct approach by Jesse Jackson, in an interview broadcast on the NPR series on AIDS and blacks. Responding to charges by blacks AIDS activists that he missed a golden opportunity to educate blacks about AIDS by neglecting to speak out about modes of HIV transmission soon after Robinson's death, Jackson provided this statement:

> Max shared with my family and me that he had the AIDS virus [*sic*], but that it did not come from homosexuality, it came from promiscuity. . . . And now we know that the number-one transmission [factor] for AIDS is not sexual contact, it's drugs, and so the crises of drugs and needles and AIDS are connected, as well as AIDS and promiscuity are connected. And all we can do is keep urging people not to isolate this crisis by race, or by class, or by sexual preference, but in fact to observe the precautionary measures that have been advised, on the one hand, and keep urging more money for research immediately because it's an international health crisis and it's a killer disease.

A number of things are notable about this statement. First of all, Jackson, like the *Newsweek* writer, is careful to reincorporate the discussion of Robinson's AIDS diagnosis into the nuclear family context, emphasizing that Robinson shared his secret with Jackson *and his family,* and thereby attempting to mitigate the effects of the association of AIDS with male homosexuality. Second, Jackson invokes the problematic and completely unhelpful concept of "promiscuity," wrongly opposing it to homosexuality (and thus implicitly equating it with heterosexuality) in such a way that he actually appears to be endorsing it over that less legitimate option, contrary to what he must intend to convey about the dangers of unprotected sex with multiple partners; and, of course, since he does not actually mention safer-sex practices, he implies that it is "promiscuity," per se, that puts people at risk of contracting HIV, when it is, rather, unprotected sex with however few partners that constitutes risky behavior. Third, by identifying IV drug use over risky sexual behavior as the primary means of HIV transmission, Jackson manifests a blindness to his own insight about the interrelatedness of various factors in the phenomenon of AIDS, for unprotected sexual activity is often part and parcel of the drug culture (especially that of crack) in which transmission of HIV thrives, as sex is commonly exchanged for access to drugs in that context. Finally, Jackson's sense of "all we can do" to prevent AIDS is woefully inadequate: "urging . . . people to observe the precautionary measures that have been advised" obviously presupposes that everyone is already aware of what those precautionary measures are, for Jackson himself does not outline them in his statement; to demand more money for research is crucial, but it does not go the slightest distance toward enabling people to protect themselves from HIV in the present; and to resist conceptualizing AIDS as endemic to one race, class, or sexual orientation is of extreme importance (though it is equally important to recognize the relative degrees of interest that different constituencies have in the epidemic), but in the context of Jackson's statement this strategy for preventing various social groups from being stigmatized through their association with AIDS is utilized merely to protect Max Robinson in particular from speculation that his bout with AIDS was related to homosexual sex. Indeed, Jackson's entire statement centers on the effort to clear Max Robinson from potential charges of homosexuality, and his intense focus on this homophobic endeavor works to the detriment of his attempts to make factual statements about the nature of HIV transmission.

Jackson is implicated, as well, in the third media response to Robinson's death that I want to examine, a response that, like those discussed above, represents an effort to silence discussion of the possibility of Max Robinson's homosexuality. In his June 1989 *Vanity Fair* article, Peter J. Boyer reports on the eulogy Jackson delivered at the Washington, D.C., memorial service for Max Robinson. Boyer cites Jackson's quotation of Robinson's deathbed request: "He said, 'I'm not sure and know not where [*sic*], but even on my dying bed . . . let my predicament be a source of education to our people.' " Boyer then asserts that "two thousand people heard Jesse

Jackson keep the promise he'd made to Robinson . . . : 'It was not homosexuality,' [Jackson] told them, 'but promiscuity,'" implicitly letting people know that Robinson "got AIDS from a woman." Apparently, then, the only deathbed promise that Jackson kept was the one he made to ensure that people would not think that Robinson was gay; no information about how HIV is transmitted or about how such transmission can be prevented has escaped his lips in connection with the death of Max Robinson, though Peter Boyer, evidently, has been fooled into believing that Jackson's speech constituted just such substantive information. This is not surprising, since Boyer's article itself is nothing more than an anxious effort to convince us of Max Robinson's heterosexuality, as if that were the crucial issue. Boyer's piece mentions Robinson's three marriages; it comments extensively on his "well-earned" reputation as an "inveterate womanizer," and emphasizes his attractiveness to women, quoting one male friend as saying, "He could walk into a room and you could just hear the panties drop," and a woman acquaintance as once telling a reporter, "Don't forget to mention he has fine thighs;" it notes that "none of Robinson's friends believe that he was a homosexual;" and it cites Robinson's own desperate attempt "to compose a list of women whom he suspected as possible sources of his disease," as though to provide written corroboration of his insistence to a friend, "But I'm not gay."

From early claims, then, that "even Robinson's family" had no idea how he contracted HIV, there developed an authoritative scenario in which Robinson's extensive heterosexual affairs were common knowledge and which posits his contraction of HIV from a female sex partner as a near certainty. It seems that, subsequent to Robinson's death, a whole propaganda machine was put into operation to establish a suitable account of his contraction of HIV and of his bout with AIDS, the net result of which was to preclude the effective AIDS education that Robinson reputedly wanted his death to occasion, as the point he supposedly intended to make became lost in a homophobic shuffle to "fix" his sexual orientation and to construe his death in inoffensive terms.

In order to ensure that this essay not become absorbed in that project, then, which would deter us from the more crucial task of understanding how to combat the AIDS epidemic, it is important for me to state flat out that I have no idea whether Max Robinson's sex partners were male or female or both. I acknowledge explicitly my ignorance on this matter because to do so, I think, is to reopen sex in all its manifestations as a primary category for consideration as we review modes of HIV transmission in

African-American communities. Such a move is crucial because the same homophobic impulse that informs efforts to establish Max Robinson's heterosexuality is also implicated in a general reluctance to provide detailed information about sexual transmission of HIV in black communities; indeed a deep silence regarding the details of such transmission has characterized almost all of what passes for government-sponsored AIDS-education efforts throughout the United States.

SINS OF OMISSION: INADEQUACY IN AIDS-EDUCATION PROGRAMS

Even the slickest, most visible print and television ads promoting awareness about AIDS consistently thematize a silence that has been a major obstacle to effective AIDS education in communities of color. Notices distributed around the time of Max Robinson's death utilized an array of celebrities—from Rubèn Blades to Patti Labelle—who encouraged people to "get the facts" regarding AIDS, but didn't offer any, merely referring readers elsewhere for substantive information on the syndrome. A bitter testimony to the inefficacy of this ad campaign is offered by a thirty-one-year-old black woman interviewed in the NPR series on AIDS and blacks. "Sandra" contracted HIV through unprotected heterosexual sex; the child conceived in that encounter died at ten months of age from an AIDS-related illness. In her interview, "Sandra" reflects on her lack of knowledge about AIDS at the time she became pregnant:

> I don't remember hearing anything about AIDS until either the year that I was pregnant, which would have been 1986, or the year after I had her; but I really believe it was when I was pregnant with her because I always remember saying, "I'm going to write and get that information," because the only thing that was on TV was to write or call the 1-800 number to get information, and I always wanted to call and get that pamphlet, not knowing that I was going to have firsthand information. I didn't know how it was transmitted. I didn't know that it was caused by a virus. I didn't know that [AIDS] stood for "acquired immune deficiency syndrome." I didn't know any of that.

By 1986, when Sandra believes she first began even to hear about AIDS, the epidemic was at least five years old.

If, even today, response to AIDS in black communities is characterized by a profound silence regarding actual sexual practices, either heterosexual or homosexual, this is largely because of the suppression of talk about sexuality generally and about male homosexuality in particular that is enacted in black communities through the discourses that constitute them. Additionally, however, this continued silence is *enabled* by the ease with which the significance of sexual transmission of HIV can be elided beneath the admittedly massive (but also, to many minds, more "acceptable") problem of IV-drug-related HIV transmission that is endemic in some black communities. George Bellinger, Jr., a "minority outreach" worker at Gay Men's Health Crisis, the New York City AIDS service organization, recounted for the NPR series "the horrible joke that used to go around [in black communities] when AIDS first started: 'There's good news and bad news. The bad news is I have AIDS, the good news is I'm an IV drug user;'" this joke indicates the degree to which IV drug use can serve as a shield against the implications of male homosexuality that are always associated with AIDS and that hover as a threat over any discussion of sexual transmission of HIV. This phenomenon is at work even in the NPR series itself. For all its emphasis on the need for black communities to "recognize homosexuality and bisexuality" within them, and despite its inclusion of articulate black lesbians and gay men in its roster of interviewees, the radio series still elides sexual transmission of HIV beneath a focus on IV drug use. One segment in particular illustrates this point.

In an interview broadcast on "Morning Edition," 4 April 1989, Harold Jaffe, from the federal Centers for Disease Control, makes a crucial point regarding gay male sexual behavior in the face of the AIDS epidemic: "The studies that have come out saying gay men have made substantial changes in their behavior are true, but they're true mainly for white, middle-class, exclusively gay men." As correspondent Richard Harris reports, however, Jaffe "doesn't see that trend among black gays." Harris notes that "Jaffe has been studying syphilis rates, which are a good measure of safe-sex practices." Jaffe himself proclaims his discoveries: "We find very major decreases [in the rate of syphilis] in white gay men, and either no change or even increases in Hispanic and black gay men, suggesting that they have not really gotten the same behavioral message." Harris continues: "White gay men have changed their behavior to such an extent that experts believe the disease has essentially peaked for them, so as those numbers gradually subside, minorities will make up a growing proportion of AIDS cases." Up to this point, Harris's report has focused on important differences between the rates of syphilis and HIV transmission among gay white men and among black and Latino gay men, suggesting the inadequacy of the educational resources made available to gay men of color. As his rhetoric shifts, however, to refer to the risk that *all* members of "minority" groups face, regardless of their sexual identification, the risky behaviors on which he focuses also change. After indicating the need for gay men of color to change their sexual behavior in the same way that white gay men have, and after a pause of a couple beats that would conventionally indicate the introduction of some narrative into the report to illustrate this point, Harris segues into a story about Rosina, a former IV drug user who has AIDS, and to a claim that "about the only way to stop AIDS from spreading in the inner city is to help addicts get off of drugs." Thus, Harris's early focus on AIDS among black and Latino gay men serves, in the end, merely as a bridge to discussion of IV drug use as the primary factor in the spread of AIDS in communities of color. Moreover, the diversity of those communities is effaced through the conventional euphemistic reference to the "inner city," which, because it disregards class differences among blacks and Latinos, falsely homogenizes the concerns of people of color and glosses over the complex nature of HIV transmission among them, which, just as with whites, implicates drug use *and* unprotected sexual activity as high-risk behaviors. The ease with which middle-class blacks can construe IV drug use as a problem of communities that are completely removed from their everyday lives (and as unrelated to high-risk sexual activity in which they may engage) makes an exclusive emphasis on IV-drug-related HIV transmission among blacks actually detrimental to efforts at effective AIDS education.

To the extent that Max Robinson hoped that his death would occasion efforts at *comprehensive* AIDS education in black communities, we must consider programs that utilize the logic manifested in Richard Harris's NPR report as inadequate to meet the challenge that Robinson posed. The inadequacy of such efforts is rooted, as I have suggested, in a reluctance to discuss issues of black sexuality that is based simultaneously on whites' stereotyped notions (often defensively adopted by blacks themselves) about the need to suppress black (male) sexuality generally, and on the strictness with which traditional forms of black discourse preclude the possibility of the discussion of black male homosexuality specifically. Indeed, these very factors necessitated the peculiar response to his own AIDS diagnosis that Max Robinson manifested—initial denial and posthumous acknowledgment. I suggested at the beginning of this essay that Robinson's final acknowledgment of his AIDS diagnosis—in the form of his injunction that we use his death as the occasion to increase blacks' awareness about AIDS—performs a sort of epitaphic function. As the final words of the deceased that constitute an implicit warning to others not to repeat his mistakes, Robinson's request has been promulgated through the media with such a repetitive insistence that it might as well have been literally etched in stone. The repetitive nature of the request ought itself to serve as a warning to us, however, since repetition can recapitulate the very silence that it is meant to overcome. As Debra Fried has said, regarding the epitaph, it is both

> silent and . . . repetitious; [it] refuses to speak, and yet keeps on saying the same thing: refusal to say anything different is tantamount to a refusal to speak. Repetition thus becomes a form of silence. . . . According to the fiction of epitaphs, death imposes on its victims an endless verbal task: to repeat without deviation or difference the answer to a question that, no matter how many times it prompts the epitaph to the same silent utterance, is never satisfactorily answered.

In the case of Max Robinson's death, the pertinent question is: How can transmission of HIV and thus AIDS-related death be prevented? The burden of response at this point is not on the deceased, however, but on us. We must formulate educational programs that offer comprehensive information on the prevention of HIV transmission. In order to do so, we must break the rules of the various discourses through which black life in the United States has traditionally been articulated. A less radical strategy cannot induce the widespread behavioral changes that are necessary in the face of AIDS, and our failure in this task would mean sacrificing black people to an epidemic that is enabled, paradoxically, by the very discourses that shape our lives.

WHATEVER HAPPENED TO AIDS?

JEFFREY SCHMALZ

from The New York Times Magazine

| **November 28, 1993** |

I have come to the realization that I will almost certainly die of AIDS. I have wavered on that point. When the disease was first diagnosed in early 1991, I was sure I would die—and soon. I was facing brain surgery; the surgeons discovered an infection often fatal in four months. I would shortly develop pneumonia, then blood clots. I was hospitalized four times over five months. But by the end of that year, I thought differently. My health rebounded, almost certainly because of AZT. I was doing so well; I really might beat it.

Now it is clear I will not. You can beat the statistics only so long. My T-cell count, which was only two when I got my diagnosis, has never gone above thirty—a dangerously low level. I have lived longer than the median survival time by ten months. The treatments simply are not there. They are not even in the pipeline. A miracle is possible, of course. And for a long time, I thought one would happen. But let's face it, a miracle isn't going to happen. One day soon I will simply become one of the ninety people in America to die that day of AIDS. It's like knowing I will be killed by a speeding car, but not knowing when or where.

I used to be the exception in my HIV support group, the only one of its eight members who was not merely infected with the virus but who had advanced to full-blown AIDS. Now, just a year and a half later, the exception in my group is the one person who does not have AIDS. All the rest of us have deteriorated with the hallmarks of the disease—a seizure, Kaposi's sarcoma, pneumonia. Our weekly meetings simmer with desperation: We are getting sicker. *I* am getting sicker. Time is running out.

Once AIDS was a hot topic in America—promising treatments on the horizon, intense media interest, a political battlefield. Now, twelve years after it was first recognized as a new disease, AIDS has become normalized, part of the landscape. It is at once everywhere and nowhere, the leading cause of death among young men nationwide, but little threat to the core of American political power, the white heterosexual suburbanite. No cure or vaccine is in sight. And what small treatment advances had been won are now crumbling. The world is moving on, uncaring, frustrated and bored, leaving by the roadside those of us who are infected and who can't help but wonder: Whatever happened to AIDS? As a journalist who has written about this disease for five years, and as a patient who has had it for nearly as long, *I* went out looking for answers.

THE DISEASE AND THE DOCTORS

Dr. Anthony S. Fauci speaks with a hint of a Brooklyn accent, which is out of sync with the elegance of his appearance—well tailored, tidy, trim. At fifty-two, he is scientist-cum-celebrity, ridiculed by Larry Kramer in the play *The Destiny of Me*, lionized by George Bush in the 1988 presidential debate as a hero.

Being the government's point man on AIDS has made Tony Fauci (rhymes with OUCH-EE) famous. He professes to be solely the scientist. But in fact, he is very much the star and the politician, one year defending modest Reagan-Bush AIDS budget proposals as adequate, the next defending generous Clinton proposals as necessary. He is the activist's enemy—"Murderer!" Kramer once called him in an essay published in the *Village Voice*. He is the activist's friend, a comrade in arms, showing up last October at the opening of the Kramer play wearing a red AIDS ribbon.

Fauci's starring AIDS role comes from the many hats he wears—among them director of the National Institute of Allergy and Infectious Diseases and director of the National Institutes of Health's Office of AIDS Research.

"Fauci deserves a lot of the blame for where we are on AIDS," said Peter Staley of TAG, the activist Treatment Action Group. But others say that is not fair. "You can't blame any one person," said Gregg Gonsalves, who wrote TAG's report on the status of AIDS research. "We've gotten to the edge of a scientific cliff."

Whatever Fauci's faults, I have never doubted his commitment. Still, he is the face of the AIDS scientific community, and twelve years into the disease there are only temporary treatments that work for a few years at most. AIDS remains a fatal illness. Approximately a million Americans are believed to be infected with the human immunodeficiency virus, the key component of AIDS, and virtually all of them are expected to develop the disease eventually. Close to half a million Americans are expected to have full-blown AIDS by the end of next year; more than 200,000 have already died. Roughly 350,000 will have died by the end of 1994. The World Health Organization puts the number infected worldwide at more than thirteen million adults and an additional one million or more children.

So far, the only treatments are nucleoside analogues, drugs like AZT, DDC, and ddI. A fourth nucleoside analogue, D4T, is expected to be approved by the spring. Fauci has focused national research efforts on these analogues, which slow the virus by fooling it with a decoy of genetic material it needs to reproduce. The analogues were of limited use, but the horrible surprise was just *how* limited. A report issued just before the meeting—the Concorde Study, conducted in England, France, and Ireland—found that, contrary to the recommendations of the United States government, use of AZT before the onset of AIDS symptoms did not necessarily prolong life. (In an extraordinary action, a United States government panel has since pulled back the earlier recommendation. AZT is still recommended for those with full-blown AIDS. But the panel left it for patients and their doctors to decide on earlier use.)

A subsequent Australian study, published in July, found that AZT, used early, did prolong life. I have always felt that it has prolonged mine. Still, what makes the fuss over AZT so stunning is not just that the drug has shortcomings—almost everyone knew that from the start. It is that AZT, flawed as it was, had become the gold standard of treatment, against which other therapies were being measured. The chilling message of the AZT dispute is this: Things are not just failing to get better; they are getting worse. We are losing ground.

"The fallout from Berlin has been devastating," said Martin Delaney, founding director of Project Inform, an AIDS-treatment information and lobbying group. "There were no surprises. But the risk now is that AIDS gets put up on the shelf along with a lot of other long-term unresolved problems. We lose the urgency for money and the scientific momentum." The bad news has left drug companies scrambling. Last spring things were so desperate that a group of fifteen announced they would pool research data.

Many scientists—and activists—are fed up with the drug companies, which seem hell-bent on pursuing more nucleoside analogues when the real future of AIDS treatment probably lies with gene therapy. The idea is to alter the genetic structure of cells to make them inhospitable to HIV. But the problem is, no one knows how to translate the occasional test-tube success into a workable treatment. In addition, most of the gene therapies are being developed by small biotechnology companies that will take years to get into full production.

So was all the time and money spent on the nucleoside analogues wasted? Fauci, who obviously has an investment in the answer, was emphatic that it wasn't. "People say the Berlin meeting was so depressing, nothing's happening," Fauci said in his office overlooking the NIH campus in Bethesda, Maryland. "I say that's not the way science works. There are little steps, building blocks. What's important is whether you're going in the right direction, and I am convinced that we are.

"Was it grossly inappropriate to do the extensive studies of AZT and ddI?" he continued. "No. Should we have done more with other drugs? If we had them, one could say, yes.

"Let's say a year and a half from now, nevirapine isn't working," Fauci said of an experimental drug undergoing trials in combination with the nucleoside analogues. "Somebody's going to say, 'Why did you waste all that time with it?' but you don't know it doesn't work until you test it."

If Fauci is defensive, it may be because he is still smarting from a political bruising. His Office of AIDS Research has been reorganized by the Clinton administration and he has been, in effect, ousted—done in by the AIDS activists through their Democratic friends in Congress. And while some of his time is being diverted to playing politics, in his own laboratory research he has now returned to basics—square one—where many AIDS researchers are working. Fauci is studying the pathogenesis of the disease, its route through the body.

I asked him the obvious: twelve years into the disease—shouldn't we know that already? "More effort looking at pathogenesis might have been appropriate in retrospect," Fauci responded. "But we were constantly being diverted—by the activists, by Congress. It was: 'What can you give me right now? Get those drugs out there as quickly as you can.'"

Not so long ago we believed that if we just could find enough money, we could make the disease manageable, like diabetes. But in a further sign of how little hope exists these days in the scientific community, money isn't seen as the main issue anymore.

"Certainly, there are more scientific opportunities than there are resources to fulfill them," Fauci said, echoing the views of other scientists. "But should we dump billions into AIDS research now? I think we'd reach a point of diminishing returns."

Fauci presents a front of optimism, at least for me. After all, there is no cure for any virus, only vaccines to prevent them—measles is an example. By the year 2000, he predicted, "we'll be into vaccine trials that show a vaccine is much more feasible than we thought, though we may not have the best vaccine then."

Other scientists are unconvinced. They point out that the rapid mutation of the AIDS virus and its many strains make development of a vaccine difficult.

"The public is frustrated; it says, 'You've been working on this for ten years,'" said Dr. Irvin S. Y. Chen, director of the AIDS Institute at the University of California at Los Angeles. Chen bemoaned the lack of money for biomedical research in general, which he said was discouraging the best and brightest from entering the field.

"We're in that in-between state," said Dr. Merle A. Sand, an AIDS expert at the University of California at San Francisco; he was head of the government panel on AZT use. "We know a lot about the virus, but we just don't seem able to translate that knowledge into significant treatment advances. It's incredibly frustrating."

Still, the frustration of the public and the scientists is nothing compared with the frustration of those of us living with AIDS or HIV. Will people still be dying of AIDS in the year 2000? Fauci didn't hesitate for a second before replying, "I don't think there's any question that will be the case."

THE ACTIVISTS AND THE GOVERNMENT

Tim Bailey was one of the Marys, and that's as close to ACT UP royalty as anybody can get.

The Marys are a subgroup of ACT UP, the group involved in the more radical demonstrations, like disruption of services at St. Patrick's Cathedral. When Bailey died in June at thirty-five, stipulating that he wanted a political funeral in Washington, ACT UP was obliged to comply.

So on a drizzly Thursday at 7 A.M., two buses filled with ACT UP members set out from New York. They were to rendezvous with the body in Washington, then carry the open coffin through the streets from the Capitol to the

White House. They would show Bill Clinton the urgency of AIDS, they would bring one of its carcasses to his doorstep.

But it was not to be. The police would not let them march, and the day turned into a sodden fiasco, as the police and activists quarreled over the body, shoving the coffin in and out of a van parked in front of the Capitol. The rage was there, but the organization was not. And when the police said no, whom did ACT UP members run to for help but the White House, the very target of their protest, getting Bob Hattoy, a White House staff member with AIDS, to intervene. In the end, ACT UP members gave up and went home, taking the body with them.

It was a perfect metaphor for the site of AIDS activism—raging in desperate but unfocused anger, one foot on the inside, one on the outside.

The AIDS movement was built on grassroots efforts. Now those efforts are in disarray. Many ACT UP leaders have died, the group's very existence was based on the belief that AIDS could be cured quickly if only enough money and effort were thrown at it—something that now seems increasingly in doubt. Besides, it is hard to maintain attacks against a government that is seeking big increases in AIDS spending. Much of the cream of ACT UP has fled, forming groups like TAG and joining mainstream AIDS organizations like the Gay Men's Health Crisis and the American Foundation for AIDS Research.

Those left behind are ACT UP's hard core. ACT UP was always part theater, part group therapy. Now, sadly, ACT UP is increasingly reduced to burying its dead.

To say all that is not to belittle the accomplishments of the group. One reason for ACT UP's decline is that it has got so much of what it wanted. ACT UP forced AIDS into the presidential race, dogging candidates. Because of ACT UP the price of AZT is lower. Drugs are approved more quickly. Today it is a given that the communities affected by a disease have a voice, and must be consulted. To a great extent, ACT UP deserves much of the credit for the increasing political power of the entire gay rights movement. But now even the gay movement has pushed AIDS to the sidelines.

Anyone questioning how AIDS ranks as an issue among gay groups need only look to the march on Washington on April 25. Six years earlier, in 1987, a similar gay march had on overriding theme: AIDS. If there was a dominant theme last April, it was homosexuals in the military. To be sure, AIDS was an element of the march but *just* an element. Speaker after speaker ignored it.

"It's like they are waiting for us to die so they can get on with their agenda," said Dr. Nicholas A. Rango, the director of New York state's AIDS

Institute, a gay man who himself has AIDS and watched the march on C-Span from his Manhattan hospital bed. [He died on November 10.]

Torie Osborn, formerly executive director of the National Gay and Lesbian Task Force, argued that the shift was inevitable with the election of a Democratic president, renewed attacks from the right wing, and just plain burnout. Increasingly, many homosexuals, especially those who test negative for HIV, do not want a disease to be what defines their community. "There is a deep yearning to broaden the agenda beyond AIDS," she said. "There's a natural need for human beings who are in deep grieving to reach for a future beyond their grieving.

"It's one thing to be fighting for treatment, believing you're going to get a cure that will have everyone survive," continued Osborn, who recently buried three friends who had died of AIDS. "But it's an incredibly depressing truth that AIDS has become part of the backdrop of gay life."

What is to some a broadening of the gay agenda, however, is to others desertion. "It's one thing for the politicians to abandon AIDS," Kevin Frost, a TAG member, said, "but for our own community to abandon the issue. . . . Who brought this issue of gays in the military out in the open? A couple of flashy queers with checkbooks. Well, what about AIDS?"

What *about* AIDS? Perhaps the greatest development affecting ACT UP, the activist community, and the entire AIDS-care world is the changing face of the disease. Homosexual sex still accounts for the majority of cases, 57 percent. But that number is dropping, down from 61 percent in 1989. Meanwhile, the percentage of cases tied to intravenous drug use is beginning to climb. It is now at 23 percent, up from 21 percent in 1989.

Black and Hispanic groups are clamoring for a greater role in running AIDS-care organizations. Their intentions seem genuine—what do gay groups know of inner-city drug use?—but also seem driven in part by a desire for money and power. In an age of government cutbacks, AIDS is where the money is—"today's equivalent of the Great Society programs of the 1960s," as Rango put it.

In Washington and Houston, gay groups and black and Hispanic groups are bickering over who should control the money and programs. In New York, the largest AIDS-care organization, the Gay Men's Health Crisis, is trying valiantly to be all things to all constituencies—it contributed $25,000 to the lobbying effort to allow homosexuals in the military even as it was helping to expand legal services in Harlem. Inevitably, focus is lost.

GMHC has recently changed executive directors, as have many of the more than 3,500 AIDS organizations in the United States. The average executive director of an AIDS service group lasts less than two years, burned out by depression and exhausted by the bickering among AIDS constituencies.

"We should be fighting the virus, not each other," said Dan Bross, the executive director of the AIDS Action Council. "We're eating our young."

Mary Fisher, who addressed the Republican National Convention in Houston as a woman infected with HIV, whom I interviewed at the time and who has since become a friend, also believes the AIDS movement is adrift. She was sitting at lunch in Manhattan with Larry Kramer, both of them bemoaning the state of AIDS activism.

"We need to agree on the goals," Fisher said.

"That's just rhetoric," Kramer shot back, "the goal is to find a cure."

Fisher sees AIDS entering a dangerous never-never land, with the day fast approaching when *no one* will be carrying the AIDS banner.

"The gay community is going to stop screaming," she said, "it is already stopping."

"I'm very despondent," Kramer said. "You don't know where to yell or who to yell at. Clinton says all the right things, then doesn't do anything."

Indeed, the Clinton administration does say all the right things, at times coming close to being patronizing about it.

"I have a real understanding that the people who feel the strongest about this, they don't have time," Carol H. Rasco, the president's top domestic policy adviser said in defense of the zealotry of ACT UP. "When a bomb is ticking inside you, you have to keep pushing."

Where once Washington doors were closed to AIDS activists, they are now open; indeed, perhaps the single biggest AIDS change in Washington under the Clinton administration has been one of tone. AIDS sufferers are no longer treated as immoral lepers. David Barr, director of treatment education and advocacy for the Gay Men's Health Crisis, recalled a May meeting with Donna E. Shalala, the secretary of Health and Human Services.

"She agreed to everything we wanted," Barr said. "I was amazed. We're so used to doing battle. But is it a ploy?"

Certainly Bill Clinton is a vast improvement over George Bush. The president proposed a major increase in spending on AIDS research, about 20 percent, coming up with an additional $227 million. That would raise the total NIH spending on AIDS research to $1.3 billion. In aid for outpatient care, the White House proposed a giant increase in what is known as Ryan White money, named for the Midwestern teenager who died of AIDS in April 1990. The current appropriation is $348 million, which the administration proposed to nearly double by adding $310 million. The House didn't add the entire amount, just a $200 million increase, but it still brought the total to $548 million. The Senate was slightly more generous, and the final appropriation was $579 million.

But is more money enough? AIDS activists say they want leadership, but they are not sure anymore what that means.

"It was much easier," said Torie Osborn, "when we could hate George Bush and Ronald Reagan, when we thought we had evil genocidal Republican presidents who weren't doing what needed to be done to get a cure."

Still, as is so often the case with Bill Clinton, he is a victim of his own lofty campaign rhetoric. He spoke eloquently about AIDS in his pitches for the gay vote. He insisted that people infected with the AIDS virus, Bob Hattoy and Elizabeth Glaser, speak at the Democratic National Convention. On election night, he mentioned AIDS high in his victory speech. It all seemed so promising. David B. Mixner, a Clinton friend who helped rally the gay vote, exclaimed in the flush of a Clinton victory, "I believe thousands of my friends who wouldn't make it, who would die of AIDS, might make it now because Bill Clinton is president."

There it is: the man from Arkansas was to be not just president but savior. He's not. Bogged down early on in a battle over homosexuals in the military, Clinton has grown wary of anything that the public might perceive as a gay issue. He delayed fulfilling his campaign pledge to name an AIDS czar, finally naming her five months into his term—and only when the National Commission on AIDS was about to attack him for not providing leadership on the epidemic.

More than anything else, what the AIDS community wants from Bill Clinton is a sense of urgency. Carol Rasco maintains that Clinton is committed. "Health-care reform and AIDS are the only thing I've worked on every day since I got here," said the domestic policy adviser. But others, even in the administration, think Clinton is doing little to help.

"Other than myself, who lives with AIDS every day, there's no one at the White House for whom this is their first-tier issue," said Bob Hattoy, who, after serving six months as a White House aide often critical of the administration's AIDS policies, was shifted to the Interior Department. He praised the president and Mrs. Clinton for having "a profoundly sensitive awareness about AIDS," but at the staff level, he said "AIDS is not on the radar screens at the White House every day." And the political advisers? Hattoy scoffed. "I don't think they'll address AIDS until the Perot voters start getting it."

THE CZAR AND THE PRESS

There was a time when it was thought that the solution to the AIDS crisis could be found in two words: AIDS czar. One omnipotent public figure with the power to marshal funds, direct research, cut through the bureaucracy—in short, to lead a Manhattan Project–size effort to force a cure for AIDS. Kristine M. Gebbie doesn't look like a czar, and she doesn't think of herself as one, either . . .

Now, she is the AIDS czar—a far cry from the stellar names that AIDS activists had fantasized about: H. Norman Schwarzkopf, Jimmy Carter, C. Everett Koop.

"We wanted 'Jurassic Park,' and we got 'Snow White,'" Larry Kramer likes to say.

"The activists wanted a war on AIDS," Gebbie said, shaking her head. "I am not one of the big names. I am someone who has struggled with systems around this epidemic since the beginning. I think I have a feel for what it takes to bring people together . . ."

And what happened to the eagerly awaited Manhattan Project? "Manhattan Project?" Gebbie said. "I don't know what that means. Both the Manhattan Project and the man-on-the-moon project involved, I think, a much more targeted goal. We know where we'd like to go—fix AIDS—but I'm not sure we can conceptualize what it would take to do that. On the other hand, if what 'Manhattan Project' conveys is: 'The government is behind you,' well, if I do my job right, we will target and have energy and direction. What we won't have is somebody in general's stripes who can walk around and order people, 'Drop what you're doing and work on HIV.'"

"There's this contradiction," said Dr. Mark D. Smith, a San Francisco AIDS expert who discussed the job with the administration but eventually withdrew, "between the public perception of great responsibility and the reality of no real organizational authority . . ."

To be fair, on that sunny Friday in the Rose Garden when he announced the appointment of Gebbie, the president sounded like the old Bill Clinton, the one in the campaign. He finally did what the activists wanted—he spoke out on AIDS as president. He labeled the virus "one of the most dreaded and mysterious diseases humanity has ever known" and "an epidemic that has already claimed too many of our brothers and sisters, our parents and children, our friends and colleagues."

But the trouble was, no one was listening. Newspapers and the networks reported the naming of Gebbie, but few carried the president's comments on AIDS. *Newsweek* magazine, in a week-in-the-life-of-the-president piece, didn't even mention the Gebbie announcement. At the news conference, there was only one question on AIDS, and that was directed to Gebbie about her qualifications. Reporters were eager to move on to the real news, like the budget and homosexuals in the military.

AIDS, it seems, had become old news.

"In the early days of AIDS, when knowledge was expanding, there were lots of very compelling things to write about," said Marlene Cimons, who covers AIDS and federal health policy out of the Washington bureau of the *Los Angeles Times*. "We were in the infant stages of making policy decisions about AIDS that had unique social and political ramifications. Now it's become harder to find angles. We've written to death most aspects of the disease. AIDS in the classroom. AIDS in the workplace. Testing. They filled the front pages. Now there's a vacuum."

Stuart Shear, a reporter for "The MacNeil/Lehrer Newshour" who covers AIDS, said the conflicts that had made for good stories—the fights between Republican administrations and AIDS advocates—were gone.

"It's become a pure science story," he said. "When it gets down to the clinical nitty-gritty, that's not what we look at. It's hard to get people to come on and complain about an administration that's increasing funding."

THE PATIENT AND THE JOURNALIST

In my interviews for this article and others, I always ask people with AIDS if they expect to die of the disease. One reason for that is a genuine reporter's curiosity; the answer is part of the profile of who they are. But I am also searching for hope for myself. Increasingly, the answers coming back are the same, even from the most optimistic of ACT UP zealots: Yes, we will die of AIDS.

I thought about that the other day in the emergency room at Lenox Hill Hospital. I had taken my boyfriend there for a blood transfusion to offset the anemia caused by the chemotherapy for his Kaposi's sarcoma. I realized on that Sunday morning in the emergency room that the moment of crisis wasn't coming tomorrow or the next day for my boyfriend. It was here today. And it will soon be here today for me, too.

Does that make me angry? Yes. I had such hope when I interviewed Bill Clinton about AIDS and gay issues for this magazine in August 1992. He spoke so eloquently on AIDS. I really did see him as a white knight who might save me. How naive I was to think that one man could make that big a difference. At its core, the problem isn't a government; it's a virus.

Still, in interviews with researchers and administration officials, it was clear that we are talking from different planets. I need help now, not five years from now. Yet the urgency just wasn't there. Compassion and concern, yes; even sympathy, but urgency, no. I felt alone, abandoned, cheated.

I asked Gebbie what she says to someone with AIDS—in other words, what she says to me. And for one brief moment, there was a glimmer of realization that delay means death.

"I say, 'I hear you and I appreciate the frustration and the sorrow and the loneliness,'" she said. "That can sound trite, but it is genuine. It's inappropriate for me to hold out a false promise to you. It would be easy to say: 'There, there. It will be better soon.' That's a disservice, so I have to be honest with you. We don't have quick answers. I can't tell you when we're going to have a cure."

I am on the cutting edge of drug testing, in a trial at New York Hospital for a new combination therapy: AZT, ddI, and nevirapine. That is the combination that drew so much publicity last February when researchers in Boston declared that they had found the combination was effective in inhibiting the virus. But at the Berlin conference, the formulator of the concept, Yung-Kang Chow, a Harvard medical student, reported a flaw in part of the original study. Other researchers challenged the findings after they were unable to confirm the results.

I was surprised at how jealous many of my fellow members of the support group were when I got into the trial—one of only twenty-five people accepted out of more than four hundred applicants. The group members felt that I had used influence. I had not. Yet admission to these trials is not purely luck either—a point driven home when a number of leading researchers called, offering to get me into one of the nevirapine trials. I did not take them up on it. If my doctors used influence to get me in, it was not with my knowledge. But I am grateful if they did. The ship is beginning to sink; the water is lapping onto the deck. I am eager for any lifeboat, however leaky.

The letters pour in from readers who know I have AIDS, which I wrote about in this newspaper last December. A Florida woman wrote detailing her son's agonizing death from AIDS. Halfway through the letter, she caught herself, suddenly blurting out, "I don't know why I am writing this to you." Like so many of the letters, it was really not so much for me as for the writer, an excuse to open up her heart and let out the pain. She ended with a line

I think of often, a line as much for her dead son, also named Jeffrey, as for me. "I intend this letter," she wrote, "as a mother's hug."

Hardly a day goes by without my getting a letter or call from someone who has the cure for AIDS. Many are crackpots. But others, I'm not so sure. Perhaps I will soon be desperate enough to pursue them.

More and more of the letters are nasty, even cruel. They are still the minority, but they make clear how deep the resentment runs against the attention given AIDS.

"As an average American," a man from Brooklyn wrote in a letter to the editor that made its way to me, "I cannot feel compassion for those who contracted AIDS through the pleasures of homosexuality, promiscuity or drug injection. The advent of AIDS sickness in the world breaks my heart—but only for those who contracted it from blood transfusion, medical skin pricks or birth. The insipid news stories and other media accounts of AIDS pain, pneumonias and cancers attempt to reach me, but they only turn me off. And I, in turn, turn them off, as I suppose that millions of your readers do. Let's permit these pleasure seekers of the flesh to live out their years in hospices or homes at minimal cost and then die."

Am I bitter? Increasingly, yes. At the ACT UP funeral for Bailey in Washington, I thought of how much the anger of the activists mirrored my own. I, too, wanted to shout—at no one really, just to vent the rage. I am dying. Why doesn't someone help us?

I didn't shout. I couldn't. All I could think about on that rainy Thursday afternoon was that a political funeral is not for me. It is at once very noble and very tacky.

What, then, is for me? I usually say that my epitaph is not a phrase but the body of my work. I am writing it with each article, including this one. But actually, there is a phrase that I want shouted at my funeral and written on the memorial cards, a phrase that captures the mix of cynicism and despair that I feel right now and that I will almost certainly take to my grave: *Whatever happened to AIDS?*

LETTERS TO THE DEAD

MARLON RIGGS

| 1993 |

AIDS

Dear Gene:

For what seemed the thousandth time I watched *Tongues United* a few days ago, this time of all places in Clemson, South Carolina. In a room filled with whites, in a small college town much like that room, I watched the screen and your image flicker by. How strange it was, in so alien an environment, to see you there, larger than life, singing, living, still. I listened closely to the music of your voice—how much you remind me of voices centuries past—your raw-edged tenor blending rhythms and inflections descended from slaves into a hymn, a doo-wop declaration of freedom.

I listened and remembered: on the night of the San Francisco premiere less than two years ago, you rested in a public hospital bed, laid low by *Pneumocystis*. Remember? I dedicated the premiere to you and your quick recovery. And when I saw you days later, your pride and glee were immediately self-evident. So clearly you spoke, so confident you seemed. Alone, you rose from the bed, and went to the bathroom. I watched and I thought, I too have been here, though for different reasons, and I know what effort—what will—so simple a task of rising to urinate requires.

I left you that day, both of us radiantly optimistic about your imminent return home. Two weeks later I was shocked by the news that you had been returned to intensive care. Relapse. At your bedside, I watched you struggle for each single, irregular breath—each breath a battle between your will and the respirator. A friend lightly clasped your bloated hand. Your eyes flickered, your lips barely moved, I watched your face. Friends bent close to hear you, to decipher your mumbled whisper. But no one understood, and so, as tactile communication, they continued to hold your hand. I watched your face. "You're hurting him," I said. "Holding his hand hurts." The friend released his grasp, and your face, ashy, drawn, immediately relaxed. Within your face I saw my own. Odd. I was not afraid. I studied you as I might study a mirror, witnessed the reflection of my own probable future, my not too dissimilar past. How close I, too, had come to being killed, not by the pneumonia, but by the virus's most lethal accomplice: silence.

"Do you think I'm going to make it?" you asked us, eyes closed, barely a whisper. We looked at one another. No one spoke. Then the man who had once been your lover and had struggled to remain your friend answered: "They're trying a new drug. But you have to rest. You have to stop fighting the respirator. Let it breathe for you. Rest so the drug can start to work."

The drug didn't work. Nor the respirator. You died the next day. And in my mind's eye I continually watch your face, study the slow drain of life from your dark-brown skin, your eyes, your chapped lips. I often see you as some superimposed photograph, you as you lay dying in the hospital that day, and you upon the screen, standing upright, tuxedoed, finger-snapping, smoothly defiant in your harmonizing doo-wop that we come out tonight.

Tell me, Gene, how is it that you could come through so much—through alcoholism, financial dependency, racial self-hatred, internalized homophobia, neglected hypertension. Tell me how you managed to master each of these demons, yet would not—could not—contend with that most insidious foe: the silence that shields us from the reality that we are at risk, that our bodies might be sites of impending catastrophe. Did you believe, as so many of us still do, that black people "don't get it"?

Dear Chris:

Didn't you say that the black community would pay dearly for denial? I heard you, but did I listen? We were sitting, the two of us, alone in your home, talking more honestly than we ever have. Sex, love, death, disease, denial: our final conversation, remember? "Black gay men," you said, "have fooled themselves into believing they are immune. The black community will pay a price." Coming from a white boy, I thought your words a little harsh. But you explained that AIDS can have a liberating effect on the tongue, lets you lash it like a whip, and get away with it. And I thought to myself: hmmmm, let's store that thought—just in case.

But that "just in case," I now know, was—as far as I was concerned—remote, theoretical. I heard you, Chris, but your message, I felt confident, was not meant for me. And the degree to which I embraced it was out of ideological and political, not personal, necessity.

Oh, don't read me, girlfriend. You know I'm not the only one, though I should have known better. I should have had some sense knocked into me by the sight of my gym buddy, Alfredo. Yes, I should have known better when I saw the peculiar rash on Alfredo's brown, muscled back, a light-colored rash which spread to his chest, his arms, his face. Should have realized something was up when his weight went suddenly down. I watched him drop as many pounds as he once pressed. I watched, while like some sick solitary elephant he wandered off from the herd to die. Alfredo quietly disappeared from the clubs, the gym, disappeared into shadows and the silence of his apartment. When did you die, girlfriend? Even now, I don't think anybody knows, you did it so—discreetly. Yes, Chris, I hear you: and we are paying a devastating price for such "discretion."

Dear Lewayne:

Funny. How crisis has a way of either deepening or disrupting our delusions. Were you watching when the German doctors told me that both of my kidneys had ceased to function, and that I was HIV-positive, to boot? Stunned, silent, yet alert, I lay in that German hospital bed, my inner eyes, at last, beginning to open. Did you see what I saw, Lewayne—Lewayne, spitting image of myself; Lewayne, whose mother/father/family declined to visit you during worsening illness; Lewayne, the first black man I personally knew to join this long, solemn procession: did you see, Lewayne, how quickly, quietly, my delusions of immunity disintegrated? Were you watching, girlfriend? Did you nod and sigh:

"It's about time!"

Sweet Lewayne, who first lost sight, then life, to the raging virus, were you nonetheless my witness? Did you see over the ensuing months of my recuperation what happened to my kidneys, my sight, my tongue? Did you see how slowly, gradually, my kidneys once started to work, how slowly, gradually I began to see the consequences of silence, and how as a consequence of this insight, my tongue unhinged from the roof of my mouth, dislodged from the back of my throat, slipped—free? And in the hospital, like some exuberant runaway escaped from slavery, I sang aloud, with all my might:

Oh Freedom
Oh Freedom
Oh Freedom over me
And before I'll be a slave
I'll be buried in my grave
And go home, yes I'll go home
And be free

Surely, I thought, some nurse would have rushed to the door and hushed me or some less polite fellow patient simply demanded that I shut up all that noise. But no one came and no one protested, so from my hospital bed I continued to sing, with all my might:

I shall not
I shall not be removed
I shall not
I shall not be removed
Just like a tree
That's standing by the water
Oh I shall not be removed

Dear Harriet:

Did you hear, Harriet, the trembling trepidation in my voice (trembling which even now in remembering threatens to repossess me)? And didn't you, like the good shepherd that you have always been, didn't you come—and take my hand?

Beneath the continuous blare of Geraldo, Joan, Oprah, Phil, "The Young and the Restless," and "All My (oh-so-tedious) Children," I heard you, Harriet, paid strict attention to your silent command: stand up and walk! Remember, Harriet? Remember while my lover, mother, grandmother, friends, walked me through the hospital hallways with IV in tow, you walked with me also, lightly holding my hand. And when we had escaped out of the woods, you pressed me on till we reached the river and you said simply, silently, with your eyes: wade in the water, child, if you want to get to the other side.

How many runaways had you so commanded? How many hung back and clung in fear to what they felt they knew, sought refuge in the woods, thick silence, darkest night? How many thought they could escape by becoming invisible? But didn't you know, Harriet, that slavery is never escaped as long as the master controls your mind? And don't you now see the chilling parallels between the means by which we were held captive in your time, and the methods of our enslavement today? Don't you see the chains, my Harriet, sweet Moses, the chains not so much of steel and the law, but more insidious: the invisible chains, linked over centuries, of silence and shame? In this latest crisis, our new master is the virus; his overseer—silence; and his whip—shame.

Were you watching when I stepped into the deep? I who have never learned to swim was certain I would drown. Chilly, troubled waters swept over my feet, rose gushingly to my ankles, my hips, waist, chest, then my neck. Troubled, angry waters whipped and tore at me, brutally washed away decades of deep-layered shame, washed away the denial, the fear, the stigma; cracked and splintered the master's lock and chain.

Before I knew it I was naked and trembling—and free. And that's when I began to sing, from the hospital bed, and I know I sang off-key, but the quality of the song didn't matter as much as the affirming act of singing:

I woke up this morning with my mind
Staying on Freedom
I woke up this morning with my mind
Staying on Freedom
I woke up this morning with my mind
Staying on Freedom
Hallelu—hallelu—hallelujah

Dear comrades, lovers, girlfriends, family:

Bless you for the blessings you've given me. I know but one way to redeem the precious gift of your lives, your deaths, and that is through living testaments, old and new, to all we have been and might become. For I know that through such testaments we are forever fortified: through such testaments we will keep on walking and keep on talking until we get to the other side.

Marlon

TO MY READERS

HAROLD BRODKEY

from The New Yorker

| 1993 |

AIDS

I have AIDS. I am surprised that I do. I have not been exposed since the 1970s, which is to say that my experiences, my adventures in homosexuality took place largely in the 1960s, and back then I relied on time and abstinence to indicate my degree of freedom from infection and to protect others and myself.

At first, shadows and doubts of various kinds disturbed my sleep, but later I felt more certainty of safety. Before AIDS was identified, I thought five years without noticeable infection would indicate one was without disease. When AIDS was first identified, five years was held to indicate safety. That changed. Twenty years now is considered a distance in time that might indicate safety, but a slight number of AIDS cases are anomalous; that is, the delay in illness is not explicable within the assumed rules, even under the most careful, cynical investigation. It doesn't matter much. I have AIDS. I have had *Pneumocystis carinii* pneumonia, which almost killed me. Unlikely or not, blood test, T-cell count, the fact that it was *Pneumocystis* means I have AIDS and must die.

There it is. At the time I was told, I was so ill, so racked with fever and having such difficulty breathing, that I hardly cared. I was embarrassed and shamed that the people who cared for me in the hospital had to take special precautions to protect themselves. Then as the fever went down I suppose my pride and sense of competition took over. When someone from social services showed up to offer counsel, I found that bothersome, although the counselor was a very fine person, warm and intelligent. I suppose I was competitive with or antagonistic toward the assumption that now my death would be harder than other deaths, harder to bear, and that the sentence to such death and suffering was unbearable.

I didn't find it so. I didn't want to find it so. Granted, I am perverse. But my head felt the doom was bearable. My body hurt. I haven't felt even halfway human for eight or nine weeks now, until the last two or three days. It was as if I had walked through a door into the most unstable physical state of wretched and greatly undesirable discomfort possible.

But, of course, blindness and dementia are worse states. And my parents suffered excruciatingly with heart trouble and cancer. Also, I was not, am not, young. I am not being cut down before I have had a chance to live. Most important, I was not and am not alone. On the second day, when the truth was known, my wife, Ellen Schwamm, moved into the hospital with me. When we began to tell the family, no one rejected me. No one. I am embarrassed to be ill and to be ill in this way, but no one yet has shown disgust or revulsion. I expect it. But in the hospital AIDS is a boring thing for interns, it is so common. And outside it arouses, at least in New York, sympathy and curiosity. I do get the feeling I am a bit on show, or rather my death is and my moods are. But so what?

So far the worst moments, in terms of grief, came about when I was visited by my grandson, aged four, a wide-faced blond, a second child, bright, and rather expert at emotional warfare. I hadn't seen him in four months, and he looked at me snottily and said, "I don't remember *you*." I said, "I used to be a pink-and-black horse." He looked at me, thought or reacted, then grinned and said, "I remember you now," and came over and took my hand and generally didn't leave my side. But the horror was I had no strength to respond or pretend after only a short while, less than an hour. I am not able to be present for him and never will be anymore. That led to a bad twenty-four hours. But that can hardly be uncommon, and I had already felt a version of it toward Ellen, although less intense, because I am able to be there in some ways still, and can find some sort of robot strength in myself still if I have to.

My doctor, who is very able and very experienced, is surprised that I am not more depressed. He says cheerfully that I am much more upset than I realize. He credits some of the medicines with shielding me, my mood, and warns me that severe unhappiness is coming, but so far it hasn't come. I have resisted it, I suppose. And my wife is with me every moment. I feel cut off from old age, it's true, but that's not like someone young feeling cut off from most of his or her possible life.

In my adult life and in my childhood, I was rarely, almost never, ill, but when I was, it was always serious, and nearly fatal. I have been given up by my doctors three times in my life and for a few minutes a fourth time. This time is more convincing but otherwise it is not an unfamiliar or unexplained territory.

I was a hypochondriac, but for a good reason—I could take no medicine, none at all, without extreme, perverse, or allergic reactions. Essentially I never got sick. I was gym-going, hike-taking, cautious, oversensitive to the quality of the air, to heat and cold, noise and odors, someone who felt tireder more quickly than most people because of all these knife-edge reactions, someone who was careful not to get sick, because my allergic reactions to medicines made almost any illness a drastic experience.

I had an extremely stable baseline of mood and of mind, of mental *landscape*. Well, that's gone; it's entirely gone. From the moment my oxygen intake fell to about 50 percent and the ambulance drivers arrived in our apartment with a gurney and with oxygen for me to breathe, from that moment and then in the hospital until now, I have not had even one moment of physical stability. I am filled off-and-on with surf noises as if I were a seashell, my blood seems to fizz and tingle. I have low and high fevers. For a day I had a kind of fever with chills and sweats but with body temperature *below* normal, at 96 degrees. I have choked and had trouble breathing. I have had pleuritis, or pleurisy, in my right lung, an inflammation of the thoracic cavity which feels like a burning stiffness of the muscles and which hurt like hell if I coughed, moved suddenly, or reached to pick something up.

And, of course, one can die at any moment or discover symptoms of some entirely new disease. My life has changed into this death, irreversibly.

But I don't *think* the death sentence bothers me. I don't see why it should more than before. I have had little trouble living with the death-warrant aspect of life until now. I never denied, never hysterically defined the reality of death, the presence and idea of it, the inevitability of it. I always knew *I* would die. I never felt invulnerable or immortal. I felt the presence and menace of death in bright sunlight and in the woods and in moments of danger in cars and planes. I felt it in others' lives. Fear and rage toward death for me is focused on resisting death's soft jaws at key moments, fighting back the interruption, the separation. In physical moments when I was younger, I had great surges of wild strength when in danger, mountain climbing, for instance, or threatened in a fight or by muggers in the city. In the old days I would put my childish or young strength at the service of people who were ill. I would lend them my will power, too. Death scared me some, maybe even terrified me in a way, but at the same time I had no great fear of death. Why should it be different now? Ought I to crack up because a bluff has been called?

As with other children, when I was very young, death was interesting—dead insects, dead birds, dead people. In a middle-class, upper-middle-class milieu, everything connected to real death was odd, I mean in relation to pretensions and statements, projects and language and pride. It seemed softly adamant, an undoing, a rearrangement, a softly meddlesome and irresistible silence. It was something some boys I knew and I thought we ought to familiarize ourselves with. Early on, and also in adolescence, we had a particular, conscious will not to be controlled by fear of death—there were things we would die rather than do. To some extent this rebelliousness was also controlled; to some extent we could choose our dangers, but not always. All this may be common among the young during a war; I grew up during the Second World War. And a lot was dependent on locality, and social class, the defense of the sexual self or the private self against one's father or in school.

Having accepted death long ago in order to be physically and morally free—to some extent—I am not crushed by this final sentence of death, at least not yet, and I don't think it is denial. I think my disbelief weeks ago gave way to the *maybe so* of the onset of belief. I am sick and exhausted, numbed and darkened, by my approximate dying a few weeks ago from *Pneumocystis*, and consider death a silence, a silence and a privacy and an untouchability, as no more reactions and opinions, as a relief, a privilege, a lucky and graceful and symmetrical silence to be grateful for. The actual words I used inwardly read ambiguously when written out—*it's about time* for silence.

I'm sixty-two, and it's ecological sense to die while you're still productive, die and clear a space for others, old and young. I didn't always appreciate what I had at the time, but I am aware now that accusations against me of being lucky in love were pretty much true and of being lucky sexually, also true. And lucky intellectually and, occasionally, lucky in the people I worked with. I have no sad stories about love or sex.

And I think my work will live. And I am tired of defending it, tired of giving my life to it. But I have liked my life. I like my life at present, being ill. I like the people I deal with. I don't feel I am being whisked off the stage or murdered and stuffed in a laundry hamper while my life is incomplete. It's my turn to die—I can see that that is interesting to some people but not that it is tragic. Yes, I was left out of some things and was cheated over a lifetime in a bad way but who isn't and so what? I had a lot of privileges as well. Sometimes I'm sad about its being over but I'm that way about books and sunsets and conversations. The medicines I take don't grant my moods much independence, so I suspect these reactions, but I think they are my own. I have been a fool all my life, giving away large chunks of time and wasting years on nothing much, and maybe I'm being a fool now.

And I have died before, come close enough to dying that doctors and nurses on those occasions said those were death experiences, the approach to death, a little of death felt from the inside. And I have nursed dying people and been at deathbeds. I nearly died when my first mother did; I was two years old. As an adult, at one point, I forced myself to remember what I could of the child's feelings. The feelings I have now are far milder. My work, my notions and theories and doctrines, my pride have conspired to make me feel as I do now that I am ill.

I have always remembered nearly dying when I was seven and had an allergic, hypothermic reaction coming out of anesthesia. When I was thirty, a hepatitis thing was misdiagnosed as cancer of the liver, and I was told I had six weeks to live. The sensations at those various times were not much alike, but the feeling of extreme sickness, of being racked, was and is the same as is the sense of the real death.

I have wondered at times if maybe my resistance to the fear-of-death wasn't laziness and low mental alertness, a cowardly inability to admit that horror was horror, that dying was unbearable. It feels, though, like a life-giving rebelliousness, a kind of blossoming. Not a love of death but maybe a love of God. I wouldn't want to be hanged and it would kill my soul to be a hangman but I always hoped that if I were hanged I would be amused and superior, and capable of having a good time somehow as I died—this may be a sense of human style in an orphan, greatly damaged and deadened, a mere sense of style overriding a more normal terror and sense of an injustice of destiny. Certainly, it is a *dangerous* trait. I am not sensible . . . At all times I am more afraid of anesthesia and surgery than I am of death. I have had moments of terror, of abject fear. I was rather glad to have those moments. But the strain was tremendous. My feelings of terror have had a scattered quality mostly, and I tended to despise them as petty. I have more fear of cowardice and of being broken by torture than I do of death. I am aware of my vulnerability, of how close I come to being shattered. But next to that is a considerable amount of nerve—my blood parents and real grandparents were said to have been insanely brave, to have had an arrogant sang-froid about their courage and what it allowed them to do. They had, each of them, a strong tropism toward the epic. My mother, before I was born, travelled alone from near Leningrad to Illinois in the 1920s, a journey that, at her social level, took nearly two months; the year before, her older brother had disappeared, perhaps murdered. My father once boxed a dozen men in a row one evening on a bet and supposedly laid all the women under thirty who lined up afterward. Another time, better attested, with two other men, he took on a squad of marching local Nazis in St. Louis, twenty-five or thirty men, and won.

I myself am a coward, oversensitive, lazy, reclusive, but the mind and spirit have their requirement of independence; and death can't help but seem more bearable than a stupid life of guilt, say.

Is death other than silence and nothingness? In my experiences of it, it is that disk of acceptance and of unthreading and disappearance at the bottom of the chute of revenant memories, ghosts and the living, the gauntlet of important recollections through which one is forced in order to approach the end of one's consciousness. Death itself is soft, softly lit, vastly dark. The self becomes taut with metamorphosis and seems to give off some light and to have a not-quite-great-enough fearlessness toward that immensity of the end of individuality, toward one's absorption into the dance of particles and inaudibility. Living, one undergoes one metamorphosis after another—often, they are cockroach states inset with moments of passivity, with the sense of real death—but they are continuous and linked. This one is a stillness and represents a sifting out of identity and its stories, a breaking off or removal of the self, and a devolution into mere effect and memory, outspread and not tightly bound but scattered among micromotions and as if more windblown than in life.

People speak of wanting to live to see their grandchildren marry, but what is it they will see? A sentimental ceremony or a real occasion involving real lives? Life is a kind of horror. It is OK, but it is wearing. Enemies and thieves don't lay off as you weaken. The wicked flourish by being ruthless even then. If you are ill, you have to have a good lawyer. Depending on your circumstances, in some cases you have to back off and lie low. You're weak. Death is preferable to daily retreat.

Certainly people on the street who smile gently at me as I walk slowly or X-ray attendants calling me *darling* or *lovey* are aware of this last thing. A woman I know who died a few years back spoke of this in relation to herself. She hated it. I don't want to talk about my dying to everyone, or over and over. Is my attitude only vanity—and more vanity—in the end? In a sense, I steal each day, but I steal it by making no effort. It is just there, sunlight or rain, nightfall or morning. I am still living at least a kind of life, and I don't want to be reduced to an image now, or, in my own mind, feel I am spending all my time on my dying instead of on living, to some satisfying extent, the time I have left.

Not constantly but not inconstantly either, underneath the sentimentality and obstinacy of my attitudes, are, as you might expect, a quite severe rage and a vast, a truly extensive terror, anchored in contempt for you and for life and for everything. But let's keep that beast in its gulf of darkness. Let's be polite and proper and devoted to life now as we were earlier in our life on this planet.

One of the things that struck me when I was first told that I had AIDS was that I was cut off from my family inheritance of fatal diseases—the strokes and high blood pressure and cancers and tumors of my ancestors. My medical fate is quite different; I felt a bit orphaned yet again, and idiosyncratic, but strangely also as if I had been invited, almost abducted, to a party, a somber feast but not entirely grim, a feast of the seriously afflicted who yet were at war with social indifference and prejudice and hatred. It seemed to me that I was surrounded by braveries without number, that I had been inducted into a phalanx of the wildly-alive-even-if-dying, and I felt honored that I would, so to speak, die in the company of such people.

Really, I can say nothing further at this point. Pray for me.

POLITICAL FUNERALS

DAVID B. FEINBERG

from Queer and Loathing

| 1994 |

I imagine what it would be like if friends had a demonstration each time a lover or a friend or a stranger died of AIDS. I imagine what it would be like if, each time a lover, friend or stranger died of this disease, their friends, lovers or neighbors would take the dead body and drive with it in a car a hundred miles an hour to washington d.c. and blast through the gates of the white house and come to a screeching halt before the entrance and dump their lifeless form on the front steps.

—David Wojnarowicz,
Close to the Knives

This past year, it seems that ACT UP is coming to terms with death.

David Robinson initiated the Ashes Action from San Francisco. His lover, Warren, had died that past spring. At first David was thinking of mailing Warren's ashes to the White House as a private gesture of anger, grief, and protest. Upon reflection, he decided a public forum would be more appropriate. There was strong support for the concept of an ashes action on the floor of ACT UP/N.Y. The Names Quilt was going to be displayed for the last time in its entirety in Washington, D.C., during Columbus Day weekend in October 1992. We decided to have the demonstration on Sunday of that weekend. We were going to shower the White House lawn with the ashes of our loved ones.

I remember seeing Warren and David dance together in a bar in Atlanta, when ACT UP/N.Y. flew down for a series of demonstrations against the CDC and the sodomy laws. Warren was gorgeous. He wore a white tank top. David Robinson had been a facilitator for the Monday-night ACT UP meetings for several years. He frequently came to meetings in postmodern drag: a skirt and a beard. David was a trained dancer. He was strong and passionate.

Warren was from the South. David and Warren moved together to San Francisco, shortly after David, as one of the "Three Anonymous Queers," penned the broadside "I Hate Straights." Warren and David were a discordant couple: Warren was positive and David was negative. After they moved to San Francisco, I heard only infrequent reports through thirdhand sources about them. Someone told me that Warren had flown to Switzerland for Dr. Roka's herb-enema treatment. My friend Sarah told me it did wonders for her friend Bo. Bo died this spring.

As time passed, more people joined the Ashes Action. They, too, were committed to bringing the ashes of their loved ones to the White House. Shane Butler coordinated the action from New York. We had a series of pre-action meetings. We formed affinity groups to march in rows at the action. Our basic objective was to protect those carrying ashes from the police until they reached the White House. My affinity group was willing to risk arrest.

We felt it wasn't our action, it was David's action, and the action of those carrying ashes of friends and companions. We were merely functioning as support. We decided to have a large, silent, dignified procession to the White House.

That Sunday, we meet at the Capitol side of the Mall. We march down the Mall to the accompaniment of the saddest drums. At first it is just the few busloads of activists from New York and the small group of maybe ten people carrying ashes. As we march silently, people join in from the sidelines. The procession grows. We are silent, for once. SILENCE = DEATH is a metaphor, after all. This is no metaphor: We carry death itself.

Frank, an activist now living in the Midwest, had smeared his face with fake blood and was chanting loudly. "It's not just their demo, it's all of us," he says when reprimanded to be quiet. David wails. Suddenly those carrying the ashes begin to chant. We all chant to the beat of the drums.

As the procession veers north from the Mall to the street, my affinity group functions as the front guard, risking arrest. We pass the pressure point unscathed.

It is impossible for me to assimilate this as it is happening. It is too immense. Our grief is literal. Does a man cease to become more than a symbol after he is dead? Yet somehow this is more than the usual "cheap theatrics," more than our street theater with strong graphics and media savvy.

A woman hands a bag of ashes, her son's, to someone as we march by. She wanted someone to use it. The crowd continues to grow, until we are almost four hundred.

We march in strength and solidarity.

We march in anger and in grief.

We march against the murderous neglect of two presidential administrations.

We march in dignity and pride.

When there is no possibility of getting to the front of the White House, we march to the backyard. The police cluster around on horses. They are planning on stopping us at the end of the driveway, before the fence.

Every action has one mad moment of uncertainty, one delirious moment of fear. We break ranks and make a mad rush, surrounding those carrying the ashes. Mounted policemen move in, forming a wedge between the group at the fence and the group on the other side of the macadam. We sit down to hold our ground. I look down and see a puddle of blood. For a moment I am hysterical. Then I realize it is more of Frank's fake blood.

Some scale the fences and start dumping their containers of ashes, to cheers. And then it is all over.

The police threaten to arrest all those on the fence side of their line. Another gauntlet is thrown. We confer and decide that we've accomplished what we came for and there is no sense in getting arrested after achieving our goal. We will disperse in groups.

We gather in the park behind the White House for a public speak-out. People tell what had happened. I learn of Alexis's grief: She had carried her father's ashes, her father who had died several years ago, and now she is finally experiencing a sense of closure. Eric Sawyer has Larry Kert's celebrity ashes. Larry was disinvited from the White House after he came down with AIDS. Well, now he's coming, invitation or not. David talks about Warren. He cries. And suddenly it rains in torrents, an intense downpour of grief. We rush to a covered grandstand at the side of the park, soaked. The ashes mix with the soil. Ten minutes earlier the Parks Service could have cleaned up our burnt offerings with ease. Now they are impossible to eradicate.

The last time I saw Mark Fisher alive was at Tim Powers's memorial. He was much thinner than I remembered. Mark was an architect from Iowa and a member of The Marys affinity group. He silk-screened T-shirts for The Marys that said "ALL PEOPLE WITH AIDS ARE INNOCENT." Mark was tall and lanky. If Eddie Haskell were gay, he would have grown up to be Mark Fisher.

For three years I sat next to Mark Bronnenberg at ACT UP meetings. He was the other Mark from Iowa. He moved to San Francisco a few years ago, as did Pam and Russell. Pam and Russell were Mark Fisher's best friends. Pam's brother died of AIDS. Pam was very hurt when the "I Hate Straights" broadsheet came out.

Mark Fisher wrote an anonymous piece published by *QW* a few weeks before his death titled "Bury Me Furiously." I'll quote the last section here:

> I suspect—I know—my funeral will shock people when it happens. We Americans are terrified of death. Death takes place behind closed doors and is removed from reality, from the living. I want to show the reality of my death, to display my body in public; I want the public to bear witness. We are not just spiraling statistics; we are people who have lives, who have purpose, who have lovers, friends, and families. And we are dying of a disease maintained by a degree of criminal neglect so enormous that it amounts to genocide.
>
> I want my death to be as strong a statement as my life continues to be.
>
> I want my own funeral to be fierce and defiant, to make the public statement that my death from AIDS is a form of political assassination.
>
> We are taking this action out of love and rage.

It is all so very terrible. Mark died of sepsis, caused by a catheter infection, on the plane coming back from Italy, less than a month after the Ashes Action. He went to Italy with Russell. During the last few days of their vacation, they were looking at hospitals. Mark was going crazy. He kept a diary. The last entry, on the morning of his death, in tiny, tiny writing, was: "Mind is clear. Feel like a complete whole." The last thing he said to Russell was "Hello." Why does dying on a plane freak me out so much?

Mark Fisher was so sweet. I tried calling Mark Bronnenberg in San Francisco three times to let him know. I found out he had died on Thursday, the day after Paul's memorial, the afternoon I found out that Richard was dead.

On Friday there is a Take Back the Night march through the East Village, sponsored by Outwatch and the Anti-Violence Project. It starts at Cooper Union. The mood is grim: Everyone is finding out that Mark Fisher had died. The Marys pass out flyers with Mark's picture on the front, and "Bury Me Furiously" on the back. There will be a political funeral next Monday, the day before the presidential election. Tom came to the demo late. He had to see Luis, who is dying of leukemia, and then his friend Chris had a hissy fit because Tom was a half hour late and Barry blurted out to Tom, "Did you hear that Mark died?" There are times when I cannot comprehend what is going on. There is too much sadness in the world. I suppose Pam knew. Russell must have told her.

I am living under a heavy sheet of sadness.

On Monday there is a ceremony at Judson Memorial Church at Washington Square. Pam has flown in from San Francisco. Russell is there in the front row, with Pam. Afterward, six people carry Mark's open casket up Sixth Avenue to Republican National Headquarters in midtown. His pale and emaciated corpse is clearly visible in the plain-pine coffin. It is raining steadily. The street is a sea of black umbrellas. A car follows the procession. James, on crutches, rides in the car for several blocks. Four people carry burning torches. I am a marshal assigned to the back of the march. I have to make sure that nobody lags behind and is picked off by police.

How many more have to die?

There is some heckling from the sidelines. Police block traffic for us. Sixth Avenue becomes a huge traffic jam. To the passengers in the cars, the drivers, the people walking home in the rain, this is a minor annoyance, just one more aggravation for living in New York. To us, a life, a death. A man on the north side of Washington Square Park yells at us, thinking it is just another pro-Clinton demonstration. It doesn't sink in. I am furious, screaming at passersby, "This is a fucking funeral, don't you get it?"

We reach our destination and have a brief ceremony. The door to the building is double-locked. People are hiding from us. Michael Cunningham speaks eloquently and angrily at the end of the procession. The casket is loaded into the car. We leave our list of demands at Republican headquarters, the same list of demands we left at Kennebunkport a year ago. These are the same demands we keep on pressing: Open the borders to HIV-positives. Distribute condoms in the schools. Fund needle-exchange programs throughout the country. Have a massive research project to find a cure for AIDS. Double the NIH budget. Put someone in charge of the crisis.

We go home. What have we accomplished? Are we any closer to ending this crisis?

Tim Bailey wanted us to throw his body over the White House fence, but we couldn't do that—"not because we didn't share his fury but because we loved him too much to treat his mortal remains that way," as Michael Cunningham said at his memorial. Instead, we chartered two buses and drove to D.C. at seven-thirty in the morning. Without a second thought, one hundred activists take off work Thursday to go to a political funeral to honor Tim Bailey. I can't sleep the night before. I am up at six. On the way down to Washington, a video on AIDS activism plays on the monitor. I huddle next to my friend Brian and try to get some sleep.

Tim was a fashion designer for the house of Patricia Field. James Baggett and Joy were his best friends. Tim was a frail bleach-blond. He had been ill for more than a year. Last summer I saw him on Fire Island. He was there for a weekend with Joy and her girlfriend. He confessed to Michael Cunningham that Fire Island was the only place on earth he truly felt safe. He had grown up to the taunt "faggot." Even in New York City, it was difficult to escape the homophobia of this culture.

We arrive in D.C. at noon. We mill around for an hour, trying not to look too conspicuous. We fail. One hundred activists with ACT UP T-shirts, stickers, and posters can't exactly fade into the reflecting pool by the Capitol. Some of us have pinned Tim Bailey's photo to our chests. Some have drums.

An hour later the van arrives with Tim's body. Several police cars have appeared in the interim. We are told to gather away from the van to form the procession. A few minutes later we hear there is trouble.

The police won't let us remove the casket from the van.

The police tell us to move away from the back of the van. We surge there and recapture our ground. Two lone police officers from the back of the van, feeling the crush of fifty activists, excuse themselves and make their exits.

This begins a three-hour standoff.

There are D.C. police, county police, federal police, and police from the Parks Service. We are simultaneously in several jurisdictions and no one is in charge. No officer is able to explain why we are being forbidden to remove the casket. A policeman has the keys to the van. He had wrestled them away from Joy during the initial confrontation. A car is parked in front of the van, blocking it.

Then we are told we need a death certificate, and the body must be examined by a coroner, in order to have a procession. The police have to make sure that Tim's death was not a homicide. Even then the police may not allow a procession. There is an arcane regulation that forbids unseemly displays.

Feeling we have made all the proper preparations, feeling we are on the right side of the law, feeling there is some respect for the sanctity of human life, we allow the police to perpetrate this humiliating charade of justice and procedure.

Joy makes the officer come to the coffin. She refuses to let the death certificate out of her hands. She demands and receives back the van keys.

The medical examiner from the coroner's office, wearing rubber gloves, examines the body. Joy and others taunt him as he performs his task. He is close to tears by the time he leaves. "Are you satisfied? Is he dead enough? This is what AIDS looks like. Are you proud of yourself?"

After the police examine the death certificate and the body has been examined, they confer and decide they still will not allow the procession to take place, on the grounds that it is an unseemly and obscene display.

In a way, the police are right.

Death is unseemly.

Death is obscene.

Death is ugly.

A light rain is falling. We haven't eaten since seven o'clock in the morning.

For close to three hours we have stood, we have sat, we have guarded the van holding the body of our friend Tim Bailey as a solid wall of police lines the perimeter of our group. We are in a parking lot. A car blocks us at the front. The cops want us to leave, but there is no possible method of egress available, even if we wanted to go.

There are ongoing negotiations. Eric Sawyer calls Bob Hattoy in the White House on his cellular phone. Someone else calls an official in the Department of Health and Human Services. Permits are waived. We are eventually offered a compromise march. We can follow the vehicle as long as we keep the casket in the van. We will be able to march with the casket for a block, two blocks away from the White House. Then we must return.

We had planned on having a ceremony at the front of the White House and leaving. We would have been long gone if the police had allowed us to proceed when we arrived. Tim's brother, Randy, is consulted. He is appalled. Eventually we accept the compromise. Perhaps we will continue with the procession after the block. Perhaps we won't. We decide that this will be the best way to proceed. We are tired and angry and hurt.

Then, as we are about to start, at three-thirty, after two and a half hours of unpleasantness and ugliness, the police change their mind. We can proceed if we wait until six-thirty, after rush hour.

The police have not acted in an honorable fashion.

The police have just been stalling us for the past three hours.

We decide to take the coffin out of the van and start our procession.

We are operating on the basic assumption that the police will respect the sanctity of death.

We are wrong.

I move with several people on the left side of the van, to give enough room to open the back door of the van. I am face to face with the cops. We open the door and several people start to take out the coffin.

"Put it back in!" scream the police. "Put it back in!"

It seems that they are afraid of death; they are that afraid of the physical evidence of the notorious neglect of this administration and the previous two presidential administrations. Tim Bailey's body is the smoking gun of the epidemic. Tim Bailey's body accuses them of murder with quiet fury.

What follows is one of the most horrible moments of my life. In a fracas that reminds me of *Day of the Locust*, police and pallbearers struggle with the coffin. I can't tell whether the police are trying to shove the coffin back into the van or steal it as evidence of our transgression. This moment of madness is captured on CNN. I can see the coffin banged on the edges. In the extreme violence of the scene, I have the impression that the wood is chipping, splintering, cracking, and breaking. To protect the body, the pallbearers return the coffin to the van. When it is over, the police have arrested Randy Bailey, brother of the deceased, for assaulting a police officer.

Randy Bailey isn't an activist. He isn't a member of ACT UP. He's had no experience with AIDS activism. He's never been arrested for a political protest. Randy Bailey is a straight man from Ohio whose brother died of AIDS.

Someone yells, "Someone volunteer to get arrested with him so he won't be alone!"

I look around. I am tired. Jim Aquino pauses, then marches straight into the police, and they immediately arrest him. He is as innocent as a lamb led to the slaughter. Two others attempt to get arrested. James Learned tries to break through a solid line of police with the fury of a caged bull, but they won't let him through. He is furious.

This is not a game. This is life and death. This is murder. This is the physical evidence. This is AIDS. This is the remains of Timothy Bailey, dead of AIDS at thirty-five.

We begin our ceremony, on top of the van. Someone sets up the sound system. Several people speak eloquently. Joy is fire and anger.

I cannot speak.

The body is to be returned to the funeral home in New Jersey. Barbara starts the van. The police allow us to have a brief procession out of the parking lot. We march and chant behind the coffin. I stand right behind the van. I do not want the police any closer; I do not want them to have any contact with the van. They desecrate everything they touch. The coffin is surrounded by bouquets of flowers from the funeral home. Jim Baggett starts passing back flowers from the van. Tim used to fill his backpack with flowers on Gay Pride Day and pass out flowers to everyone he saw. In his honor, we pass flowers back until each of us has a flower. At the end of the driveway, the cops push us all aside and form a line between us and the van. Vincent was going to be dropped off at a D.C. hotel with the sound equipment. The police tell them to dump Vincent and the sound equipment on the street. The police give the van an escort all the way to Baltimore, Maryland.

Throughout the entire standoff, an officer stands to the side with a shit-eating grin on his face. "Don't you understand, this is a funeral? Wouldn't you give this much respect to any warrior who died fighting bravely? He's dead! Show some respect!" I am close to hysterical. Barry is infuriated. He wants to go to D.C. the next time a policeman dies in the line of duty to laugh at the funeral service.

What do you plan on doing with your body after your death? Do you want your body burned in effigy at the offices of the Pharmaceutical Manufacturers Association? Do you want it impaled on the White House fence as an indictment of the current administration? Do you want to donate your HIV-infected organs to the Archdiocese of New York, members of the religious Right, militant antiabortionists, members of the National Rifle Association, feminists against pornography, and right-wing Republicans?

I stand in awe of those like Mark Lowe Fisher and Tim Bailey who are able to commit their bodies for political funerals.

The concept is unfathomable, incomprehensible, as difficult to grasp as death.

FROM MY OWN COUNTRY

ABRAHAM VERGHESE

| 1994 |

I remember as an intern in 1981 reading a *New England Journal of Medicine* article with the curious title "*Pneumocystis carinii* Pneumonia and Mucosal Candidiasis in Previously Healthy Homosexual Men—Evidence of a New Acquired Cellular Immunodeficiency." It described the seminal AIDS cases in Los Angeles. Companion articles described cases in New York and San Francisco. Three things about these reports stayed in my mind: gay men, immune deficiency, and death.

I knew precious little about gay culture.

In college I had picked up and parroted the snide asides and took part in the buffoonery and condescension that constituted the heterosexual response to homosexuality.

For me, reading about ritualized meeting places like bathhouses and gay bars and understanding the extent of gay culture was astonishing and eye opening. It was as if a whole megalopolis had existed around me, intertwined with my city, and yet invisible to me. I was intensely curious.

I knew no *openly* gay men. I only knew the stereotype. I sensed the stereotype might be as untrue as the stereotype of the southerner, the redneck. If the southerner was a born racist and terribly intolerant, I—a brown-skinned foreigner—had never experienced this. In fact, the first time I experienced racism, felt it as a palpable presence in my daily life, was in Boston, not Tennessee.

The month the first papers on AIDS came out, the disease became a topic for late-night, idle discussion in the Mountain Home VA and Miracle Center cafeterias. AIDS seemed so far away, so bizarre: New York and San Francisco were its epicenters. We were seeing in our lifetime, so we told ourselves, yet *another* new disease. And surely, just like Legionnaire's, Lyme disease, toxic shock—all new diseases—we felt this new disease, this mysterious immune deficiency, would soon be understood and conquered.

To say this was a time of unreal and unparalleled confidence, bordering on conceit, in the Western medical world is to understate things. Only cancer was truly feared, and even that was often curable. When the outcome of treatment was not good, it was because the host was aged, the protoplasm frail, or the patient had presented too late—never because medical science was impotent.

There seemed to be little that medicine could not do. As a lowly resident, I was inserting Swan-Ganz catheters into the vena cava and the right side of the heart. Meanwhile, the cardiologists were advancing fancier catheters through leg arteries and up the aorta, then using tiny balloons to open clogged coronary arteries or using lasers in Roto-Rooter fashion to ream out the grunge.

Surgeons, like Tom Starzl in Pittsburgh, had made kidney, liver, heart, and heart-lung transplantation routine, and they were embarking on twelve- to fourteen-hour "cluster operations" where liver, pancreas, duodenum, and jejunum were removed en bloc from a donor and transplanted into a patient whose belly, previously riddled with cancer, had now been eviscerated, scooped clean in preparation for this organ bouquet.

Starzl was an icon for that period in medicine, the pre-AIDS days, the frontier days of every-other-night call. My fellow interns and I thought of ourselves as the *vaqueros* of the fluorescent corridors, riding the high of sleep deprivation, dressed day or night in surgical scrubs, banks of beepers on our belts, our tongues quick with the buzz words that reduced patients to syndromes—"rule out MI," "impending DTs," "multiorgan failure." We strutted around with floppy tourniquets threaded through the buttonholes of our coats, our pockets cluttered with penlights, ECG calipers, stethoscopes, plastic shuffle cards with algorithms and recipes on them. The hemostats lost in the depths of our coat pockets were our multipurpose wrenches and found uses from roach clips to earwax dislodgers. Carried casually in sterile packaging in our top pockets were seven-gauge, seven-inch needles with twelve-inch trails of tubing. We were always ready—should we be first at a Code Blue—to slide needle under collarbone, into the great subclavian vein, and then to feed the serpent tubing down the vena cava in a cathartic ritual that established our mastery over the human body.

There seemed no reason to believe when AIDS arrived on the scene that we would not transfix it with our divining needles, lyse it with our potions, swallow it and digest it in the great vats of eighties technology.

I had made up my mind that I wanted a career in academic medicine. If there was glory in medicine, then I was not satisfied with the glory of saving a patient and having the family and a few others know about it. The rewards of private practice—money, autonomy, the big house, the big car, the big boat, the small plane, the bubble reputation in a provincial hospital—were not enough for me. I loved bedside medicine, the art of mining the patient's body for clues to disease. I loved introducing medical students to the thrill of the examination of the human body, guiding their hands to feel a liver, to percuss the stony dull note of fluid that had accumulated in the lung, to be with them when their eyes shone the first time they heard "tubular" breathing or "whispering pectoriloquy" and thereby diagnosed pneumonia. The acclaim of the lecture hall, the lead article in the *New England Journal of Medicine*, the invitations to be a keynote speaker at gatherings of my peers—these were the coins I wished to hoard.

My mentor in Tennessee was Steven Berk, an infectious-diseases specialist fresh out of training at Boston City Hospital. Boston City Hospital was for many years the premier infectious diseases (ID) training program in the country. Steve, a quiet, unassuming, and shy man, had already published several important papers prior to coming to Tennessee. His ability to see research opportunities in the wards, nursing home, and domiciliaries of the VA excited me. Steve was quietly cataloguing the causes of pneumonia in the elderly, a domain in which he would become the world's expert. And I was along for the ride. I came to value a good sputum specimen that was not contaminated with saliva as much as I valued gold.

I became Steve's shadow. I worked long hours in the library looking up references, painfully composing the first draft of a manuscript that he would then take and revise and hand back to me for further work.

I took Steve's rationale for why he had gone into ID as a specialty and made it my own. Infectious diseases, he said, was the one discipline where cure was common. In the battle of man against microbe, man was winning. Astute diagnosis was rewarded by a return to perfect health. Death from infection used to be common on bone-marrow-transplant wards and on leukemia wards. Now, he pointed out, with newer, more powerful antibiotics, better diagnostic tools, and a new understanding of immunology, ID physicians were getting the upper hand.

But I also had a selfish reason for picking infectious diseases. Most medical residents flocked to cardiology or gastroenterology or pulmonary medicine—specialties rich in invasive procedures (and therefore very lucrative). Fellowships in these areas were very competitive. Unlike the internship year (where foreign graduates were in much demand and were critical to the survival of many inner-city hospitals), both foreign and American medical graduates were competing for the limited number of fellowship slots across the country.

Comparatively few people went into ID. My chances of going to a top-notch university to train were best if I opted to specialize in ID.

Steve was delighted when I told him my decision. We mapped out a strategy: I would apply for a fellowship in infectious diseases at Boston City Hospital as well as at Yale, Tufts, Stanford, and San Francisco General Hospital. We hoped that Steve's strong letter of recommendation, as well as the three scientific papers I had now published, would erase my foreignness.

When, after my round of interviews, William McCabe, the chief of Infectious Diseases at Boston City Hospital and a legend in the field, called me and offered me a position, preempting the other places, I jumped at it.

My first days in Boston were anxious and disorienting. When I was on call, I had to cover three hospitals: the Veterans Hospital in Jamaica Plain, Boston City Hospital, and University Hospital, both in the South End. Each hospital had its own protocol for parking, for where the patients' charts were kept, for where you could safely leave your things without being ripped off, for the format of the consultation.

The first weekend I was on call, I was summoned to Boston City Hospital to see a gay male with fever and pneumonia.

This would be my first patient with possible AIDS, my first encounter to my knowledge with a gay patient. It was July of 1983. I had read the burgeoning literature on AIDS and told myself I should not agonize over my own safety. The virus seemed to spread in the manner of hepatitis B: by body fluids and blood. None of the doctors in San Francisco and New York who had taken care of scores of patients with AIDS had as yet contracted it. On the other hand, the incubation period and the asymptomatic phase of the disease could be very long. Still, simply examining the patient did not call for gloves or any other precaution.

I was excited and a little nervous.

Osler, the dean of American medicine who had died in the early part of this century, said that to study medicine without textbooks was to go to sea without charts. But to study medicine without patients was to not go to sea at all.

I was ready to test the waters.

I found parking near the Thorndike Building. A female physician was behind me as I walked down one of the dark, dingy tunnels that ran under Boston City Hospital and connected the different buildings. We both flattened ourselves against the wall as the clatter of an eccentric wheel and a rattly frame grew louder behind us. An electric cart brushed closer to me than I would have liked. It pulled two wagons of laundry. Only the back of the driver's Afro was visible. I could smell the ammoniacal odor of soiled linen mingling with the tunnel's faint reek of wet insulation from the pipes overhead.

We rounded a corner and came to a dead end at an incinerator. The doctor behind me laughed. She introduced herself as a new nephrology fellow. She confessed that she had been following me, hoping that I knew where I was going. As we backtracked to safety, we talked about the energy we were expending trying to look unfazed in this new and intimidating environment.

The medical wards were in the oldest section of Boston City Hospital. The stairs were uneven and wire mesh extended up six floors to enclose the stairwell and keep anyone from jumping over the banister. The bottom of the stairwell was dirty, dusty, and littered with cigarette butts that had been pushed through the chicken wire from the floors above.

I found Tony Cappellucci's room. An "isolation" sticker on his door warned of the need for "blood and body fluid precautions."

The rooms in the older part of Boston City Hospital were not known for being bright and airy; this room was no exception. The drawn curtains left the room pitch dark. There were two beds in the room. I could make out that one bed was empty and a figure was curled up in the second.

When I approached, a pair of close-set eyes looked at me with suspicion from behind a purdah of sorts: he had coiled the bedsheet around his head and across his face.

I introduced myself and Tony gradually emerged from the bedclothes, shielding his eyes as I drew back the curtain. Tony was in his twenties. He had close-cropped blond hair except at the back where he had grown it out. He was about five foot six and had the compact appearance of a gymnast.

His face was pockmarked with acne and his teeth were in poor repair; I remember his nails were grubby and the room had a stifling, old-socks odor to it.

His tone was defensive and combative. He said he had been visiting Boston from New York when he fell ill. He was irritated with the treatment he was getting and commented on how much better things were at Bellevue.

"I *told* them I was gay," he said. "I was up front about it. And so I'm being treated like a leper. As if I have AIDS. I don't have AIDS, do I?"

I promised him I would try to answer that after I had a chance to go over him thoroughly. Certainly there was nothing to warrant that diagnosis thus far.

The physicians and nurses had treated him well; his present mood was a result of a trip back from radiology, which in Boston City Hospital required a journey through the tunnels. The male attendants from the transport service who took him to radiology and back had worn gloves and masks and grumbled their displeasure at being pressed into this service. As far as they were concerned he had AIDS.

Fever and a nagging cough that had gone on for three days had brought him to the hospital. His chest X-ray had been suspicious for pneumonia in the base of the left lung. His arterial blood gases showed his blood oxygen to be quite normal, a finding against his having *Pneumocystis carinii*. He had noted lymph node enlargement all over his body for a year now, for which he was being followed at Bellevue. "Before I came to Boston, I was fine," he said, as if this illness was yet more evidence of the city's shortcomings.

He told me he had contracted rectal gonorrhea twice before, as well as venereal warts and syphilis. He knew people who had died of AIDS.

I examined him carefully. There were white patches of thrush in his mouth and moderate enlargement of the lymph nodes in his armpits and groin. I could detect a few crackles in the base of his left lung. His genitalia were circumcised and normal. He had a small venereal wart around his anus that he was unaware of. I searched his skin carefully, looking for the purple, violaceous lesions of Kaposi's sarcoma. I found none. I asked him if anyone had ever told him what the two coin-shaped corrugated skin lesions were on his abdomen, exactly six inches below his nipples on either side. They were brown and barely noticeable.

"These?" he asked, scrunching his head down to peek, looking worried. "I've had them forever."

"They're accessory nipples."

"What? You're kidding!"

"They're very common. This line from your nipples down to your pelvis is the mammary line. Embryologically, mammary glands develop in mammals along this line. Almost any skin blemish you see along this line is an accessory nipple. In your case there isn't any doubt about it because they are quite symmetrical, and look: they have the shape of an areola with a tiny nipple in the center."

"Damn! Do you suppose they are sensitive?" I said I had no idea.

I took a specimen of his sputum to stain and look at under the microscope, leaving him to continue his study of his accessory nipples. The sputum showed many white blood cells in it and a predominance of purple, lancet-shaped bacteria. His pneumonia was being caused by a bacterium—the pneumococcus. The pneumococcus is the commonest cause of pneumonia in people without AIDS. Osler had spoken of it as "the captain of the men of death, the old man's friend."

I telephoned my attending physician, discussed my findings, and we agreed on what we would recommend to the house staff.

I came back to Tony's room to answer his, Do I have AIDS? question.

As I write this, it is difficult to imagine that unreal time, 1983, in the history of AIDS. Not only did we not know what caused AIDS, there was no test to say who did and who did not have the mysterious disease.

The best that doctors across the country could do was to agree on a "definition" to ensure that everyone was talking about the same entity: if one was previously healthy and, for no obvious reason, developed an infection with an organism like *Pneumocystis* or else developed Kaposi's sarcoma, one had acquired immune deficiency syndrome. AIDS.

(After HIV was discovered to be the cause of AIDS, it made sense to discard the cumbersome appellation "AIDS." We could simply say "mild," "moderate," or "severe" HIV infection. But the metaphor of AIDS is so powerful, it appears impossible to eradicate the term. Eligibility for Medicaid and Supplemental Security Income revolve around the definition.)

I was able to tell Tony that he did not have AIDS. On the chart I wrote that he did not "fulfill" the definition. His pneumonia did not look like *Pneumocystis carinii* pneumonia. He was very pleased to hear this and shook my hand vigorously.

What I didn't tell Tony was that his lymph node enlargement and the thrush in his mouth suggested that he might be infected with the agent—whatever it was—that caused AIDS. There was mounting evidence that young men like Tony who had the risk factors—in his case, unprotected anal intercourse—and who had lymph node enlargement, often evolved into full-blown AIDS. I had a feeling he knew this already.

I never saw Tony again. As I write this, I have little doubt that Tony was infected with HIV. And that he is dead now.

Tony, my first gay patient, had been quite pleasant after he got past his initial hostility and annoyance. In the ensuing two years in Boston, I saw a steady increase in the number of AIDS cases presenting to the Boston University hospitals. Not the vast numbers that were being seen in New York or San Francisco or even at the New England Deaconess Hospital where many of the gay men in Boston seemed to go. Still, we were seeing enough patients to accumulate experience with AIDS and to develop some confidence in predicting what certain symptoms meant. At Boston City Hospital, we saw mostly Haitians and intravenous drug users. At the Boston VA we saw intravenous drug users and gay men in equal proportions. At University Hospital we saw predominantly gay men but not in any significant numbers; University Hospital seemed anxious not to develop a reputation like the Deaconess that would attract droves of persons with AIDS to it.

Near the end of my training in Boston, Steve Berk, who was now chief of Medicine at the Mountain Home VA in Tennessee, offered me a staff position at the VA and an appointment as assistant professor at East Tennessee State University School of Medicine. About the same time I was made an offer of a junior faculty position at Boston University. The two jobs could not have been more different.

If I stayed in Boston, the pay would be no better than my fellowship stipend, and within a year I would be expected to generate most of my salary by writing and receiving grants. Basic or bench research and National Institutes of Health funding were the currency of success in Boston. Therefore I would spend ten or eleven months of the year in the labs—"protected time"—and just one or two months on the wards. Most academic departments in Boston were top-heavy with researchers. In Tennessee it would be the reverse: I would spend most of my time on the clinical wards with a small amount of protected time for research; the pay would be much better and not as tenuous.

Rajani, who had completed her M.B.A. in Tennessee, was now working with a commercial real estate company in Boston. She enjoyed her work and I was proud of what she had accomplished in her short time in America. But she was pregnant now and was planning to quit the workforce for an extended period so that she could have and enjoy our first child. We wrestled with the choices: Stay in Boston? Return to Tennessee and raise our baby in a safe, rural, pastoral setting?

Going from India to Johnson City, Tennessee, had been a bit of a culture shock for both of us: the Appalachian accents were twangier, more singsong than we could possibly have imagined. Not even reruns of "The Beverly Hillbillies" that we had watched in India prepared us for this. But that culture shock was a mere tremor compared with the shock of going from Tennessee to Boston. On a fellow's stipend in Boston, a roach-infested, third-floor walk-up in Brighton off Commonwealth Avenue was the best we could do. Break-ins were so common that every time I returned to the apartment, my gaze went quickly to the TV and stereo to see if they were still there.

Three years in Tennessee had gotten us used to making eye contact with people anywhere and automatically exchanging a "How you all doing?" or at least a nod. But in Boston, neighbors discouraged this sort of familiarity. The only time we spoke with ours was when a burglar in broad daylight knocked a hole in the neighbors' wall, reached through it to open the front door and then robbed them. The neighbors came to ask if we had seen or heard anything. We hadn't.

My academic ambitions had become less lofty. I had worked hard for two years developing an animal model of pneumonia. I had learned how to anesthetize a hamster and then slide a tiny hollow tube past the epiglottis, between the vocal cords and into the trachea—much like the intubation of a patient during a Code Blue. I would then shoot a dose of bacteria into the hamster's lung. At the end of a morning, thirty-two hamsters would be lined up flat on their backs, their paws in front of them, snoring, looking like a bunch of drunken soccer fans sleeping off a hangover. I sacrificed four hamsters a day, ground up their lungs, painstakingly counted the number of bacteria surviving and plotted a "clearance" curve for staphylococci. Each clearance experiment took one week. I did many clearance experiments. Later in my fellowship I began to work with macrophages, the lung scavenger cells, testing their ability to ingest bacteria in the test tube.

But my experimental results were slow in coming and it was a long time before I had enough data to publish a paper. And despite all my effort, I was merely scratching the surface of a biological system. Basic research had become so complex: no one cared if in a certain disease you discovered that some protein in the blood was either high or low. The question being asked was what *gene* was controlling this protein? And how quickly could you clone it? Science had gone molecular. An investment of a couple of years after fellowship training was necessary just to learn the *methodology* of molecular biology.

I accepted Steve's offer to return to Tennessee. Sorting out the real-time, real-world puzzles of living people seemed to be what I wanted. Steve would generously provide me with a lab and a technician so I could continue my hamster research. But I was returning to Tennessee to be a teacher and a clinician, not a researcher.

The impending arrival of our first child had changed our view of life. We wanted now to settle in one place for a while. We looked forward to returning to Appalachia; we were ready for a less frenetic existence in a corner of rural America that we loved.

Toward the end of my fellowship came the exciting news that Gallo and Montagnier (or Montagnier and Gallo depending on whom you believed—this too was part of the excitement: the personalities and the rivalries) had discovered that AIDS was caused by a virus: HIV.

A test to screen blood for HIV was rapidly developed, and it was confirmed that all those who had AIDS carried the virus in their bodies.

As more people were tested there came the sad confirmation that the Tony Cappelluccis of the world—people with minor symptoms of oral thrush or lymph node enlargement—were also infected with the virus. And even worse, many persons with no symptoms who appeared to be in perfect health but were either gay or intravenous drug users showed evidence that the virus was sitting silently in their immune system, biding its time. Safe-sex maxims and warnings about not sharing needles had come too late for many. The virus seemed to have saturated the population of urban gay men even as they became aware of its very existence.

Still, the mystery of *causation* had been solved.

Surely, the cure was just around the corner.

THE NINTH DIVE

GREG LOUGANIS WITH ERIC MARCUS

from Breaking the Surface

| 1995 |

The preliminaries were going off almost as well at the '88 Olympics as they had in 1984: Thirty-five divers from around the world were competing for one of twelve spots, and after eight dives, I was leading. Only three more dives and I'd be on my way to the finals and a chance at my third gold metal.

Several thousand people were packed into Seoul's Chamshil Pool, and the atmosphere was electric. As I waited at the bottom of the ladder for my turn, I went through the dive in my mind, visualizing each step and playing music in my head to the beat of the dive. Most of the time I dove to "If You Believe," from *The Wiz,* because of its message: "If you believe within your heart you'll know / That no one can change the path that you must go. Believe what you feel, and know you're right / Because the time will come around when you'll say it's yours."

Once the diver ahead of me was in the air, I climbed up the ladder to the 3-meter board. My next dive, the ninth, was a reverse two-and-a-half pike, usually one of my best dives. The crowd was still cheering the previous diver as I walked out onto the board and set the fulcrum, the movable bar you adjust to give the board more or less spring.

My dive was announced, and I walked to my starting point on the springboard, got into place, took a deep breath, and told myself to relax. I took the first step, the second step, the third step, and the fourth step, all to the beat of the music from *The Wiz* that only I could hear. On the fifth step, I swung my arms in a smooth arc and started bending into the hurdle, pushing the board down. As I pushed into the hurdle, I inhaled, reaching up with my arms straight over my head, bringing my right knee up toward my chest, and extending my left leg down toward the board. I listened to hear the board bounce once against the fulcrum, then a second time, and then came down on the board with both feet. I pushed down on the board with the full weight of my body, bending into the board in preparation for the takeoff.

To take off from the board, I reached up with my arms and pushed off with my legs at the same time, allowing the board to kick me into the air. As I pulled my shoulders back a bit and pushed my hips up and out, I could feel right away that my weight was back in the direction of the board, which meant that I was going to be close. When that happens, you worry about hitting your hands on the board, so my concern as I went through the dive was to get my hands out of the way.

Ron O'Brien, my coach, was standing at the side of the pool farthest from the board. From the moment I pushed off, he later said, he could feel in his stomach that I was going to hit, but he didn't know whether I was going to tick my head, hit my head, tick my hand, or break my hand. He said he hoped I was going to slide by the board like I'd done in the past when I was close. I'm usually able to make split-second adjustments to get out of the way of the board when I know I'm going to be close.

So, as I brought my legs up into the pike position to initiate the somersault, I exhaled and held my breath. Spinning through the somersaults, I saw the water once, then a second time, and then I came out of the pike position with my arms wide so I wouldn't hit my hands on the board. I thought I'd cleared it, but I heard this big hollow thud and felt myself landing in the water in a really strange way.

I was underwater before I realized that I'd hit my head. Once I did, the first emotion I felt was embarrassment: This was the Olympics, I was a gold medalist, and here I'd gone and hit my damn head on the board. I'd had accidents before, but never at the Olympics.

While I was still underwater, I tried to figure out how to get out of the pool without anybody seeing me. I guess I was in shock. Ron ran to the side of the pool where the diving board was, watching to see if I was coming up. If I wasn't coming up, he was going in after me. Ron's wife, Mary Jane, was up in the stands holding her breath. She knew better than most people how bad that thud could be. She also knew that a springboard is pretty forgiving compared to a 10-meter platform. Nine years before, I'd hit my head on a platform in Tbilisi, in the former Soviet Union, and was knocked out for twenty minutes: They had to pull me out of the water. I had a concussion and had to drop out of the competition, but I was lucky I wasn't killled.

So there I was underwater in Seoul, humiliated. I couldn't stay under there forever, so I came up and started swimming to the side of the pool. Looking out into the crowd and at the people standing on the deck, I could tell that everyone was shocked and concerned. They could probably tell that I was upset, too. My first reaction was to get angry with myself for hitting the board—my first reaction is always to get angry with myself. But the anger passed quickly, because I was terrified about something that I'm sure never crossed the mind of anyone in that hall.

As I swam toward the side of the pool, all kinds of thoughts raced through my head: What if I cut my scalp? What if I'm bleeding? Is there blood in the pool? What happens if I get blood on someone? In normal circumstances that wouldn't have been such a big deal, but these were anything but normal circumstances. I was in a total panic that I might cause someone else harm. It was sheer terror. I didn't even pause to think that I might be badly injured. But whatever was going through my mind, I had to get out of the pool.

As I climbed onto the deck, I felt around my scalp to see if I was bleeding. Ron was coming toward me, but before he got to me, one of the other coaches, Jan Snick, started digging through my hair to see if I had a cut. I held up my hand to get him to back off and to keep everyone else away. I was angry at Jan for trying to help, but he wasn't doing anything unusual. He just didn't know that he was dealing with HIV. I didn't want anyone to touch me—except Ron, who knew the whole story.

Several months before, I'd finally gotten my courage up to go for an HIV test. My lover of six years had already been diagnosed with AIDS; it wasn't surprising that I was HIV-positive. But hitting my head on the diving board was a complete shock. I know it must seem irresponsible now, but I hadn't considered the possibility that I could injure myself in that way. Since my diagnosis, I'd focused entirely on my training for the Olympics and was in almost complete denial about my HIV status. Now, having hit my head, there was no denying the terrifying truth.

Ron got to me, and he put his arm around me and walked me out of the pool area toward a waiting room just beyond the pool. He asked me how I felt, if I was okay, trying to see if I was alert or not. I told him how embarrassed I was, and then, just as we were walking past where most of the divers and coaches were sitting in the stands, Ron saw a trickle of blood coming down the back of my neck. He used his hand to push it back up under my hairline and out of sight. Ron didn't want anyone to see it because he thought it would upset people even more if they saw I was bleeding. But there was also another reason: The Chinese divers and coaches, who were very competitive with me, were standing right there, and he was sure they were thinking, Here's our chance now. Ron always wanted the Chinese to think I had ice water in my veins.

We got to the waiting room and the team doctor, Jim Puffer, met us there. I sat down on the edge of a massage table, and Dr. Puffer started digging around, trying to find the wound.

So many things went through my mind. One stream of thought was: Did I get any blood in the pool? Is the filtration system working? Did they allow ample time before the next diver dove? Did any blood spill on the pool deck? Could I have infected Ron? Then I worried about Dr. Puffer, who wasn't wearing gloves. Was I putting Dr. Puffer in danger?

I was too panicked in that moment to think clearly, but eventually I had a chance to think it through, and then later I talked with Dr. Anthony Fauci, who is the director of the National Institute of Allergy and Infectious Diseases and one of the nation's foremost experts on HIV and AIDS. Dr. Fauci explained: "Even if you started bleeding before you got out of the pool, there would have been an extraordinarily low risk of infecting anyone who used the pool following your accident. There are two reasons for this. First, there's the profound dilutional effect—at most, there may have been a minuscule amount of blood in a pool filled with tens of thousands of gallons of water. Second, the chlorine in the pool would have killed the virus." I was relieved to learn that I hadn't put any of the other divers at risk.

The only people who were at any risk, it turns out, were those who came in direct contact with my blood, and according to Dr. Fauci, the risk was extremely small. He explained: "Even if Dr. Puffer had a syringe that contained some of your blood and accidentally injected himself beneath the skin, there would still only be a 0.3 percent chance of infection. In this case, Dr. Puffer was not using a syringe, but a [solid] needle, to stitch the wound, so if he had punctured his own skin, the risk would have been much lower than 0.3 percent. As far as Ron O'Brien and Dr. Puffer both coming in direct contact with your blood, the risk was also extremely low, but how low depends on a number of factors. If they got the blood on intact skin—in other words, they had no abrasions or cuts on their hands—then the risk was very, very low. In fact, there are no well-documented cases existing of somebody becoming infected from having HIV-infected blood splashed on intact skin. If there were an abrasion or a nick or a cut, that would increase the risk, but it would still be a small risk." Since 1988, both Ron and Dr. Puffer have been tested for HIV and both are negative.

Before we left for the '88 Olympics, I had debated telling Dr. Puffer about my HIV status. I realize that it was irresponsible for me not to inform him, but I didn't want him to have the burden of keeping such a difficult secret. We knew a lot of the same people, and I was afraid it might put him in a position to have to lie to somebody. I had entrusted only a handful of people with that information—Ron, my coach, and Tom, my lover, were the only two people at the Olympics who knew. And now I wanted to warn Dr. Puffer, but I was paralyzed.

Ron was standing beside the table where I was sitting, and I looked at him, and I broke down. I wanted to say something about the HIV, but all I could do was cry. Everything was all so mixed up at that point: the HIV, the shock and embarrassment of hitting my head, and an awful feeling that it was all over. The Olympics, I thought, were over for me.

Ron held me as I cried and said, "Greg, you have a wonderful career to look back on. You don't have to do this. You don't have to do anything. No matter what you decide, I'm behind you a hundred percent." Between sobs, I managed to say, "I got halves and zeros on that dive. I can't still be in the contest."

Ron knew I wasn't out of the running, and he was just trying to figure out if I was physically and emotionally up to going on. Actually, I had a strong enough lead when I hit the board to make it into the finals as long as I did reasonably well on the last two dives. Ron went out to check my standings and came back with the news that I was in fifth place. The top twelve divers make the finals. So it wasn't over as long as I had the strength to compete. Ron asked me what I wanted to do.

It was easier for me to focus on diving than it was to think about the possibility of having put Dr. Puffer in danger of contracting HIV. Diving had always been my refuge, and once again it gave me something to focus on in a moment of crisis: It was my way of escaping, just as it had always been.

Once I knew I was still in the running, I never considered giving up. I thought about my friend Ryan White, the teenager from Indiana who had become a national spokesman on the AIDS epidemic. I knew Ryan would never give up, and that gave me the extra push I needed. So I said to Ron, "We've worked too long and hard to get here. I'm not going to give up now."

LIGHTS, CAMERA . . . DEATH

ELINOR BURKETT

from The Gravest Show on Earth

| 1995 |

Teenagers hanging out on Washington Avenue pointed and stared as twenty-six-year-old Sean Sasser sauntered around Miami's South Beach. Twentysomethings on rollerblades—the terrors of the sidewalks—stopped to say hello. Strangers in restaurants sent waitresses over to ask for his autograph.

"How's Pedro?" everyone wanted to know.

Sean gritted his teeth and muttered, "Hanging in there."

The truth was that that moment in October 1994 his partner, Pedro Zamora, was lying in bed in a corner room at Mercy Hospital, paralyzed on his left side. He could no longer speak. He would no longer eat. Sometimes his friends and family could pull him out of his semiconscious state, but only with difficulty. Even then, when he opened his eyes and held on to the nearest hand, no one was entirely sure that Pedro knew where he was or who his visitors were. His physician said that only 10 percent of his brain was functioning.

The kids on rollerblades and in trendy cafés already knew the full details of Pedro's condition when they accosted Sean. Pedro's imminent demise was the lead story on the local news, complete with the kind of graphic that stations design for continuing coverage of an event. "Pedro's Final Battle," Channel 4, the NBC affiliate, called it. The accompanying photograph of his once devastatingly handsome visage bore no resemblance to the gaunt death mask Pedro's face had become.

Despite Pedro's ordeal, no one in a neighborhood where Sylvester Stallone and Sandra Bernhardt are regulars hesitated to pursue Sean. So what if Sean was in town for a wake and a funeral, not a day at the beach and a night posturing at the nation's hippest clubs? They could touch him, feel connected to a myth and go home and brag to their friends. Sean and Pedro weren't people, after all. They were stars. And this was the price they were paying for that stardom, a stardom based on Pedro's imminent death.

Pedro Zamora and Sean Sasser were America's first tragic romance of AIDS. Both men had spent years of their young lives trudging from classroom to classroom, from PTA meeting to political caucus warning young people of the dangers of AIDS. Pedro, a high school track star and honor student with a poise and sense of public duty decades beyond his years, got his start the afternoon he walked into the office of his high school counselor and suggested that Miami's Hialeah High School should begin AIDS education.

"That's a really good idea, Pedro," said the counselor, trying to be supportive of student initiative but unable to conceal entirely the condescension creeping into his voice. "But it's not necessary. We don't have that problem here."

Pedro, always polite and dignified, responded in a calm voice. "Yes, we do," he said. "I have it."

Sean's career as an AIDS educator began the day he was due to ship out for training in the U.S. Navy's nuclear program. He stopped by the recruitment office to pick up his file and board the bus for the airport. His papers weren't with those of the other men. The woman behind the desk found them in a different box and, with a pained look on her face, sent him into another room. "You're not eligible for enlistment," a medical officer told him sternly. "We found HIV in your blood."

Sean had been having sex with older men, but with the brash self-confidence of an adolescent who believes himself invulnerable to disaster, the bright young man—he was a student at the University of Chicago—he had never considered the possibility that he might become infected. The Detroit high school from which he had graduated in 1986 never bothered to mention AIDS in its sex education or health classes.

Once they had turned their personal tragedies into an opportunity for education, both Pedro and Sean drew honor and praise from the small communities of the AIDS-aware across the nation. Pedro spoke before the U.S. Congress. Sean was photographed by the celebrity photographer Annie Leibovitz. That portrait became an AIDS poster in San Francisco that read: "Testing HIV positive was a wake-up call for me. Today I have a clearer idea of who I am and what I want from life. I think everything will be okay. I have no plans of disappearing any time soon."

At some point along the way, Pedro and Sean also became commodities, in a process so subtle and seductive they could neither fully register nor resist it, a process that sometimes distorted or completely obscured their initial message.

Maybe that point came when MTV realized that an HIV-positive gay man might sell more Ikea furniture than just another nouveau clubby, and invited Pedro to join the rotating cast of the hip and glam station's *Real World*, a cross between a documentary and a soap opera, created by throwing seven people in their twenties into a house and chronicling their interactions and adventures. Pedro's courtship of Sean was filmed in full color and aired to an audience of 1.5 million viewers whose demographics made advertisers drool. His visits to schools were broadcast, as was his growing illness. When Pedro went to the doctor, MTV was in the examining room. When Pedro was diagnosed with pneumonia, MTV was in the hospital.

He was featured on the cover of *Poz* magazine, molded into a sexy symbol that HIV does not equal ugly. Before he fell ill, a modeling agency had been looking for the ideal product match. *Real World* aired Pedro and Sean's commitment ceremony—the best a Cuban refugee and an African-American from Detroit could manage in a country still unable to cope with the concept of two men marrying. After Pedro was hospitalized, agents and producers began planning the made-for-TV movie.

Pedro never had any money. After graduating from high school, he sold suits at Burdine's department store, then lived on a \$300-a-week stipend from Body Positive, a Miami AIDS resource center. When he arrived in San Francisco to begin filming *Real World*, his wallet was empty. His salary from MTV came in a lump sum at the end of his five-month contract.

He could hardly begin to spend it in the few months before he found himself dying in a bed at Mercy Hospital in Miami, and his growing celebrity brought benefits he could no longer enjoy. Mercy Hospital moved another patient out of the prime corner room on its AIDS wing to give their most famous patient the most commodious accommodations. President Bill Clinton called. The local archbishop, a fervent anti-homosexual zealot, dropped by. Mary Fisher, who barely knew the young man and whose distant affection for him was decidedly not returned, flew in from Washington. After coming out as HIV-positive at the Republican National Convention in 1992, she had fashioned herself a kind of Miss Congeniality of the AIDS pageant. This duty went along with the crown.

So many strangers called and stopped in for a chance to see a bona fide celebrity buckling under a big-time disease that the hospital had to give Pedro an alias. Middle school students who had heard Pedro's speeches pooled their lunch and video-game money to send to his trust fund. Hollywood dressed up in red ribbons and held a gala fund-raiser.

Curiously absent were the MTV cameras. The station would hardly air scenes of nurses changing Pedro's diapers hourly to remove the diarrhea that poured out of his body, or scenes of family members gasping and crying as Pedro suffered yet another set of convulsions. They would hardly have complemented his image as the nation's HIV poster boy, so his death seemed as melodramatically unreal as the final swoon of Marilyn Monroe.

Pedro Zamora, a shy kid who left Cuba on a trawler in 1980 and became the Person With AIDS that young America embraced, died on November 11, 1994, five years and one day after he learned he was infected with HIV. It marked the loss of an extraordinary individual, but not an end to his ruthless commodification.

Congresswoman Ileana Ros-Lehtinen took public credit for Pedro's deathbed reunion with his Cuban relatives. His physician, Dr. Corklin Steinhart, held yet another press conference, enjoying the best free advertising a doctor could imagine. Two of his MTV co-stars hired an agent to help them build mini-careers on the lecture circuit off their friendship with Pedro. Reverend Fred Phelps, a Baptist rabble-rouser who had been disavowed by most of his fellow fundamentalists, staged a protest at Pedro's memorial service. And millions of Americans cried, convinced that because they'd had a crush on Pedro, they had compassion for AIDS.

I guess I could say that I discovered Pedro Zamora in that strange way that Columbus discovered America or a Hollywood talent scout takes credit for the existence of a nubile, young starlet.

I learned about Pedro from a tip, the kind of lead that feeds hungry newspaper reporters in competitive markets. "Have I got a story for you," Joel Rapoport announced one Saturday afternoon in the fall of 1990. Joel was the city's most knowledgeable AIDS activist, but he was infamous for his hyperbole. That afternoon he outdid himself. A gorgeous young man—"and I mean GORGEOUS" Joel said—had joined the support group he attended at Body Positive, a resource center for people with HIV. He was a powerful speaker: composed, articulate, and funny. He was Cuban, just eighteen years old.

I'd been looking for a teenager with HIV to put a face and a family on the growing problem among south Florida's youth. No one in Miami was talking about the number of young adults turning up with AIDS—thus the number of adolescents being infected. Joel was sure he had found THE ONE.

The next day I waited anxiously on the patio of a café by the ocean, wondering if I'd be able to pick Joel's wunderkind out of the crowd of greased, oiled, and meticulously maintained bodies. A young man with perfectly chiseled features walked up the steps and glanced over the crowd. He was wearing a purple Izod shirt. His eyes were penetrating. Every head turned toward him. Perfect, I thought, already imagining the color photograph on the front page of the features section.

It was the beginning of the packaging of Pedro Zamora, and I plead guilty to a hand in it. A photographer from the newspaper adjusted Pedro's clothing and placed him in just the right light to capture both his beauty and his power. I crafted my lines carefully to make Pedro into a captivating Everykid. It wasn't hard. Even in his accented English, he knew what to say to reach out to an audience. He took to a camera like a pro.

I could never have imagined that I was helping to turn Pedro Zamora into a star. I could never have imagined that the person—the sweet boy who missed his mother desperately, who had long, intimate talks with his father, who found love just as death was beginning to find him—would get lost in the hype.

Pedro Zamora was hardly born for fame. No one from his decaying neighborhood on the outskirts of Havana had ever made it to national prominence, even on that island. And rags-to-riches, or rags-to-fame, stories are hardly the true-to-life fare of late-twentieth-century America.

He was just another anonymous immigrant among the 125,000 Cubans who were packed into yachts and trawlers in the spring of 1980 when Fidel Castro opened the port of Mariel and invited the island's "scum" to depart for capitalism's shores. Pedro's father, Hector, who worked in a warehouse, accepted the invitation for himself and his wife, Zoraida, for eight-year-old Pedro, fifteen-year-old Milagros, twelve-year-old Jesus, and their grandmother.

Pedro often said that May 30, 1980, the day of his journey, was the worst of his life, even worse than the day a nurse sat him down and told him he was HIV-positive. It wasn't just the press of thieves, rapists, and crazies who were his fellow passengers on the thirteen-hour trip to Key West on the *Cynthia D.* It was saying good-bye to the five brothers and sisters who stayed behind, to the familiar, to the warmth of enormous family dinners and parties and outings.

It will be all right, Hector had reassured his youngest. By next year Castro will be gone and we'll all be together again.

It never became all right. Castro didn't fall, in one year, in five, or ten. Pedro mastered English and became yet another of the thousands of Miami Cuban kids who translate the realities of America for their parents. They all delighted in the luxury of knowing that the supermarkets always had food on their shelves, but the breakup of the family was a gnawing pain. When Pedro's mother had one of her crying spells, it fell to her baby to dance with her.

Then, in the spring of 1983, the pretty mole that Hector had long admired on Zoraida's face began to change. In June she was diagnosed with cancer. Two years later, without cooking any more of her famous dinners, she was dead.

Four years later, Pedro received a letter asking him to call the Red Cross about the blood he'd donated during a drive at Hialeah High School. He ignored it. He received another letter. He ignored that as well. He finally screwed up his courage and went to the family doctor. He'd heard of AIDS; he vaguely remembered a lecture on the disease from when he was in seventh grade. But it seemed to have nothing to do with the lives of junior high school students in suburban Hialeah. He'd put the handout on AIDS with his other classroom notes and forgotten it.

He was stunned when the doctor told him the news, although he shouldn't have been. Soon after his mother's death, promiscuity became his escape from reality, and embraces from strangers became a sad substitute for hugs from his mother. In Pedro's case, the strangers were the older men he found in the bars and bathhouses that he used as refuges from grief.

An awareness of AIDS did not accompany him there. "I could never connect a face with the disease," he said in an interview just months after his diagnosis. "No one ever sat me down and talked about AIDS. Our parents and teachers told us to have safe sex, but no one ever explained to me how. If they had, maybe I wouldn't be in this situation now."

Several weeks later, Pedro delivered the news to his father. "I looked at my son, my beautiful son, and saw a corpse," said Hector Zamora, who had spent his entire time in the United States caring for his dying wife, worrying about his children in Cuba, and cutting grass, working construction, and struggling in factories. "I thought, why can't it be me. I'm old. I've lived my life. Please, God, let us trade places."

After his mother's death, Pedro had buried his sorrow in a frenzy of school activities. If he kept himself busy, he could sometimes forget his mother's death. By the time he turned thirteen, he was a star athlete and student—president of the science club, Student of the Month in the city of Hialeah, captain of the cross-country team, member of the honor society. The teachers loved him. The girls were crazy for those eyes that seemed both wise and incredibly sexy. He'd become the family's hope. Pedro would never dirty his hands with the manual labor that had kept the Zamoras going. He'd go to college and be a doctor, a lawyer, an executive.

By the time he received that fateful letter from the Red Cross, Pedro had adjusted to the loss of his mother. He was no longer spending his evenings looking for somebody, anybody, to give him affection.

But it was already too late. For Pedro, AIDS meant death, so he prepared himself for the end. Within four months, the seventeen-year-old had worked himself into such anxiety that he wound up in the hospital—not with any AIDS-related ailment but with shingles, from the stress.

By the end of his two-month hospital stay, he discovered an antidote to the stress and the despair—anger, "at the government for not caring, at people for not seeing us as real people with a real disease, at society for not teaching us anything about AIDS," he said.

Pedro never planned to leverage that anger, or his diagnosis, into celebrity status. He didn't make any plans at all. Things just seemed to happen to a boy who was extraordinarily handsome and couldn't abide ignorance. During summer school just before his graduation, Pedro sat in a classroom and heard one of those typical student discussions of gays. The word "faggot" cropped up. Pedro tensed. One boy bragged about gay bashing. Pedro exploded, although in the hushed tones his intensity always demanded.

"I'm gay," he announced. He began talking about his life as a gay man, about being HIV-positive. He didn't stop for the remaining four years of his life.

Pedro had no talent for the kind of righteous indignation that fueled most activists. Yelling simply wasn't his style. Talking was. He was acutely aware of his heavily accented English, of being an immigrant kid who'd lost his mother and his family, who'd been sexually abused as a young child and sexually used by forty-year-old men at the most vulnerable time in his life.

But when he opened his mouth to speak to journalists, elementary school students, even members of Congress, he was dazzling. "He never clears his throat, repeats the question, or employs any of the standard stalling-for-time tactics," said Hal Rubenstein, the *New York Times* reporter who interviewed him for *Poz* magazine in 1994. "His speech is devoid of hmms, huhs, let-me-thinks, and, sometimes, when he's really zooming, even breath."

Pedro was pulled into a vortex that overwhelmed him. At first the pull was merely local. Pedro would take time off from his job selling suits at Burdine's to talk to public school kids about HIV and AIDS. Warning them was both a mission and personal therapy. "The anger, the pain," he said. "I don't want anyone else to have to feel this way." After his story appeared in the *Miami Herald*, the demands on his time overwhelmed the suits and Pedro became a professional AIDS educator, receiving a salary from Body Positive to expose himself to public view. He was in constant demand at schools, synagogues, and churches. He spoke to civic groups, to businesses and their employees' children. Gradually, the requests began coming from farther afield, from northern Florida and Georgia, then Washington, D.C., and overseas.

He thought about going to school so he could learn to be a counselor for the dying, about creating some balance in his life so that he'd be more than "Pedro Zamora, wonder teen with AIDS." But the bookings kept coming, the honors rolled in. He was asked to appear before Congress. He was invited to give plenary addresses. The U.S. Public Health Service selected him as a poster boy, to deliver the national AIDS message.

For the most part, Pedro partly revelled in the celebrity status, as anyone his age would. He'd always wanted to meet President Jimmy Carter, the man who opened America to the young Cuban refugee; AIDS paved the way. He loved flying around the country, staying at fancy hotels and being cheered. But acutely aware that his immune system was deteriorating, he also fought desperately to find a way to fit the fragments together, to have a normal life like a normal young man. He tried to carve out time to watch *Star Trek* in the apartment he shared with his boyfriend Angel or spend time with his family. But there wasn't really any time. There was always another plane to catch, another speech to prepare, another interview to give. Time was running out, and racing around blurred that truth as effectively as promiscuous sex had blunted the reality of his mother's death.

Finally, in 1993 a new director at Body Positive tried to transform Pedro from a full-time speaker into a part-time clerk. He balked. That wasn't what he wanted to do, needed to do. He turned in his resignation. Lost and broke, Pedro tried the commercial lecture circuit. It wasn't his world. Then he heard that MTV's *Real World* was looking for new cast members. He was chosen from among the 30,000 other applicants. An articulate, handsome, HIV-positive gay man was almost too much to hope for on a program that thrived on the conflict bred by diversity.

"His message was, 'Look at me. I'm twenty-two years old, I look healthy, I look vibrant . . . but there's a killer lurking inside of me and it can come up and grab me at any moment,'" said Doug Herzog, MTV's executive vice president of programming and production. The drama was beyond MTV's wildest dreams. They even spiced it up some more by refusing to tell the cast members which one of them had HIV. The producers decided that the revelation, when it came, would look great on film.

When Pedro moved from Miami to the house on Russian Hill in San Francisco that MTV used as the real-life stage set for the program, he moved from one fantasyland to another. Life as Wonder Boy with AIDS became life as Wonder Boy with AIDS being filmed almost twenty-four hours a day.

Cameras followed him to his speaking engagements. They captured his clash with his roommate Puck, a scab-picking bike messenger who refused to eat with utensils. They were there on his first date with Sean Sasser. For five months Pedro enjoyed a love-hate relationship with the camera. He was a dyed-in-the-wool ham who turned on a magical electricity when the red light came on. But when he fell ill with pneumonia, taping became a nightmare. His mission was to project a positive image of having HIV—the image of living with the virus, not dying from it. He escaped to Sean's apartment for two weeks. But then it was back to the cameras, to the speaking engagements, to the pressures of being the perfect AIDS poster child.

When the filming wrapped up, Pedro flew to New York for an interview on the CBS morning show. He'd been complaining about headaches and promised Sean that he'd slow down. Like most twenty-two-year-olds, he wasn't much good at pacing himself. He had to visit his family in Miami, to confront their confusion about his marriage to Sean and his decision to move to San Francisco. He had a full booking of speaking engagements and offers from a modeling agency.

The night before his CBS interview, however, he was more than just stressed. His head was throbbing. He was strangely upset that he had to change rooms in the hotel, that his shirt wasn't pressed, and that the hotel laundry service was shut down for the night. He called Sean in California. "Cancel the interview," Sean told him. "Just tell them you're sick."

The next morning, Pedro didn't appear at CBS. He didn't call. He just disappeared. When he returned to the hotel, his room key wouldn't open the door. With uncommon aggressiveness he demanded that a cleaning woman let him into his room. She gave in to the request, and reported the incident. The hotel manager thought he was dealing with yet another weirdo and he called the police, who charged Pedro with trespassing. Finally an MTV producer showed up. "Look, he's Pedro Zamora, a guest in the hotel," he explained. Pedro had been trying to get into the wrong room. It seemed like an odd mistake, but mistakes happen, he figured. Then Pedro asked to make a phone call before leaving for the airport. He didn't come out of his room. When the MTV producer went in, he found Pedro sitting staring at the phone, unable to remember the number he wanted to call.

By the time he was admitted to St. Vincent's Hospital, he had no memory of anything that had happened—where he had gone in the morning, his altercation with the maid, his failed attempt to make a phone call. Something was seriously wrong. Doctors examined the confused young man, checked out his blood, and ran scans on his brain. They couldn't be sure, but they suspected that Pedro had two simultaneous brain infections.

Sean flew in from California. Toxoplasmosis would almost be good news, he knew, since it was relatively easily cured. But PML would be a disaster, the nightmare of every AIDS patient. A poorly understood viral infection of the brain, PML causes confusion and seizures, blindness, paralysis, and death. There is no effective treatment. There is no known cure.

One Monday morning a neurologist shaved the side of Pedro's head and stuck a needle deep into his brain. Pathologists examined the results of the biopsy. The PML diagnosis was confirmed.

Two days later, accompanied by Sean, his cousin Oscar, and another *Real World* cast member, Pedro flew home to Miami—to the bosom of a family that still saw him as their little boy, to the bosom of a community that still thought of him as their wonder teen.

At first, it was easy to maintain the illusion that Pedro would be OK. He still looked gorgeous. He wasn't wasted or feeble. He could still samba with his friends. He took walks with Sean through his family's neighborhood. But one night his friend Ernie came over at dinner time. Pedro looked intently at the piece of ham on his plate, then picked it up with his hands and began to chew it. "Do you want me to cut it up for you?" Ernie asked. "Oh—eh, no, *gracias*," Pedro answered, picking up the knife and fork he had forgotten. Another night his friends panicked when Pedro locked himself in the bathroom and wouldn't come out. They agonized over his apparent anger, not realizing that their friend had forgotten how to unlock the door.

As Pedro became increasingly helpless, he became increasingly dependent, and the fight for control was waged. His old friends wanted to surround him; his new friends from MTV flew in from California. His family wanted him back in their nest; Sean wanted to lie next to him, to enfold him in his arms. The family spoke little or no English; Sean spoke no Spanish at all. One day Pedro's hand began to swell from the IV dripping into his vein. His sister Milagros removed his wedding ring. Sean never saw it again.

Pedro's speaking schedule had been planned for months before he fell ill. Judd Wineck, another member of the *Real World* cast, replaced him. He didn't speak about AIDS. He couldn't. He spoke about Pedro. While he lay dying, there was yet another AIDS benefit at a fancy Miami Beach restaurant. Pedro was the star—in absentia. His friend Alex was asked to speak. Members of the *Real World* cast were called up to the stage. No AIDS activist talked about Pedro's work. Sean sat, virtually unnoticed, in the audience.

During those last steamy days of fall in Miami, Sean Sasser lived suspended between the reality of the death watch over Pedro's withering body and the fantasyland of chic cafés and sleek bodies on Miami Beach, where he was staying. As he moved back and forth between the two, he was haunted by a distant image, a flashback to his last speaking engagement in a middle school in San Francisco. He'd told his story, yet again, about studying at the University of Chicago, taking time off for a long trip to France and Italy, about joining the Army and testing positive. The kids recognized him from his bus shelter photograph and from his constant appearances on *Real World*.

One of the eighth graders sat in the back of the room and scowled. "I don't understand," the boy finally blurted out. "I thought you were trying to scare us about AIDS. Instead, you tell us about going to Europe and becoming television stars because of HIV. You make it seem so wonderful and glamorous."

Pedro had been dead nine days. The anger and grief were still raw as hundreds of friends and family, strangers who had heard him speak, and fans who'd fallen in love with the young man on *Real World* made their way to an old theater on Miami Beach's Lincoln Road Mall. MTV Latino had provided a stage manager and an audio system for the event. MTV footed most of the rest of the bill for the memorial service.

Nine months earlier Pedro had gone to the memorial service held for journalist Randy Shilts in San Francisco. It was his first view of the viciousness of Reverend Fred Phelps, whose mission was to expose the evil ways of people with AIDS. Phelps had a long history of picketing the funerals of AIDS patients with signs reading "Fags = Death" and harassing grieving families with letters calling their sons "filthy dead Sodomites." Pedro had been sickened at the sight of Phelps and the family members who always accompanied him parading in front of Glide Memorial Church with signs condemning the filthy face of fag evil. What kind of country is this? Pedro wondered. He hadn't been raised to that kind of hatred.

But the crowds and the passion, the energy of the protest and the tribute paid to Shilts moved the young man who still thought himself immortal. "That's what I want," he said in an offhand comment. A protest, not a solemn wake.

His best friend in Miami, Alex Escarano, had taken the comment literally and supervised the arrangements, because Sean, feeling snubbed and displaced by some members of Pedro's family, fled to a friend in New Orleans. Escarano would grant Pedro his final wish, or at least what he understood it to be. He began making the calls, spreading the word.

The bigwigs and bandleaders didn't need a special invitation. Patsy Fleming, President Clinton's new AIDS czar, flew in from Washington, along with the leaders of Washington's AIDS bureaucracy and other members of the AIDS social A-list. The *Real World* cast was there, along with its groupies. Fred Phelps came from Kansas.

Phelps stood outside the theater, behind police barricades. The filthy face of fag evil he protested that day belonged to Pedro Zamora. Community leaders intent on avoiding violence, and on demonstrating Gay America's moral superiority, wandered through the angry crowd. "Turn your back on him," they murmured. "It's more powerful not to say anything."

As Ivan Bernstein, a Miami AIDS activist, surveyed this pageant and all the pilgrims who had journeyed to it, he was struck by an infuriating realization: he was the only one on the mall that day who had spent hour after hour, night after night at Mercy Hospital, watching Pedro die. The rest of them knew Pedro in only the most heady of times, if they knew him at all.

Most of them hadn't known him, as Ivan had, when he began his passionate public speaking in Miami, with no aspirations for a glamorous makeover on national TV. Most of them hadn't seen him when the glamour ebbed and he lay catatonic on the brink of death. This service, Ivan fumed, was not about Pedro the activist or Pedro the casualty of a hideous disease. It was about Pedro the star.

Pedro hadn't been in the ground two weeks, and his history was already being rewritten, Ivan thought, burning.

"Fuck you," he screamed at the protesters in particular, but really at everyone. "Go fuck yourselves."

THESE WAVES OF DYING FRIENDS:
Gay Men, AIDS, and Multiple Loss

SIMON WATNEY

from Imagine Hope: AIDS and Gay Identity

| 1996 |

Cities are our gardens, with their stench
and contagion and rage, our memory, our
sepals that will not endure
these waves of dying friends
without a cry.

—MICHAEL LYNCH, 1989

A witness accomplishes things that were not intended.

—CZESLAW MILOSZ, 1991

INTRODUCTION: THEORIZING LOSS

Those with sharp eyes attending the Eighth International AIDS Conference in Amsterdam in June 1992 might have noticed, among the material promoting the many thousands of talks and papers, a small but significant cluster of posters and other presentations dealing with the growing experience of multiple loss among gay men (Amsterdam 1992). For example, from San Francisco, Michael Gorman and others reported on suicide as the leading cause of non-AIDS mortality in a cohort study of local men, regarding suicide in the dry, defensive language of the social sciences as one aspect of "the natural history of outcomes secondary to HIV itself" (Gorman *et al.* 1992). In other words, we are invited to distinguish between the *primary* medical symptoms of HIV infection, which are by now well established, and the *secondary* social symptoms caused by proximity to illness and death among one's friends and acquaintances on a constant, recurrent basis, over time.

A paper from Washington suggested from U.S. data that young men who have attempted suicide "engage in twice as many risk behaviours as those who have not attempted suicide" (Cunningham 1992). Another paper from Los Angeles identified a wide range of characteristics, understood to constitute what is now increasingly understood as "Multiple Loss Syndrome" (Jacoby Klein 1992). These include: feelings of numbness, anger, isolation, guilt, abandonment, disbelief, depression, etc.; inability to emote; the expression of feelings of loss, by pessimism, cynicism, fatalism, or insecurity; socially irresponsible behaviour with self-destructive overtones; withdrawal from support systems; preoccupation with one's own mortality; pathological grief symptoms; panic, self-doubt, loss of control; and resentment over never-ending memorial services. The "coping mechanisms" also recorded in the paper seem almost pitifully inadequate for the scale of suffering in the situations with which they are supposed to help individuals to cope. They include involvement with support systems; lighting a candle to represent loss; volunteering to help the less fortunate; attention to self-care, grooming, exercise, nutrition and so on; and finally establishing a "new place in life for the deceased."

Writing from the perspective of a gay man living with AIDS, Leon McKusick identified three distinct processes involved in Multiple Loss Syndrome (a term discussed below) (McKusick 1992). First, grief and bereavement, "feeling pain, disengaging from the dead and re-engaging with the living"; second, a process akin to Post-traumatic Stress Syndrome, involving either the intense re-experiencing of tragic events, or conversely, a protective dissociation, with symptoms of excessive coolness and numbing. Third, he describes burn-out, concluding on the subject of the need fully to feel and explore loss, in order to be able to readjust to the world of the living, and to redirect a sense of hope from the dead, as it were, to those who are still alive. This reinvestment involves new ideas, new people, a whole new start to life. It is thus implicit that mourning on such a constant and protracted scale constitutes a completely transformative personal experience, after which one will never again be the person one was "before."

Writing this article, and others, is for me a part of an ongoing process of mourning, and in turn part of the far wider attempt on the part of so many of my generation to "make sense" of what has happened to us (Watney 1994). This requires us to overcome reticence. Indeed, the strong feeling that one should not speak in public about questions of personal loss might be seen as one of the primary symptoms of multiple loss, whether or not one considers this a discrete, clinical syndrome. Here I want to explore some aspects of the ways in which multiple losses may be experienced, and to suggest that while distinct patterns of emotional and behavioural responses may indeed be established and classified, these do not necessarily lock together in any immediately apparent and uniform fashion. For example, the same scale of loss which may drive one gay man into workaholism and unsafe sex, may render another incapable of work or sex of any kind. Furthermore, such symptoms may change unpredictably over time. While there may at first sight seem to be some advantage in drawing an immediate parallel between the primary medical symptoms of acquired immune deficiency syndrome (AIDS), and the secondary socio-psychological symptoms of a closely associated Multiple Loss Syndrome, the analogy strikes me as initially misleading, and part of a wider contemporary tendency to conceptualize supposedly distinct syndromes (Air Hijack Victim Syndrome, Falklands War Syndrome), rather than considering and confronting death and disease as necessary aspects of the human condition. Neatly classifying our various responses to the AIDS crisis as a syndrome, we run the risk of finding yet another way *not* to talk about pain (Scarry 1985; Sedgwick 1993; Hacking 1995).

SEROPREVALENCE AND MULTIPLE LOSS

In Britain we are still in many respects in the "early stages" of the full-scale experience of high AIDS mortality rates. It is thus of some practical significance to consider multiple loss as an experience which will predictably sadly affect increasing numbers of gay men, and others, in the coming decade, in order to be able to plan and resource adequate service provision and other forms of community-based support for those in need. At the same time it is equally important not to exaggerate the scale of multiple loss in the United Kingdom, compared to countries such as the United States, Canada, or France, where HIV is far more widely prevalent among the various well-known risk groups, and where levels of immediate loss are already being experienced among gay men on a scale which we are, fortunately, most unlikely to experience in the United Kingdom.

Within the United Kingdom, the effects of AIDS-associated mortality have been overwhelmingly concentrated among gay men (King 1993). Thus, as of the end of 1993, 76 percent of all reported AIDS deaths had been of gay and bisexual men, a total of 4,291 fatalities. The next single largest number of deaths in any other social constituency was the 381 heterosexual women and men infected by "high risk" partners. These made up 7 percent of the total. In other words, in the United Kingdom HIV/AIDS have had an impact among gay and bisexual men which is incommensurate with the effects in other risk groups, let alone among heterosexuals (Public Health Laboratory Service AIDS Centre 1994). Of the 9,218 cases of AIDS diagnosed in the United Kingdom since the beginning of the epidemic, 7,334 resulted from unprotected sex between men, or 80 percent of the total figure (Public Health Laboratory Service AIDS Centre 1994). No less than 74 percent of these cases have been among gay and bisexual men aged between twenty-five and forty-four, and it is therefore in this group that we may also reasonably expect the experience of multiple loss to be most concentrated, bearing in mind that another 21 percent of HIV and AIDS cases have been among men over forty-five.

With some 75 percent of all British AIDS cases being in London, it is also clear that multiple loss is fundamentally an urban phenomenon, closely related to the networks of friendships established over many decades in the lives of gay men in London. Taking the North West Thames region of London alone, we may note that 840 men aged between fifteen and sixty-four died of AIDS in the years 1991–2, compared to fifty-four women (Ward and Hickman 1994). The great majority of these men were gay or bisexual, and it is within their immediate social environment that multiple loss is most frequently experienced, often by men living themselves with HIV or AIDS. It should, moreover, be understood that AIDS thus threatens to corrode the most fundamental level of social "belonging" in most gay men's lives, namely those bonds of friendship and shared personal histories that constitute our sense of gay identity. All too often it is imagined that gay identity functions in this crisis like some kind of magical prophylaxis, whereas in reality self-confidence and self-esteem may be radically undermined rather than strengthened by the prolonged experience of illness, suffering, and death all around one. For AIDS devours not only one's past, in the sense of ex-lovers and friends from one's earlier life, but also one's future, especially perhaps in the loss of so many of those younger friends who in happier times one might casually imagine as the friends of one's own middle and old age. That is, if you are not yourself infected. In this context I well remember the words of an old friend of mine, now in his late forties, while nursing his first lover (with whom he had lived for many years two decades ago) through his final illness in the early 1990s. Describing to colleagues at work within an academic institution that a "friend" was dying, he was met with little understanding or sympathy. "Friendship" among gay men is not frankly widely understood outside our own communities, just as the scale of our losses is rarely acknowledged by most heterosexuals, who seem often to prefer to imagine that HIV is some kind of "equal opportunities" virus, affecting everybody equally, as so much official AIDS education continues misleadingly to insist.

Thus, for example, we may note a widespread cultural concern about so-called killer viruses and their theoretical implications, in films such as *Outbreak*, and the writings of Richard Preston concerning the Ebola virus, while the actual, extensive impact of HIV among gay men is never publicly acknowledged, let alone regarded as tragic, or even regrettable (Preston 1995). Indeed, AIDS is frequently presented to heterosexuals as a "warning" of other potential threats in such a way that the direct impact of HIV itself is displaced or ignored. Hence it is still possible for a leading British medical journalist to write casually of HIV as a virus which is:

> not particularly infectious, but its delayed action combined with its transmission during the most compulsive human activity can cause the complacency and denial that make it such a great threat.
>
> (Connor 1995)

For most heterosexuals in the United Kingdom, HIV is indeed a most remote statistical possibility, and this is precisely why they are generally so ill-equipped to understand or comment upon the situation confronting gay men, as the third decade of the epidemic in our midst looms into sight. Thus throughout the extensive social scientific and popular medical literature of AIDS we may find frequent references to the supposed dangers of "denial", referring to the imagined refusal or inability of gay men to recognize the "realities" of the epidemic, and to avoid *all* possible risk of infection. By this logic, gay men are thus deemed personally responsible for contracting HIV, while at the same time there is no consideration whatsoever of the possibly contradictory impact the epidemic has had in our lives. Nor is there any consideration of the many years of irresponsible journalism which has repeatedly insisted that there is no association whatsoever between HIV and AIDS, and even in effect that there is no such thing as an "AIDS epidemic" at all (King 1993).

Rarely is there any understanding of the great difficulties facing gay men entering intimate personal relationships against the background of epidemic illness, which for many remains largely anecdotal and distant. Nor is there much interest in how we sustain our relationships over time, or the specific difficulties of ending relationships. So-called denial is sternly admonished, but there is rarely any question of how gay men manage to "get through" the epidemic, or any note of sorrow or loss concerning those who don't. "Complacency" is a marvellously convenient term for those who have not felt or exhibited the slightest concern for gay men's lives throughout the entire history of the epidemic. Writing of the 270,000 military fatalities among British armed service personnel in the Second World War, and the 60,000 civilians killed in air raids and so on, historian David Cannadine has observed that death in postwar, peacetime Britain tends to be thought of as "either general and in the future, or individual in the present" (Cannadine 1981). AIDS has been posed as a largely abstract, imaginary horror for most heterosexuals, and there has been little attempt to consider it "from the inside" as it were, as it affects those for whom HIV has long been a complex everyday reality, continually changing in its significance and meaning. Besides, "denial" is a singularly inappropriate and insensitive term with which to try to make sense of the wide range of ways in which fallible human beings may respond over time to the escalating prevalence of HIV and AIDS within a relatively small social constituency such as gay male society. Who is to say what the "reality" of HIV should be to a teenager "coming out" in 1996, or to an older gay man who may have already lost over forty personal friends and long-term acquaintances, who are likely to include many ex-lovers and ex–sexual partners who subsequently became "friends," with all the ordinary complexity the word implies. How is one supposed to live an ordinary, "healthy" gay life with the knowledge that up to 20 percent of one's community may already be infected, and that the worst years, in terms of deaths from AIDS, still lie ahead? It seems to me that these things are not currently being sufficiently discussed within the field of gay culture, from theatre and film to the gay press.

Such problems are exacerbated at a time when some gay intellectuals can still claim that AIDS is merely "one issue among many" facing gay men, as if questions of reducing HIV transmission, and dealing with illness and death on an unparalleled scale in modern times were somehow strictly comparable with such issues as anti-gay discrimination in public housing or in the workplace (Annetts and Thompson 1992). Such issues are of course of great importance, but they are not commensurate with AIDS. These same attitudes are also reflected in the fashionable Wanna-Be-Julie-Burchill school of so-called post-gay and anti-gay journalism, which significantly flourishes in publications such as *Time Out* and the *Independent* and the *Guardian* newspapers, which are only too predictably happy to publish "post-gay" or "queer" journalists attacking the very idea of gay collectivity, or community values of any kind. In an epidemic, such attitudes also amount to cultural symptoms of the crisis in our midst, complex displacements of anxiety, uncertainty, and so on. Such attitudes also usually stem from those who have happily been largely spared the full impact of disease and death in their immediate social environment, and for whom spurious comparisons between incommensurate issues may often form their own type of personal defence against an otherwise unbearable reality.

The challenge here is not so much that of dealing with "denial," imagined as a voluntary personal fault, as of meeting the dangers posed by the very psychological mechanisms that may serve to make life tolerable in the context of unevenly experienced illness, when the direct experience of asymptomatic HIV infection is far more common among gay men than that of death. Indeed, the crude social amnesia and exaggerated emotional detachment on the part of those gay men who complain that "too much" is said about AIDS are themselves probably best understood also as displaced cultural symptoms of the epidemic, as it unfolds in our midst. This unevenness of experience of *all* aspects of HIV/AIDS is one of the major characteristics of the situation in the United Kingdom, unlike that in countries with much higher levels of seroprevalence. Thus the probability of multiple loss may be roughly calculated from local seroprevalence rates as they translate unpredictably into the daily lived experience of individuals and groups. With approximately twelve thousand cases of AIDS in Britain up to mid-1995, and around six thousand deaths, it is impossible accurately to assess how many gay men are currently experiencing multiple loss, though it is certainly several thousand. To this figure should be added the many thousands who have many friends living at various stages of HIV infection and related pre-AIDS illness. As the epidemic develops in time we may thus detect a common narrative, involving the gradual multiple experience of HIV illness, and AIDS, prior to the experience of death on a large scale. It is thus of the greatest importance that we recognize the essentially *slow-motion* impact of the epidemic among gay and bisexual men, bearing in mind that the average rate of progression from HIV infection to symptomatic illness is ten years, with a further uncertain future involving many potential different sequences and combinations of illnesses in the lives of people with AIDS.

We should therefore expect widespread cumulative emotional distress from the largely unpredictable course of illness and death surrounding us. At the same time, we should recognize the wide disparity of the experience of illness, death, and mourning among gay men in Britain. Furthermore, it is statistically unlikely that younger gay men will have shared the same experience of illness and death as older gay men. This may serve to make death harder to talk about, and to share. In the coming decade, however, death will increasingly affect those moving through their twenties and into their thirties, as infected contemporaries sicken and die. It should be noted that for several years approximately 1,000 gay men annually are discovering that they are infected. Indeed, one reason for criticizing those who wilfully exaggerate the actual numbers of gay or homosexually active men in Britain is that exaggerations such as "one in ten" obscure our understanding of the likely future impact of the epidemic. While many of those who find themselves infected each year will not necessarily be cases of recent infection, it is none the less only too tragically clear that in the absence of more effective antiretroviral treatment drugs, a steady rate of symptomatic illness and death will remain dispersed among gay men for at least another twenty years. The cumulative effects of such terrible losses can hardly be imagined, which is precisely why we need good research at this stage of the epidemic, in order to be able to respond to future needs.

The steady death rate from AIDS among gay men is also likely to have important consequences for HIV education and prevention work, not least in relation to the growing potential for personal fatalism which the long-term experience of the epidemic may induce. And since illness and death are not evenly distributed among gay men, especially outside London, it is also likely that HIV and AIDS will remain largely theoretical for many gay men, whether or not they are actively involved in the social gay scene. Thus individuals experience the risk of HIV in very different ways, according to complex changing personal experience. For some this may result in feelings of magical invulnerability. For others it may conversely lead to the feeling that with so many of one's friends infected, or ill, or dead, one has no right to be alive and uninfected oneself. Future health-promotion campaigns will need carefully to monitor and evaluate the changing perceptions and experience of the epidemic in the gay community, since it is clear that no single strategy can be adequate. If gay men think that such work is already taking place on an adequate scale, they are sadly deluding themselves. Education which was effective at one stage of an epidemic may be irrelevant or even counterproductive at later stages. In this context, the likelihood that multiple loss may increase some gay men's potential vulnerability to HIV must be considered very seriously.

At the same time we may be confident that nothing will be clarified or adequately explained by those who claim there is a type of "death-wish" intrinsically connected to homosexual desire, and always of course conveniently unconscious (Guibert 1991; Gehler 1994). How gay men managed to survive before the advent of HIV is never of course considered by such fatalistic theories, which present illness and death as the direct by-products of individual or collective gay pathology, "problems" only for those who are innately "predisposed" to premature death. From such a perspective the entire personal impact of the epidemic among gay men can be largely, if not entirely, ignored, together with any serious consideration of ongoing HIV education or treatment research, since presumably nothing can be done to help the innately "predisposed" to protect themselves or one another. Such attitudes are frequently combined with the assertion that safer sex is really very simple and easy, and that vast amounts of well-researched, effective education work have been developed for and by gay men. Nothing could be further from the truth.

REPRESENTING LOSS: NEGOTIATING LIFE

No two deaths are ever the same. To live through the slow, and frequently painful, deaths of close friends, one after the other, and sometimes at the same time, over many years, is an experience for which nobody can be adequately prepared. For many of us, the epidemic has unfurled in more or less distinct stages, including stages in our experience of death. First, the early deaths, isolated, inexplicable, shocking, surrounded by mystery. These were the deaths that motivated many into HIV/AIDS-related work in the voluntary sector in the early and mid-1980s. Then deaths began to accumulate, though still scattered: sudden deaths, entirely unexpected deaths, as well as deaths which were fought long and hard, to the very last breath. Many now have quietly prayed for many friends to die. Many have marvelled at the strength of young hearts in prematurely aged and emaciated bodies. Deaths overlap. Sometimes the death of a comparative stranger is felt more deeply than that of an old flame. Names disappear, and surely few have time to honour all the anniversaries of deaths. Many weeks and even months would be packed with little else. Sometimes entire groups of friends are swallowed up as if they had never existed. Looking through old photos one becomes aware of a growing army of the dead. You learn to avoid certain streets, certain towns, certain cities. Often bars and clubs feel intolerably thick with ghosts, though they usually encourage one to have a good time. To avoid ghosts it is necessary to find new social haunts, but nowhere remains ghost-free for long. Then you learn to stop trying to avoid them, for their messages are important. I keep a kind of personal iconostasis where I work, with photographs of the living and the recently dead, and some now long-dead. We develop our own private rituals. There are some deaths, or dyings, one just cannot deal with. As a gay man in my mid-forties I find I am currently most deeply upset by the continued new infections and illness among younger friends and colleagues, from the generations which followed mine, which had been the generation of Gay Liberation in the early 1970s. They feel in a way like our children, and it sometimes seems that our most brilliant children were also the most vulnerable. Thus one also comes to mourn for futures that can never be, as much as for the "pre-AIDS" past, which now seems all but unimaginable—locked far away behind gates guarded by angels holding blazing torches. For many, drugs serve their efficient narcotic function, blocking off the intolerable—for a while.

And sometimes, when death has become more or less completely normal, and is almost taken for granted and continuous with everyday life, death may, as it were, "reach out" in ways that we have hardly begun to consider. Certainly morbidity and frankly self-destructive behaviour are likely to be frequent symptoms of cumulative loss. Some may indeed become wholly stupefied by the scale of death around them, while others painfully learn to adapt, make new friends, retain their sexual appetites, their self-confidence, and so on. As we move through the last years of the second decade of the epidemic, it is more apparent that the long-term emotional impact of HIV and AIDS is likely to be increasingly deeply felt among more gay men, as the direct impact of illness and death becomes inexorably wider, and the gaps in experience begin to narrow, like the isolated rings of ripples from individual raindrops on the surface of a pond, gradually overlapping as the rain sets in.

It is precisely in order to avoid fatalism and morbidity that we need to be thinking and talking more about death and dying in our communities at this stage of the epidemic. We have not chosen this terrible catastrophe. We do our best to control it. But it is there, and it is not going to vanish overnight. Somehow we have to come to be able to live with AIDS deaths without letting death overwhelm us. Alongside the struggles for effective health promotion, and better treatment drugs and services, we should also recognize the serious danger of widespread HIV/AIDS-associated clinical depression and other forms of mental illness throughout our communities. Bland talk about "burn-out" does not begin to do justice to the complexity of the issues involved, not the least of which concerns the ways in which cumulative loss may undermine gay identity, returning individuals to private hells of shame and loneliness from which we thought we had long since escaped. Yet our contemporary gay and "queer" culture seems to find it infinitely easier to deal with body-building than with soul-searching. Nor does the world of lesbian and gay politics seem to have anything much to say on these growing problems associated with cumulative loss in our communities, and has more or less surrendered the whole issue of "feelings" to a motley crew of New Age gurus, who doubtless provide some people with some help.

For example, I have been struck by the reading of a late Victorian prayer by Henry Scott Holland at three funerals or commemoration ceremonies I have attended in the past year:

> Death is nothing at all. I have only slipped away into the next room. I am I, and you are you. Whatever we were to each other, that we still are. . . . Put no difference in your tone, wear no forced air of solemnity or sorrow. . . . Why should I be out of mind because I am out of sight? I am waiting for you, for an interval, somewhere very near, just round the corner. All is well.
>
> (Scott Holland 1992)

I think this is an appalling prayer. I think it makes mourning impossible, because it so trivializes and sentimentalizes death. At each of the three occasions on which I heard it read, in relation to the lives of socially active, politically committed gay men I wanted to shout out loud: "*No*! Death is *not* 'nothing at all.' It's the pits, the worst. You are not who you were, as I am not who I was. You are dead, and I am devastated. All is not well at all. They are not just there having a quick smoke in 'the next room' before opening the door to come back in. And I will be as embarrassingly 'emotional' as I fucking well choose!" Providing only false consolation, the Scott Holland prayer (and the New Age culture that it typifies) strikes me as a positive barrier to mourning, and the slow, painful acceptance of loss that mourning involves, if it is not to turn into melancholia, unable to "cut off," unable to incorporate the dead person into one's new, changed, diminished life.

Thus the cultural challenge of adequately memorializing the dead is always intimately connected to the widely shared yet generally private, individual experience of grief and cumulative multiple loss. Yet what kind of memorials might we need? Certainly it would be a disaster if we were to drift into a kind of victim mentality, along the lines of vague and generally misleading metaphors of the Holocaust. Surely lesbian and gay culture already suffers from more than its share of "victim politics," with regular ritual shamings of the "impure," and so on, and its upside-down hierarchies of victimhood status. Yet with so much grief in our private lives, we need opportunities for its shared expression, as well as the need to celebrate and affirm the significance of the lives of those who have died. We may perhaps eventually be able to rescue something meaningful from the annual platitudes of World AIDS Day, but at present our only two major national memorializing projects are both imported traditions from the United States—the Candle-lit Vigil, and the UK Quilts Project, and while both have doubtless provided many with a means of public mourning, neither has seized the national imagination at the level of national cultural symbols. Indeed, it may well be that they were, as it were, "premature," arriving in Britain from a country which has experienced a vastly higher death rate from AIDS than the United Kingdom.

Perhaps some of our most effective memorials will be essentially local, like the light shop in New York's West Village, whose windows contain an ever-changing display of photographs and obituaries and personal tributes to local people who have recently died from AIDS, or like the images and texts by Derek Jarman which appeared in shop-windows up and down Old Compton Street in the heart of London's West End gay "village" the day after he died. A street that he had travelled almost daily for many decades now mourned his passing, and even today, more than two years later, there is still a shrine with fairy-lights behind the counter at his favourite Soho café, the Maison Bertaux which he, like me, had known since the 1960s, when it had been under the formidable rule of old Madame Bertaux herself, and next door there was a very proper hardware store, with neat, diligent apprentices. Derek would fight his way to the upstairs tea-room even after he could hardly walk (Watney 1994).

Many will by now be familiar with the types of secular funeral and commemorative ceremonies which are such a feature of the immediate social gay response to the epidemic. For example, I suddenly recall walking through West London two years ago behind a magnificent horse-drawn glass catafalque carrying an ex-lover to the crematorium, and the wonderful release in the chapel as Barbra Streisand belted out "Comin' in and out of Your Life," using our culture to affirm our lives and our feelings. Or, more recently, walking into another packed chapel, to the wonderfully appropriate and infinitely moving strains of Lou Reed's "Take a Walk on the Wild Side." In this context it is perhaps also worth considering the way in which so much recent techno music has, in effect, revivified and reconstructed so many of the gay disco "standards" and anthems of the pre-AIDS era as new re-mixes, insisting as it were on the unbroken continuities of pop music and dance culture. Such continuities affirm the underlying tenacity of gay culture, and its deeper will for life and happiness, in spite of the growing presence of death all around us.

In such circumstances we should probably at least try to observe the anniversaries of our friends, or else life itself can begin to seem unreal and devoid of value or purpose, because we have been unable to integrate our dead into our new, changed lives. Questions of spirituality are much in the air, and it seems important not to "give" this ground over wholly to purveyors of psychobabble, or to spurious New Age religiosity. One of the measures of the strength of our culture will be reflected in the ways we learn to take care of ourselves and of one another, emotionally, and in every other way. Gay culture and self-confidence is very young, and we have little to draw upon by way of models. Nor can it be sufficiently pointed out that nothing quite like this has ever happened before—the steady haemorrhaging of a significant percentage of a marginalized social constituency which is itself widely blamed for the disaster in its midst.

At a time when mental health care and service provision is under fire throughout the statutory sector and the National Health Service, existing institutions should recognize the strong likelihood of steadily increased demand for both emergency service provision and for long-term counselling, group work, and so on. For just as we were initially most at risk from HIV at the beginning of the AIDS crisis at a time when nobody knew HIV was out there, so today we are also most vulnerable to the long-term emotional and psychological consequences of living cheek by jowl with death in an epidemic of such duration, from all the varieties of clinical depression, to frankly suicidal behaviour. I can only conclude that it is our capacity to seize onto life and joy and happiness that will be most needed to carry us through the grim years ahead. We go clubbing on Friday night not out of "denial," but in order, among many other things, to mourn. This is the complex nature of urban gay life in the 1990s, and it is already inseparable from the epidemic in its midst. How we are to share all this, and come through, only time will tell.

REFERENCES

Amsterdam (1992) Eighth International AIDS Conference Abstracts, *Track D: Poster Social Impact and Responses,* D465.

Annetts, J. and Thompson, B. (1992) 'Dangerous activism', in K. Plummer, (Ed.) *Modern Homosexualities: Fragments of Lesbian and Gay Experience,* London: Routledge, pp. 227-36.

Cannadine, D. (1981) 'War and death, grief and mourning in modern Britain, in Joachim Whaley, (Ed.) *Mirrors of Mortality: Studies on the Social History of Death,* London: Europa, p. 238.

Connor, S. (1995) 'The terror is infectious', *Independent,* section two, London Thursday 20 April 1995, p. 31.

Cunningham, R. *et al.* (1992) 'AIDS risk behaviour: a new way of committing suicide?', Eighth International AIDS Conference, Amsterdam.

Gehler, M. (1994) *Adam et Yves: enquête chez les garçons,* Paris: Grasset.

Gorman, M. *et al.* (1992) 'Suicide as the leading cause of non AIDS mortality in a cohort of men in San Francisco', Eighth International AIDS Conference, Amsterdam.

Guibert, H. (1991) *To The Friend Who Did Not Save My Life,* London: Quartet.

Hacking, I. (1995) *Rewriting the Soul: Multiple Personality and the Sciences of Memory,* Princeton, NJ.

Jacoby Klein, S. (1992) 'AIDS related gay grief: an update including multiple loss syndrome', AIDS Project Los Angeles, Eighth International AIDS Conference, Amsterdam.

King, E. (1993) *Safety in Numbers: Safer Sex and Gay Men.* London: Cassell; New York: Routledge, 1994.

Lynch, M. (1989) 'Cry', *These Waves of Dying Friends,* New York, Contact Publications, p. 82.

McKusick, L. (1992) 'The epidemiology and psychology of multiple loss in our communities', session 61, Eighth International AIDS Conference, Amsterdam.

Milosz, C. (1991) *The Late Show,* BBC-2, Monday 25 November.

Preston, R. (1995) 'Back in the hot zone', *New Yorker,* 22 May, pp. 43-5.

Public Health Laboratory Service AIDS Centre (1994) *AIDS/HIV Quarterly Surveillance Tables,* 25, Data To End September.

Scarry, E. (1985) *The Body in Pain: The Making and Unmaking of the World,* Oxford: Oxford University Press.

Scott Holland, H. (1992) 'Death is nothing at all' in Liz Stewart (Ed.) *Daring to Speak Love's Name,* London Hamish Hamilton, pp. 141-2

Sedgwick, E.K. (1993) 'Epidemic of the will', *Tendencies,* Durham, NC, Duke University Press, pp. 130-43.

Ward, H. and Hickman, M. (1994) *The Epidemiology of AIDS and HIV in North West Thames,* London: Academic Department of Public Health, St Mary's Hospital Medical School.

Watney, S. (1994) 'Acts of memory', *Out Magazine, 15,* New York p. 92.

A VISION OF THE QUILT

CLEVE JONES AND JEFF DAWSON

from Stitching A Revolution: The Making of an Activist

| 2000 |

AIDS

After eight months on Maui I was back in the Castro. I had no job, no money, and was sleeping on a friend's couch (Jim Foster had taken me in). But I had a plan. I'd written a speech that I hoped would reignite the will to fight. I would give my speech at the candlelight march commemorating the day Harvey Milk and George Moscone had been shot. After that, who knows? I never really worried about career and fortune in those days. I was surviving, and that seemed quite a lot.

It's hard to communicate how awful it was in the fall of 1985. I'd left town out of my own fear and frustration. And somehow that sabbatical had been recuperative. Physically I felt fine. The shingles had left with only lingering tingles. And I'd gotten myself out of the coke and drinking routine thanks in part to Randy Shilts, an old friend from the Haight-Ashbury days. He, alone among my friends, had encouraged me to go to an AA meeting. It was hard as hell to attend those first meetings. Then, slowly, I broke the pattern and eventually learned to sleep without numbing myself with drink.

But there was something different in the San Francisco I returned to. Everyone seemed exhausted, almost fatalistic about AIDS. I understood that, certainly; but I also detected signs of hope within the despair. For one, the media had caught on to what was happening. Randy, who'd been a staff writer for the *Advocate*, was hired full-time by the *Chronicle* to write weekly AIDS columns, and he was extremely dogged in his attempts to puncture all the myths. There was a piece on the fallacy of AIDS being transmitted by mosquito bites, by tainted water, by waiters handling dinner plates. He went into AIDS wards and interviewed the nursing staff and doctors, and the truth was coming out.

Other newspapers followed his lead, and the public began to learn, if not always to accept, that this disease was not divine retribution. And other "points of light" flared up. Bobbi Campbell and his lover sat smiling on the cover of *Newsweek* in an article on the new disease—appearing shockingly alive and productive. There were respected physicians speaking out and against the panic. These were all important achievements, but still it was just so much whistling in the dark. We desperately needed an immediate fix, and it wasn't even on the horizon.

Seven years before, on the night of Harvey Milk's murder, I swore to myself that he would not be forgotten and began organizing a candlelight march to mark the day of his and Mayor Moscone's deaths. It had become a ritual, with thousands attending every year. A few days prior to the 1985 march, my friend Joseph Durant and I were walking the Castro handing out leaflets reminding people of the candlelight memorial. We stopped to get a slice at Marcello's Pizza and I picked up a *Chronicle*. The front-page headline was chilling: "1,000 San Franciscans Dead of AIDS." I'd known most of them from my work with the KS Foundation. Virtually every single one of them had lived within a ten-block radius of where we were standing at Castro and Market. When I walked up Eighteenth Street from Church to Eureka, I knew the ugly stories behind so many windows. Gregory died behind those blue curtains. Jimmy was diagnosed up that staircase in that office behind the venetian blinds. There was the house Alex got kicked out of when the landlord found an empty bottle of AZT in his trash can: "I'm sorry, we just can't take any chances." I wasn't losing just friends, but also all the familiar faces of the neighborhood—the bus drivers, clerks and mailmen, all the people we know in casual yet familiar ways. The entire Castro was populated by ghosts.

And yet, as I looked around the Castro with its charming hodgepodge of candy-colored Victorians, there were guys walking hand in hand, girls kissing each other hello, being successfully, freely, openly who they were. So much had been accomplished since the closeted days when the community met furtively in a back-alley culture. The Castro was a city within the city, an oasis and harbor for thousands who lived there and millions of gay men and lesbian women around the world for whom it symbolized freedom. And now, in what should have been its prime, it was withering.

Angrily, I turned to Joseph: "I wish we had a bulldozer, and if we could just level these buildings, raze Castro. . . . If this was just a graveyard with a thousand corpses lying in the sun, then people would look at it and they would understand and if they were human beings they'd have to respond." And Joseph, always the acid realist, told me I was the last optimist left standing: "Nobody cares, Cleve. This thing doesn't touch them at all."

November 27, 1985, the night of the memorial march, was cold and gray. As we waited for people to gather, Joseph and I handed out stacks of poster board and Magic Markers, and through the bullhorn I asked everyone to write down the name of a friend who'd been killed by AIDS. People were a little reluctant at first, but by the time the march began we had a few hundred placards. Most of the marchers just wrote first names, Tom or Bill or George; some of the signs said "My brother" or "My lover," and a few had the complete name—first, middle, and last—in bold block letters.

That Thanksgiving night we marched as we had for six years down Market Street to city hall, a sea of candles lighting up the night. One of the marchers asked me who else would be speaking this year and I said, "No one else. Just me. People are tired of long programs anyway." I was an angry, arrogant son of a bitch. The candles we'd been carrying were stumps by the time we'd gathered at Harvey Milk Memorial Plaza at city hall.

". . . We are here tonight to commemorate the deaths of Supervisor Harvey Milk and Mayor George Moscone, victims of an assassin's bullets seven years ago this very day . . ." I talked of Harvey and how even back then he was not really our first martyr, that we'd lost many people to murder and suicide and alcohol and AIDS. "Yes, Harvey was our first collective martyr, but now we have many more martyrs and now our numbers are diminished and many of us have been condemned to an early and painful death. But we are the lesbian women and gay men of San Francisco, and although we are again surrounded by uncertainty and despair, we are survivors and we shall survive again and the dream that was shared by Harvey Milk and George Moscone will go forward. . . ."

Then we moved down Market to the old federal building. At that time it housed the offices of Health and Human Services—not such an effective rallying point as city hall, but perfect for our next demonstration, one that turned out to have more impact than I ever imagined. Earlier in the day, Bill Paul, a professor at San Francisco State University, and I had hidden extension ladders and rolls of tape in the shrubbery around the building's base. As the federal building came into view, I ended the chanting ("Stop AIDS now! Stop AIDS now!") and explained through the bullhorn that we were going to plaster the facade with the posters inscribed with our dead. And that's what happened. The crowd surged forward, the ladders were set in place, and we crawled up three stories, covering the entire wall with a poster-board memorial.

It was a strange image. Just this uneven patchwork of white squares, each with handwritten names, some in script and some in block letters, all individual. We stared and read the names, recognizing too many. Staring upward, people remarked: "I went to school with him" . . . "I didn't know he was dead" . . . "I used to dance with him every Sunday at the I-Beam" . . . "We're from the same hometown" . . . "Is that our Bob?"

There was a deep yearning not only to find a way to grieve individually and together but also to find a voice that could be heard beyond our community, beyond our town. Standing in the drizzle, watching as the posters absorbed the rain and fluttered down to the pavement, I said to myself, *It looks like a quilt.* As I said the word *quilt,* I was flooded with memories of home and family and the warmth of a quilt when it was cold on a winter night.

And as I scanned the patchwork, I saw it—as if a Technicolor slide had fallen into place. Where before there had been a flaking gray wall, now there was a vivid picture and I could see quite clearly the National Mall, and the dome of Congress and a quilt spread out before it—a vision of incredible clarity.

I was gripped by the same terror and excitement that I'd felt standing before other large works commemorating other large issues. Not long ago I'd seen Christo's running fence in Sonoma County. It was a beautiful and moving sight, and I was struck by the grandeur of those vast expanses of shimmering opalescent fabric zigzagging up and down the golden hills. How it billowed in the breeze with the light playing off it, like a string of azure tall ships sailing on a golden sea. And there was the memory of Judy Chicago's *The Dinner Party*. This was a long table, maybe one hundred feet in length, with each place setting designed by a different artist. Both Christo and Judy Chicago had taken commonplace items, sheets drying on a line in his case, plates and utensils in hers, and by enlarging them had made the homely a dramatic, powerfully moving statement. It seemed an apt synthesis: individual quilts, collected together, could have the same immense impact.

When I told my friends what I'd seen, they were silent at first, and as I tried to explain it, they were dubious: "Cleve, don't you realize the logistics of doing something like that? Think of the difficulty of organizing thousands of queers!" But I knew there were plenty of angry queens with sewing machines. I wouldn't be working alone, I told my friends. Everyone understands the idea of a quilt. "But it's gruesome," they said.

That stopped me. Was a memorial morbid? Perhaps it was. And yet there is also a healing element to memorials. I thought of the Vietnam Veterans Memorial wall. I did not expect to be moved by it. I was influenced by the Quakers, who are suspicious of war memorials, which they believe tend to glorify war rather than speak to the horror of it. But I was overwhelmed by the simplicity of it, of that black mirrorlike wall and the power it had to draw people from all across America to find a beloved's name and touch it and see their face reflected in the polished marble and leave mementos.

So I thought about all these things and also about how quilting is viewed as a particularly American folk art. There was the quilting bee with its picture of generations working together, and the idea that quilts recapture history in bits of worn clothing, curtains, jackets—protective cloth. That it was women who did the sewing was an important element. At the time, HIV was seen as the product of aggressive gay male sexuality, and it seemed that the homey image and familial associations of a warm quilt would counter that.

The idea made so much sense on so many different levels. It was clear to me that the only way we could beat this was by acting together as a nation. Though gays and lesbians were winning political recognition in urban centers, without legitimate ties to the larger culture we'd always be marginalized. If we could somehow bridge that gap of age-old prejudice, there was hope that we could beat the disease by using a quilt as a symbol of solidarity, of family and community; there was hope that we could make a movement that would welcome people—men and women, gay or straight, of every age, race, faith, and background.

To this day, critics ignore one of the most powerful aspects of the Quilt. Any Quilt display, no matter how small or large, is filled with evidence of love—the love between gay men and the love we share with our lesbian sisters as well as love of family, father for son, mother for son, among siblings. Alongside this love, the individual quilts are filled with stories of homophobia and how we have triumphed over it. There's deep and abiding pain in letters attached to the quilts from parents bemoaning the fact that they didn't accept their dead son. And there's implacable anger in the blood-splashed quilts blaming President Reagan for ignoring the killing plague. All these messages are part of a memorial that knows no boundaries. We go to elementary schools, high schools, the Bible Belt of the Deep South, rural America, Catholic churches, synagogues, and wherever we unfold this fabric we tell the story of people who've died of AIDS.

That night, standing with those few men and women in the damp and dark, I saw a way out for all of us, a method of surmounting our fears and coming together in a collective memorial of our experience: all the sadness, rage, and anger; all the hope, all the dreams, the ambitions, the tragedy.

Eleven years later, this picture in my mind's eye became reality. But that night in November 1985 it was just an idea, and on the 8 Market bus up to the Castro, my friends Joseph Durant and Gilbert Baker and Joseph Canalli were unimpressed. Reagan will never let you do it, they said. Straight families won't join any cause with a bunch of San Francisco queers. It was late, they were tired. An AIDS quilt was a sweet idea, but it was morbid, corny, impossibly complicated. Give it up. But I was on fire with the vision. The idea made so much sense, in so many ways—the irony and truth of it. I couldn't get it out of my head.

THE ART OF LOSING

ANDREW SOLOMON

from Loss Within Loss: Artists in the Age of AIDS

| 2001 |

There is always the Mozart story out there: someone died young with a whole lifetime already achieved. Then there are the rest: those who slowly, over perhaps threescore years and ten, built up bodies of work informed by experience. Beethoven? If he'd died in his thirties, there would for all intents and purposes be no Beethoven. Verdi? My father used to shake his head with wonder when he told me how Verdi had composed *Falstaff* at the age of eighty. I loved the story of Verdi, because it seemed to me that the only way one could tolerate time was to believe that life was getting steadily better, to imagine growing rich in the mind even as the body went creaky. There are elements of youth that are hard for any of us to let go, but a true artist, I thought, achieved not only the immortality of his work, but also the persistent burgeoning of his genius. When I decided to be a writer, it was my idea to arrive at fulfillment simply by continuing myself indefinitely. I was a kid, and patient. There were so many days left. I was shocked when it turned out that there weren't necessarily so many days, that there might in fact be almost no time at all. All around me, artists whose enterprise required thousands of hours started dropping a hundred hours in. If you weren't Mozart, you had no chance; there would never be a *Falstaff* again. The brilliance of maturity was a thing of the past. I watched artists struggling to pack into their dense work not only the experience they had had but also the experiences they had once expected to have, and now wouldn't: people dying in the throes of their own potential. Nipped in the bud, many of these young sick people were bereft of voices before they knew what their voices were. It is all very well to mourn the distinguished men whose genius had manifested itself early, the ones interrupted halfway through; but I weep at the tomb of the unknown soldiers, the ones whose work, hardly begun, would with just a decade or two more have become something that we cannot imagine well enough to miss. We mourn the dinosaurs who perished in a sudden ice age, but our dead young artists are not pterodactyls; they are dragons whose would-be accomplishments never passed beyond the barrier of myth. We do not have enough information to begin to catalog the losses imposed on us. Writing panegyrics for individual artists whose names we know, we forget how much actually went with the acquired immunodeficiency syndrome. Here is the tragedy: we have no idea what passed. We are never told what might have been.

The crisis consumed us. We got used to living with fear, and its chill effect changed everything for us: how we lived, what we made, and, of course, how we loved. Though some remarkable art was inspired by the intensity of ever-present accumulating deaths, we mostly lost in the battle against fear. Terror freezes creativity, and none of us had the purchase on gladness that should be the essence of young work. Coming of age in AIDS's cold climate, I lived with a perpetual residual neuropathy, a compromised mind. There are so many people who would have been my friends if they had not died before I had a chance to meet them, much less love them. There are so many who would have inspired me in my own work and thoughts. There are so many who would have changed the world. Who can forgive these losses? How is it that they failed to break the heart of God, when they broke the hearts even of those among us who were spared the plague?

I first heard of AIDS (GRID at the time) in the office of my ophthalmologist, Dr. Maurice G. Poster, at 71 Park Avenue South on a Wednesday afternoon in 1981 at about 4:45. I was in eleventh grade, and had just decided to wear contact lenses instead of glasses, so it was before I cut my hair shorter and after I got my Frye boots. It was then I'd resolved that I wanted to be attractive, and it was indeed that quest for attractiveness (a quest whose object I had not yet defined to myself) that had led me to the waiting room of Dr. Poster, who specialized in soft contact lenses for people with sensitive eyes. I do not have a good visual memory, but I can recall in living sepia that waiting room, the other myopic people reading copies of *National*

Geographic, the nurses coming out from time to time to escort someone with dilated pupils to the doctor's room. I remember the brownish sofas and the yellowed lampshades and the hush that obtains in waiting rooms even when the patients are not particularly ill. I had leafed through several magazines and had haphazardly picked up a copy of *Time*. There, I happened on a brief description of a mysterious illness that killed Haitians and homosexuals.

The gay part didn't entirely surprise me. There were already so many bad things about being gay that the additional information that some people were dying from it seemed almost logical to me. On the other hand, I found the mortality of the Haitians somewhat bewildering. I couldn't think of any Haitians I knew; I'd had a protected liberal New York childhood and though I had black friends, they were all American blacks with approximately middle-class lives. My mother said, when I asked her later that day, that there were lots of Haitians in New York. She mentioned Mr. Leon (as we called him), who worked in the garage and drove a big Cadillac with a license plate that said MRLEON. I wondered whether Leon was going to disappear any time soon. Leon was in general grumpy and a little scary and I had always suspected that he did cultish voodoo with strangled chickens in some hidden part of the Bronx, but on good days he had a huge gold-toothed smile, and though he made me nervous, he was also the first person who ever called me Mr. Solomon (perhaps just because he'd forgotten my name, but when I was seven it made me feel wildly important). I had known him for a long time and I was sorry to think of him going. I was sorrier still about the gays of my life: my art history teacher and a pair of old family friends whom I thought of as surrogate uncles. Why would any illness be threatening Leon, Mr. Yates, and Willie and Elmer? The logic of it kept me up night after night, ruminating.

I remember wondering what I was going to do. I was not ready at the time to opt out of safe virginity. Still, it was a considerable disappointment that I would never be able to have sex with a man, though I had already sort of decided that I would never have sex with a man anyway, since gay men were social outcasts, sad figures, lonely, prone to undignified aging, childless, and null. I had, a few months earlier, been approached by a man (he told me his name was Dwayne, and showed me his credit card to prove it) while I was walking the family dog, and he had been unusually aggressive, taking my hand and putting it in his trousers. Dwayne lived in the big new building that had gone up on the corner of Seventy-second and Third. I had acutely wanted, for a few seconds at least, to go home with him, but I couldn't bear the fact that we might have to walk past the building where I lived and the doormen who knew me; and I knew that it would be complicated for the dog, who didn't really like new places, and that my parents would wonder what had happened to me, and that Dwayne might be a crazed ax-murderer. I left Dwayne and his pederastic ambitions on the corner. I hoped at that time that with practice and a little coaching, I would learn how to have sex with women, and I thought that *not* having sex with men was a good opening measure. I knew that women's sexuality scared me; I hoped that that would pass, as my childhood fear of the color orange had passed. I knew that I found men attractive, but I didn't find homosexuality itself attractive. Well, it was a puzzle. I'd perhaps never have sex at all; I had a spinster great-aunt who had lived a good life in the world, and it seemed to me that one could do worse than she had done. This illness described in the pages of *Time* seemed to me relatively insignificant in this grand scheme of things, though I felt awfully sad for Leon and Mr. Yates and Willie and Elmer.

In the months that followed, I scanned newspapers for mentions of this illness. It fascinated me and scared me, and it also seemed to add to the alluring madness and evil and sensuality and pleasure of men loving men. I thought about the people who had done forbidden things and were now paying the price, and the images were curiously erotic. Everything was even more forbidden, even more dangerous, even more fascinating than I had dared to suppose. I didn't know much about sexually transmitted diseases (then called venereal diseases), and the question of what bodily fluids mixed with what other bodily fluids under what circumstances was one that no one in the press had yet thought to ask. What I understood was simply the fatal consequence of difference, and I wondered what other illness might strike some other world within my world. The groups it affected might be as haphazard as the legionnaires who had suffered Legionnaire's Disease. I concentrated on fear of the erratic to distract myself from terror of the erotic.

The first time I had sex was later that year, in the Metropolitan Museum of Art, where I was a summer intern. By that time, I knew a lot more about venereal diseases, though much of it was vague and some of it was wrong. I had sex with one of the museum guards, in the medieval sculpture court, after the museum was closed. I wanted him to do the things he wanted to do to me, but I did not allow it. Instead of violating the limitations imposed by the possibility of disease, I violated the security regulations of the Metropolitan Museum of Art and maintained some bodily integrity. As I reached that eternally memorable, never-equaled release, I saw saints and angels gazing down on me with expressions of pure benevolence. I was suddenly terrified by this sculpture that had witnessed my giving way to temptation (Christ on his cross, in the far corner of the room, had resisted temptation—and was much admired for it, I knew). I pulled up my khakis and I ran from that place as though there were eight winds at my back.

During my undergraduate years, I prayed a lot. It was kind of an abstract notion for me, since I didn't really believe in God and hadn't grown up with anything much like faith. I prayed to my own future, that it not allow me to turn into one of those people who wore tight jeans and smoked cigarettes and were snidely girlish and died. I had a series of girlfriends with whom I didn't really have sex, though with one I felt excitement and with another I felt an adoration never equaled since. I had lots of gay friends, and I envied them their public freedom and wildness, though I never wanted to participate in it. My friendships were emotional, intellectual, monumental, physical in the embrace—but not sexual. I was safe against my will, so I was promiscuous in keeping with my yearning. Was promiscuity itself not a violation of the code of restraint and ethics to which AIDS made us subject? I often met men, really often, maybe six times a day, and had some kind of contact with them. I would let them suck me or feel me. Under duress, I would touch them. No fucking ever. I sucked once or twice but was too upset afterward. It was not about love or even about desire; the guys were often old or ugly or both. I expected that I would die from it, but I couldn't manage to believe that enough to change what I did.

I wondered what it would be like to be Brett, a year ahead of me in college, gay as Christmas, friends with James or Max (who were not really out of the closet but who were a lot closer to out than I was). Brett's mother was gay too, and they both had that strange and kind of ugly red hair. Brett was off having sex with everyone and taking drugs and talking about it. I found him vulgar and alarming and fascinating. He was a good singer and really cynical and came from Texas, and he had a garish limp-wristedness that didn't seem to bother him much. He tried to cheer on everyone whom he thought might be gay; he was a kind of mascot for gayness. I also wondered about what it would be like to be Hugh, haughty and imperious and beautiful, who was gay as though it were a birthright, who was so bitter, and so nasty, and who regarded the rest of us struggling with our identities as ludicrous and faintly embarrassing—if he regarded us at all. It was a time of wondering. I wondered, also, who would die. I retained with some pride an unconvincing facade of relatively unscathed asexuality.

Senior year, I went to see a sexual surrogate from the back-page ads of *New York* magazine because I wanted to practice having sex with girls and felt I should get the basics down before trying the experiment at home. That went better than I'd anticipated, and I kind of liked my surrogate, a blond Southern woman who eventually told me that she'd been a prostitute for a while but that her real thing was necrophilia. She told me I was pretty good and alive and reminded her of whoring days, but that a lot of the guys she met were "kind of like dead people but so *sweaty*. And a lot of them are gays who are just *not* going to manage to put it in me, no matter how much they want that." We talked about whether she was afraid of AIDS, and she said she assumed she'd been exposed and if she was gonna go she was just gonna go. We used condoms together, though who was being protected from what was never really clear. I was glad for what I'd learned with her, but I couldn't yet translate it into a convincing passion.

Shortly after the end of college, I told a good friend all about my sexual history and she had said, "Listen, it doesn't matter that much whether it's girls or boys. It *really* matters whether it's inside or outside, and whether it's with people you know or with total strangers. And it *really* matters whether it's *totally* safe." By the time I was in graduate school, there were tests for HIV; and you had to be crazy to take risks. My mother spoke only occasionally about grandchildren, about having a family, about all the ways she would have liked my sexuality to fall in line with hers. She spoke to me instead about how scary it was to be gay—scary now not only because one would grow old alone and unloved, but also because one would not grow old at all. I went to get a test and I expected bad news and I thought that I might deal with it by killing myself. When I heard I was negative, I thought they must have made a mistake; I'd been careful, but I'd been careful with two thousand people, and I couldn't see how that was careful. I went to a party in New York at around that time and met a friend of a friend, a cheery fellow, Nick, who was cute as a button. "I just thought you should know," another friend whispered, watching us flirt, "that he's positive." I was shocked—this guy was about twenty, and well educated, and if I had known enough so soon, hadn't he known enough too? A little later I heard that Brett had AIDS. I hadn't seen him in years, but I thanked whatever God I had once beseeched for freedom that I had been too repressed to do damage to myself when I had wanted so badly to do all the dangerous things. Time passed.

I was not in a gay world when I started living with Michael, my first serious boyfriend, a year later. I was not infected. He and I knew about the epidemic mostly from the press, since we had no ill friends. Nonetheless, AIDS was one of the dominant realities of our life. I took the test again and again to make sure about the results, and I waited for the bomb to go off.

Friends of mine had joined ACT UP. I was living in England then; I never went to ACT UP events, but I watched the protests happen.

I never once had sex with anyone the way I wanted. I never once did everything I wanted when and as I wanted. I was unacquainted with that reckless abandon that sounded like it had been so much fun a generation earlier. All the struggle to be frank and open about sexuality—and for what?

When Michael and I broke up, I was released back into peril. I remet a friend from grad school, Mark, some eight months later, the week my mother died. He was someone I'd almost slept with when I was in grad school, but at that time he'd been sharing an apartment with the guy with whom I was in love, and in my doe-eyed grad school way, I had chosen to pine after the roommate instead of seizing the moment with Mark. I'd afterward regretted the lost opportunity, since the roommate was repressed as all England, and Mark was hotly available. When I met Mark again, when my mother was newly dead and I wanted to die myself, I was exhilarated by his sexual energy. He lived on all the edges. He'd grown up in South Africa and was now attracted exclusively to inner-city black men, whom he picked up at night in neighborhoods where I was afraid to drive by day. He let them do anything to him. He was bruised with that, and he was also HIV-positive. I kind of wanted to be him.

I fell in love with a friend of his (I liked his friends), and we all went away for a weekend in Montauk. We were all the same out there until I dropped a glass in the bottom of our rowboat and Mark stepped on it. Blood came out of his foot and began to pool on the bottom of the boat. "Jump," he said to us. "Jump!" he said again, and I realized that there was broken glass all over the bottom of the boat, that I could have cut my foot too, that our bloods could have mixed. I jumped. So did the other guy. We swam as if there were piranhas in Long Island Sound. From the shore, we watched Mark picking up the pieces of broken glass and dumping them over the side of the boat. On the safe soft sand, I felt a wave of nausea. I hadn't thought to jump myself. If Mark hadn't told me to jump, I could have died. You needed a life preserver *in* the boat, not out of it.

I went out, then, with Talcott, and after that with Carolina. I loved these women and I loved the escape from everything I disliked about being gay. I loved too how far we were outside the bleak world of AIDS. But I felt as though I had abandoned my comrades—as though this route I was taking had become, ironically, the easy way out.

Brett died. I'd never liked him much and had never much respected him, and though I bore him no malice, I felt sorry more for friends who had been fond of him than for him. At the time, I thought he was the first of a cascade of losses, and that made me very sad. I involved myself in the cause. I gave money to all the AIDS charities. I marched. I worried about my friends, and about people who weren't even friends. I mourned for the tens of thousands dead. I read about and wrote about the breakdown of the community. I made friends with people who were ill and waited to be called on, waited to stand by their deathbeds. I knew a thousand people who were positive. I said, dramatically, when one of them was difficult, "But he's dying," and I thought that was true. I went on like that for years. I heard that this person had converted, or that one, and I reached out to them and tried to give comfort. I hoped that if I learned how they lived, I'd be able to live when my turn came, and that if I helped them as they died, I'd be able to die when it was my day to go. I gave money to AmFar and GMHC as a talisman against my own demise.

I remet Hugh, the haughty guy from college, and he was now an *artist* and keen to be friends. That chill austerity of his was gone. Hugh Steers. He joked, "Well, maybe HIV has made me nicer"—as though he didn't remember that he had been absolutely and deliberately and grandly the least nice person in the world. I thought it was tragic. I don't think he was a great artist, but his art became all of what he had learned from being ill. That slight sadistic superiority remained, mediated now by a touching empathy. I was glad and sorry to see that art, and to know that it was about a process never fully realized, though what fascinated me in Hugh was still the horrible way he had been rather than the poignant way he was, the alive part of him and not the dying part.

I went through a depression and had unprotected sex a bunch of times during it. Even at the bottom of my emotional pit, I had to be the top if I was being unsafe because to be unprotected and the bottom seemed too much like suicide. All I wanted was to tempt fate, to give the gods a chance to knock me off if they'd really decided I wasn't worth it. I gave them ample opportunity and I thought, when the depression cleared, that I'd be dying soon. Then I tested negative again. The routine for the test, the forms to fill out, the vial with the purple top into which my blood spurted, the waiting, the phone calls, the paralytic fear between giving the blood and getting the result—it was a commonplace of my life. I took a test every year or so. I lived in terror of the tests even when I knew there was nothing to fear, because they were to my mind still tests of how angry fate was on a given day. I lived a life of tempered passions, mostly. When I got into a relationship I always went in for an extra test. Unfathomably, I was always fine.

I never bothered with safe sex in relationships; that much real intimacy I insisted on having. I was terrified that I was going to make girlfriends ill with the illness I didn't have, that doctors told me I didn't have, but—who could be so sure? I was terrified of my fluids. I worried less with boyfriends; our risk seemed mutual, part of a covenant that neither party should have entered. I met Søren and had a grand romance for two years, until I walked in on him as he was having unsafe sex with a stranger. I broke his nose and his jaw with my bare hands, and, feral with rage, bit a chunk of flesh out of his cheek. That was all about AIDS. I remember all that rage, all that blood, drenching his clothes and mine. Then I met brilliant, cherry-lipped, full-bosomed Julie, and fell really in love, and nearly married her. Shortly after that plan failed, I met Ernö. Eventually, we moved in together. Later, he rediscovered God and took up the cause of Christ, renouncing the body that had given us both so much pleasure.

The losses for which I prepared myself never happened. My friends were too young or too cautious or too lucky. The positive guy, Nick, Mr. Cute-as-a-Button, eventually got on protease inhibitors and he's still cute as a button. Mark is doing fine. Mr. Yates is still teaching art history at my high school. Willie and Elmer eventually died in their eighties of old age. Leon is still working in my father's garage. The guys who were in on my house share one summer, my HIV-positive friends, are also on the meds of our time, and they look great. The rest of my crowd—well, they aren't even positive. If I hadn't been so cautious, so constantly restrained, would I have died? Would we all have died? Would it have been worth it, to forget ourselves entirely? In fantasy, it would have been worth it; in reality—who could even think it?

4

GOING GLOBAL

AIDS: THE AGONY OF AFRICA

MARK SCHOOFS

from The Village Voice

| 1999 |

THE VIRUS CREATES A GENERATION OF ORPHANS

November 3–9, 1999

Penhalonga, Zimbabwe—They didn't call Arthur Chinaka out of the classroom. The principal and Arthur's uncle Simon waited until the day's exams were done before breaking the news: Arthur's father, his body wracked with pneumonia, had finally died of AIDS. They were worried that Arthur would panic, but at seventeen years old, he didn't. He still had two days of tests, so while his father lay in the morgue, Arthur finished his exams. That happened in 1990. Then in 1992, Arthur's uncle Edward died of AIDS. In 1994, his uncle Richard died of AIDS. In 1996, his uncle Alex died of AIDS. All of them are buried on the homestead where they grew up and where their parents and Arthur still live, a collection of thatch-roofed huts in the mountains near Mutare, by Zimbabwe's border with Mozambique. But HIV hasn't finished with this family. In April, a fourth uncle lay coughing in his hut, and the virus had blinded Arthur's aunt Eunice, leaving her so thin and weak she couldn't walk without help. By September both were dead.

The most horrifying part of this story is that it is not unique. In Uganda, a business executive named Tonny, who asked that his last name not be used, lost two brothers and a sister to AIDS, while his wife lost her brother to the virus. In the rural hills of South Africa's KwaZulu Natal province,

Bonisile Ngema lost her son and daughter-in-law, so she tries to support her granddaughter and her own aged mother by selling potatoes. Her dead son was the breadwinner for the whole extended family, and now *she* feels like an orphan.

In the morgue of Zimbabwe's Parirenyatwa Hospital, head mortician Paul Tabvemhiri opens the door to the large cold room that holds cadavers. But it's impossible to walk in because so many bodies lie on the floor, wrapped in blankets from their deathbeds or dressed in the clothes they died in. Along the walls, corpses are packed two to a shelf. In a second cold-storage area, the shelves are narrower, so Tabvemhiri faces a grisly choice: He can stack the bodies on top of one another, which squishes the face and makes it hard for relatives to identify the body, or he can leave the cadavers out in the hall, unrefrigerated. He refuses to deform bodies, and so a pair of corpses lie outside on gurneys behind a curtain. The odor of decomposition is faint but clear.

Have they always had to leave bodies in the hall? "No, no, no," says Tabvemhiri, who has worked in the morgue since 1976. "Only in the last five or six years," which is when AIDS deaths here took off. Morgue records show that the number of cadavers has almost tripled since the start of Zimbabwe's epidemic, and there's been a change in *who* is dying: "The young ones," says Tabvemhiri, "are coming in bulk."

The wide crescent of east and southern Africa that sweeps down from Mount Kenya and around the Cape of Good Hope is the hardest-hit AIDS region in the world. Here, the virus is cutting down more and more of Africa's most energetic and productive people, adults aged fifteen to forty-nine. The slave trade also targeted people in their prime, killing or sending into bondage perhaps twenty-five million people. But that happened over four centuries. Only seventeen years have passed since AIDS was first found in Africa, on the shores of Lake Victoria, yet according to the Joint United Nations Programme on HIV/AIDS (UNAIDS), the virus has already killed more than eleven million sub-Saharan Africans. More than twenty-two million others are infected.

Only 10 percent of the world's population lives south of the Sahara, but the region is home to two-thirds of the world's HIV-positive people, and it has suffered more than 80 percent of all AIDS deaths. Last year, the combined wars in Africa killed 200,000 people. AIDS killed ten times that number. Indeed, more people succumbed to HIV last year than to any other cause of death on this continent, including malaria. And the carnage has only begun.

Unlike ebola or influenza, AIDS is a slow plague, gestating in individuals for five to ten years before killing them. Across east and southern Africa, more than 13 percent of adults are infected with HIV, according to UNAIDS. And in three countries, including Zimbabwe, more than a quarter of adults carry the virus. In some districts, the rates are even higher: In one study, a staggering 59 percent of women attending prenatal clinics in rural Beitbridge, Zimbabwe, tested HIV positive.

Life expectancy in more than a dozen African countries "will soon be seventeen years shorter because of AIDS—forty-seven years instead of sixty-four," says Callisto Madavo, the World Bank's vice president for Africa. HIV "is quite literally robbing Africa of a quarter of our lives."

In the West, meanwhile, the HIV death rate has dropped steeply thanks to powerful drug cocktails that keep the disease from progressing. These regimens must be taken for years, probably for life, and they can cost more than $10,000 per patient per year. Yet in many of the hardest-hit African countries, the total per capita health-care budget is less than $10.

Many people—in Africa as well as the West—shrug off this stark disparity, contending that it is also true for other diseases. But it isn't. Drugs for the world's major infectious killers—tuberculosis, malaria, and diarrheal diseases—have been subsidized by the international community for years, as have vaccines for childhood illnesses such as polio and measles. But even at discounted prices, the annual cost of putting every African with HIV on triple combination therapy would exceed $150 billion, so the world is letting a leading infectious killer for which treatment exists mow down millions.

That might be more palatable if there were a Marshall Plan for AIDS prevention to slow the virus's spread. But a recent study by UNAIDS and Harvard shows that in 1997 international donor countries devoted $150 million to AIDS prevention in Africa. That's less than the cost of the movie *Wild Wild West*.

Meanwhile, the epidemic is seeping into central and west Africa. More than a tenth of adults in Côte d'Ivoire are infected. Frightening increases have been documented in Yaoundé and Douala, the largest cities in Cameroon. And in Nigeria—the continent's most populous country—past military dictatorships let the AIDS control program wither, even while the prevalence of HIV has climbed to almost one in every twenty adults.

Quite simply, AIDS is on track to dwarf every catastrophe in Africa's recorded history. It is stunting development, threatening the economy, and transforming cultural traditions.

Epidemics are never merely biological. Even as HIV changes African society, it spreads by exploiting current cultural and economic conditions. "The epidemic gets real only in a context," says Elhadj Sy, head of UNAIDS's East and Southern Africa Team. "In Africa, people wake up in the morning and try to survive—but the way they do that often puts them at risk for infection." For example, men migrate to cities in search of jobs; away from their wives and families for months on end, they seek sexual release with women who, bereft of property and job skills, are selling their bodies to feed themselves and their children. Back home, wives who ask their husbands to wear condoms risk being accused of sleeping around; in African cultures, it's usually the man who dictates when and how sex happens.

Challenging such cultural and economic forces requires political will, but most African governments have been shockingly derelict. Lacking leadership, ordinary Africans have been slow to confront the disease. Few companies, for example, have comprehensive AIDS programs. And many families still refuse to acknowledge that HIV is killing their relatives, preferring to say that the person died of TB or some other opportunistic illness. Doctors often collude in this denial. "Just the other day," says a high-ranking Zimbabwean physician who spoke on condition of anonymity, "I wrote AIDS on a death certificate and then crossed it out. I thought, 'I'll just be stigmatizing this person, because no one else puts AIDS as the cause of death, even when that's what it is.' "

Why is AIDS worse in sub-Saharan Africa than anywhere else in the world? Partly because of denial; partly because the virus almost certainly originated here, giving it more time to spread; but largely because Africa was weakened by five hundred years of slavery and colonialism. Indeed, historians lay much of the blame on colonialism for Africa's many corrupt and autocratic governments, which hoard resources that could fight the epidemic. Africa, conquered and denigrated, was never allowed to incorporate international innovations on its own terms, as, for example, Japan did.

This colonial legacy poisons more than politics. Some observers attribute the spread of HIV to polygamy, a tradition in many African cultures. But job migration, urbanization, and social dislocation have created a caricature of traditional polygamy. Men have many partners not through marriage but through prostitution or sugar-daddy arrangements that lack the social glue of the old polygamy.

Of course, the worst legacy of whites in Africa is poverty, which fuels the epidemic in countless ways. Having a sexually transmitted disease multiplies the chances of spreading and contracting HIV, but few Africans obtain effective treatment because the clinic is too expensive or too far away. Africa's wealth was either funneled to the West or restricted to white settlers who barred blacks from full participation in the economy. In apartheid South Africa, blacks were either not educated at all or taught only enough to be servants. Now, as the country suffers one of the world's most explosive AIDS epidemics, illiteracy hampers prevention. Indeed, AIDS itself is rendering Africa still more vulnerable to any future catastrophe, continuing history's vicious cycle.

Yet AIDS is not merely a tale of despair. Increasingly, Africans are banding together—usually with meager resources—to care for their sick, raise their orphans, and prevent the virus from claiming more of their loved ones. Their efforts offer hope. For while a crisis of this magnitude can disintegrate society, it can also unify it. "To solve HIV," says Sy, "you must involve yourself: your attitudes and behavior and beliefs. It touches upon the most fundamental social and cultural things—procreation and death."

AIDS is driving a new candor about sex—as well as new efforts to control it, through virginity testing and campaigns that advocate sticking to one partner. And slowly, fitfully, it is also giving women more power. The death toll is scaring women into saying no to sex or insisting on condoms. And as widows proliferate, people are beginning to see the harm in denying them the right to inherit property.

The epidemic is also transforming kinship networks, which have been the heart of most African cultures. Orphans, for example, have always been enfolded into the extended family. But more than seven million children in sub-Saharan Africa have lost one or both parents, and the virus is also killing their aunts and uncles, depriving them of foster parents and leaving them to live with often feeble grandparents. In response, communities across Africa are volunteering to help orphans through home visits and, incredibly, by sharing the very little they have. Such volunteerism is both a reclaiming of communal traditions and their adaptation into new forms of civil society.

But even heroic efforts can't stop the damage that's already occurred here in the hills where Arthur Chinaka lost his father and uncles. The worst consequence of this epidemic is not the dead, but the living they leave behind.

Rusina Kasongo lives a couple of hills over from Chinaka. Like a lot of elderly rural folk who never went to school, Kasongo can't calculate how old she is, but she can count her losses: Two of her sons, one of her daughters, and all their spouses died of AIDS, and her husband died in an accident. Alone, she is rearing ten orphaned children.

"Sometimes the children go out and come home very late," says Kasongo, "and I'm afraid they'll end up doing the same thing as Tanyaradzwa." That's the daughter who died of AIDS; she had married twice, the first time in a shotgun wedding. Now, the eldest orphan, seventeen-year-old Fortunate, already has a child but not a husband.

Few people have conducted more research on AIDS orphans than pediatrician Geoff Foster, who founded the Family AIDS Caring Trust (FACT). It was Foster who documented that more than half of Zimbabwe's orphans are being cared for by grandparents, usually grandmothers who had nursed their own children to the grave. But even this fragile safety net won't be there for many of the next generation of orphans.

"Perhaps one-third of children in Zimbabwe will have lost a father or mother—or both—to AIDS," says Foster. They are more likely to be poor, he explains, more likely to be deprived of education, more likely to be abused or neglected or stigmatized, more likely to be seething with all the needs that make it more likely that a person will have unsafe sex. "But when they get HIV and die, who cares for their children? Nobody, because they're orphans, so by definition their kids have no grandparents. It's just like the virus itself. In the body, HIV gets into the defense system and knocks it out. It does that sociologically, too. It gets into the extended family support system and decimates it."

Foster's chilling realization is dawning on other people who work in fields far removed from HIV. This year, South African crime researcher Martin Schönteich published a paper that begins by noting, "In a decade's time every fourth South African will be aged between fifteen and twenty-four. It is at this age group where people's propensity to commit crime is at its highest. At about the same time there will be a boom in South Africa's orphan population as the AIDS epidemic takes its toll." While some causes of crime can be curtailed, Schönteich writes, "Other causes, such as large numbers of juveniles in the general population, and a high proportion of children brought up without adequate parental supervision, are beyond the control of the state." His conclusion: "No amount of state spending on the criminal justice system will be able to counter this harsh reality."

More AIDS and more crime are among the most dramatic consequences of the orphan explosion. But Nengomasha Willard sees damage that is harder to measure. Willard teaches eleven- and twelve-year-olds at Saint George's Primary School, located near the Chinakas and the Kasongos. Fifteen of Willard's forty-two pupils have lost one or both of their parents, but he's particularly worried about one of his students who lost his father and then, at his mother's funeral, cried inconsolably. "He doesn't want to participate," says Willard. "He just wants to be alone."

"I see thousands of children sitting in a corner," says Foster. "The impact is internalized—it's depression, being withdrawn." In Africa, says Foster, the focus on poverty eclipses research into psychological issues, but he has published disturbing evidence of abuse—emotional, physical, and sexual. Meanwhile, the orphan ranks keep swelling. "We're talking 10 percent who will have lost both parents, maybe 15 percent. Twenty-five percent who will have lost a mother. What does that do to a society, especially an impoverished society?"

Among his students, Willard has noticed that some of the orphans come to school without shoes or, in Zimbabwe's cold winter, without a sweater. Sometimes their stepfamilies put them last on the list, but often it's because grandmothers can't scrape together enough money.

Among economists, there has been a quiet debate over whether HIV will harm the economy. Some think it won't. With unemployment rates in sub-Saharan Africa between 30 and 70 percent, they reason that there are plenty of people to replenish labor losses. One scenario is that economic growth might slacken, but population growth will also dwindle, so per capita GNP might hold steady or even rise. Then, says Helen Jackson, executive director of the Southern Africa AIDS Information Dissemination Service (SAfAIDS), Africa might face the grotesque irony of "an improvement in some macroeconomic indicators, but the exact opposite at the level of households and human suffering."

But evidence is mounting that the economy will suffer. Between 20 and 30 percent of workers in South Africa's gold mining industry—the mainstay of that country's economy—are estimated to be HIV-positive, and replacing these workers will cut into the industry's productivity. In Kenya, a new government report predicts that per capita income could sink by 10 percent over the next five years. In Côte d'Ivoire, a teacher dies every school day.

Then there are the effects that can't be quantified. "What does AIDS do for the image of Africa?" asks Tony Barnett, a veteran researcher on the economic impact of AIDS. To lure investors, the continent already has to battle underdevelopment and racism, but now, he says, many people will see Africa as "diseased, sexually diseased. It chimes in with so many stereotypes."

Beneath the corporate economy, millions of Africans subsist by cultivating their own small plot of land. When someone in the family comes down with AIDS, the other members have to spend time caring for that person, which means less time cultivating crops. And when death comes, the family loses a crucial worker. Studies have documented that among rural AIDS-stricken families, food production falls, savings dwindle, and children are more likely to be undernourished.

For Kasongo and her ten orphans, food is a constant problem, but now it has become even harder. On her way back from the fields, carrying a basket of maize on her head, Kasongo tripped and fell. Her knee is swollen, her back is aching, and cultivating the fields is close to impossible. Here, under the radar of macroeconomic indicators, Kasongo's ordeal shows how AIDS is devastating Africa.

This is the context in which one of Africa's most agonizing debates is taking place: Should doctors administer drugs to pregnant women that sharply reduce the chances that a baby will be born with HIV? So far, the debate has centered on the cost of the drugs, but a new, inexpensive regimen has pushed thornier arguments to the surface. The "vaccine for babies," as it is sometimes called, does not treat the mother and so does nothing to reduce the chances the baby will become an orphan. That's why Uganda's Major Rubaramira Ruranga, a well-known activist who is himself infected with HIV, opposes it.

"Many children in our countries die of malnutrition, even with both parents," he argues. "Without parents, it's almost certain they'll die." Isn't it impossible to know the fate of any given child and presumptuous to decide it in advance? "That's sentimental," he snaps. Even Foster, who believes "every child has a right to be born without HIV," wonders whether the money is best spent on the "technical fix" of giving drugs to the pregnant women. The medicine is only a part of the cost, for women can infect their children during breast feeding, which raises expensive problems such as providing formula and teaching mothers how to use it safely in places where clean water may not exist. Would all that money, Foster wonders, be better spent alleviating the root causes of why women get infected in the first place? "It's very difficult to stand up and make such an argument because you get portrayed as a beast," he says. In fact, such arguments testify to how the epidemic is forcing Africans to grapple with impossible choices.

Weston Tizora is one of thousands of Africans who are trying to give orphans a decent life. Just twenty-five years old, Tizora started as a gardener at Saint Augustine's Mission and threw himself into volunteering in the mission's AIDS program, called Kubatana, a Shona word meaning "together."

Next year he will take over the program's leadership from its founder, British nurse Sarah Hinton. Kubatana's thirty-seven volunteers care for homebound patients, and they help raise orphans by, for example, bringing food to Rusina Kasongo's brood.

Just a few steps from Kasongo live Cloud and Joseph Tineti. They're fourteen and eleven, respectively, and the oldest person in their home is their fifteen-year-old brother. They are, in the language of AIDS workers, a child-headed household. Who's in charge? "No one," Joseph answers—and it shows. Their one-room shack is strewn with dirty clothes, unwashed dishes, broken chairs. On the table, a roiling mass of ants feasts on pumpkin seeds and some kind of dried leaves.

The troubles run deeper. Their father, who had divorced their mother before she died, lives in nearby Mutare. Does he bring food? "Yes," says Joseph, "every week." It's not true, Tizora maintains. Kubatana members have even talked with the police in their effort to convince the father to take in his children or at least support them. But the police did not act, explains Tizora, because the father is unemployed and struggling to provide for the family of his second wife. Once a month—sometimes not even that often—he brings small amounts of food, so the orphans depend on donations from Kubatana volunteers. But if little Joseph's version isn't true, it's what an orphaned kid would want: a father who at least brings food, stops by frequently, and acts a little like a dad. And his mother: What does Joseph remember of her? The question is too much, and he starts crying.

Kubatana volunteers are supposed to look after the Tineti orphans, so why is their home so unkempt? There used to be two volunteers in this area, explains Tizora. One has been reassigned to work in the nearby mining village, ravaged by AIDS. The other has been away at her parents' home for two months, attending to a family funeral and to her own late-stage pregnancy.

And everyone in these villages has their hands full. Standing in a valley, Tizora points to the hillsides around him and says, "There are orphans in that home, and the one over there, and there by the gum trees. And see where there's that white house? They're taking care of orphans there, too." By the time he finishes, he has pointed out about half of the homesteads. When the Kubatana program started, in 1992, volunteers identified twenty orphans. Now they have registered three thousand. In many parts of Africa, notes Jackson of SAfAIDS, "It has actually become the norm to have orphaned children in the household rather than the exception."

Foster makes some quick calculations: Given the number of volunteers in the Kubatana program, there's no way they can care for all their orphans. So when a volunteer gets pregnant, has a family emergency, or gets sick, kids like Cloud and Joseph fall through the cracks. Says Foster: "You can't lose a quarter of your adult population in ten years without catastrophic consequences."

In his office, Tizora has a wall of photographs showing the original twenty orphans. One is a girl who looks about twelve. She lost her parents and then she lost the grandma who was caring for her. At that point, she started refusing to go to school, hiding on the way there. Now, she's run away and, Tizora says, "we don't know where she is."

SOUTH AFRICA ACTS UP

Building a Movement on the Ruins of Apartheid

December 22–28, 1999

KwaMashu, South Africa—It's a hot, gray Sunday afternoon in March, and the sprawling Durban train station is almost deserted—hardly the best stage for an AIDS demonstration. Yet sitting on the floor is a small woman named Mercy Makhalemele, one of South Africa's foremost AIDS activists. And she is protesting. Makhalemele found out she was HIV-positive in 1993. When she told her husband, he shoved her into a pot of water boiling on the stove, scalding her arm. She went to her job selling shoes "as if everything was OK," but her husband showed up telling her to go back home, get her things and leave him, because how could he live with someone infected with HIV? That was at 10:00 in the morning. At 3:00 that afternoon she was fired from her job. Her youngest child, Nkosikhona, meaning "God is there," was born infected. Makhalemele remembers taking her to the hospital and having nurses say, "She is HIV-positive, there is nothing we can do." And Makhalemele would insist, "I'm not asking you to treat her HIV, I'm asking you to treat her bronchitis." Her child died at two and a half.

For most of this time, Makhalemele tried to push her government—the new government of Nelson Mandela, the most progressive in Africa and maybe the world—to fight AIDS.

It looked like it would be easy. Quarraisha Abdool-Karim is one of South Africa's leading HIV researchers, and she was the first to head the country's AIDS-control program. She remembers an AIDS conference in 1992, when Mandela gave the keynote. Abdool-Karim was to speak after him, but, she recalls, "there was very little to add. He knew all the issues, everything that had to be done."

But then there was silence. Until the end of 1998, when the prevalence of HIV among South African women attending prenatal clinics surged beyond 20 percent, the only major AIDS speech Mandela gave was to an economic forum in Switzerland. Why he waited so long to confront AIDS remains one of the most maddening enigmas of the epidemic. Mandela declined requests from the *Voice* for an interview, but even his friend and personal physician, Nthato Motlana, can't plumb it.

"I get so angry," Motlana said in an interview earlier this year. "I go to Mandela—I had breakfast with him this morning—and I give him hell." Exasperated, he adds, "The response by the previous apartheid government was a national disgrace. The response by my government—and I'm a very loyal member of the ANC, have been since the age of eighteen—has also been disgraceful."

In fact, the new administration made colossal blunders. First, the headstrong health minister, Nkosazana Zuma, authorized a $2.2 million AIDS prevention play, called *Serafina II*, that hogged a huge portion of the AIDS budget and was widely criticized for being ineffective. Then came Virodene, a locally developed treatment for AIDS. In fact, it contained an industrial solvent, harmful to humans. But Zuma—and Thabo Mbeki, then deputy president and now president of South Africa—championed the drug. When objections were raised by the Medicines Control Council, the South African equivalent of the Food and Drug Administration, Zuma dismissed their concerns, suggesting the council was in league with big pharmaceutical companies that didn't want competition from Virodene.

Finally, in October 1998, the government unveiled its Partnership Against AIDS, a public-private effort that has won high praise for prompting companies, churches, and civic organizations to tackle AIDS. But even as it was being launched, Zuma announced that the government was nixing the so-called vaccine for babies, a regimen of AZT given to HIV-positive pregnant women that can greatly reduce the chance that babies will be born with HIV. Unaffordable, insisted Zuma, despite a government-funded study showing that giving AZT to pregnant women would save money in the long run, because treating babies with AIDS is very expensive.

Because of her infected daughter, Makhalemele was especially outraged by the AZT decision. But she was also heartsick about what she saw as the larger issue: "How do we, as people already infected, fit into the government's program? We don't fit in any way because it's all about prevention." So she helped start the Treatment Action Campaign, an AIDS activist group patterned partly on ACT UP but also on South Africa's own tradition of protest politics, a tradition epitomized, of course, by Mandela.

Indeed, Mandela may not have done much for AIDS, but he did give his country a political system that responds to ordinary citizens. In a very real sense, he made AIDS activism possible.

But even Mandela couldn't make it easy. While activists everywhere must push politicians, South African AIDS activists must also cope with a society thrown horribly out of joint by modern Africa's most authoritarian, exploitative white regime. In building an AIDS movement, the legacy of apartheid is the biggest obstacle, even more onerous than errant leaders. Apartheid poisoned people with rage, resentment, and despair, creating a culture of violence and stigma that still haunts people with HIV. That's a problem because, before the infected can band together to fight, they must acknowledge they carry the virus. That's hard everywhere, but in South Africa, people who come out as HIV-positive risk physical assault, even murder.

Makhalemele's home region, KwaZulu-Natal, suffered some of the worst terror, because here a three-way war raged between the white regime, the African National Congress, and the Zulu Inkatha Freedom Party. AIDS activist Musa Njoko grew up in KwaMashu, a forbidding township outside Durban, the kind of place where people seem so beaten down that they are looking for someone weaker to kick. "The boys treated me very roughly," Njoko recalls. "I thought someone would get hurt for being HIV-positive." So she was "shocked but not surprised" when last December a woman named Gugu Dlamini declared that she was HIV-positive and got beaten to death three weeks later because, as some of her assailants were heard to say, her honesty shamed the township.

Three months after Dlamini's murder, the Treatment Action Campaign was kicked off with a nationwide petition drive, and Makhalemele, who had worked with Dlamini, decided to confront AIDS stigma by sending her petitioners to KwaMashu. Wearing T-shirts emblazoned with the photo of the slain activist and the slogan "Never Again," about twenty activists arrived in the township shopping center, a dusty place with bars on all the windows. The activists had requested a police escort, but with no police in sight, they fled.

Makhalemele never made it to KwaMashu. A few days earlier she had asked for the train company to provide the activists free transportation from Durban to KwaMashu. She asked again when she got to the station, and again the answer was no—and something inside her snapped. She sat down in the middle of the station, launching a fast that would last for seven days.

Sitting on the floor of the train station, she starts to weep. "I'm going to a Catholic mission," she says. "I'm going to stay there to heal the sorrow, the pain, the rage I have from working for seven years as an AIDS activist in this country."

Apartheid was never merely a racial system, but also an economic one that created copious wealth. It is possible to travel to Capetown or Johannesburg and believe one is in London or New York. The mansions are palatial. The phones work. The roads are good. All this gives the country a critical mass of educated, prosperous, urban inhabitants—no longer all white—who have a sense that they are entitled to a democratic society that works as well as any nation anywhere. The comparatively strong economy also means that people with HIV can dare to hope for at least some medication to extend their lives.

Of course, South Africa's wealth was created by ruthless exploitation, so the country is also blighted with poverty on a staggering scale. Illiteracy is rampant. Millions lack electricity and running water. This is what people mean when they talk about South Africa as a country of extremes or, as Mbeki puts it, two countries within the same borders. But this does not begin to describe the far-reaching devastation wreaked upon the nation.

To understand apartheid, go not to KwaMashu or even Soweto, but instead descend in a mine-shaft elevator deep below the surface of the Witswatersrand region to the reef, a band of sediment created millions of years ago by prehistoric rains. It's hard to see the gold, but it's there—tons upon tons of it scattered through the reef in mostly microscopic particles. Here is the simple geological fact has shaped modern South Africa more than anything else: Each ton of Witswatersrand earth yields only a few ounces of gold, and the richest deposits lie buried under eons of newer geological layers. So South African mines must plunge deeper than any others—as far down as five kilometers—and miners have to haul up colossal aggregations of earth. Without very cheap labor, it would have been impossible to make a profit.

Yet gold has long been the country's largest revenue producer. For example, the West Driefontein mine in Carletonville has extracted more than 4.5 million pounds of gold. The company has provided splendid housing for the mine manager: a gated mansion complete with manicured garden. The ordinary laborers also live in company housing. Typical is a room about twenty by twenty feet, crammed with fourteen bunk beds and lockers no bigger than those in a school gym. The men who live in this room come from across southern Africa, and they are all married. But their wives are back home. The miners see their families only every two or three months, usually for just a few days at a time. It is a system that was invented nearly a century ago by the diamond and gold industries. Africans were crowded into reservations, where hut taxes forced them into wage labor. Chiefs were paid to supply men—but only men. Housing black families would cost money, and letting black workers settle permanently in mining towns would make it easier for them to organize resistance. So workers were housed in all-male barracks, called hostels, much like the ones at West Driefontein.

Apartheid's mesh of more than one hundred interlocking laws basically nationalized the pattern devised by the mining industry, which at its height employed more than a fifth of black South African adults. Apartheid's hated pass laws, which restricted the movement of blacks, grew out of company policies designed to shuttle workers between their homes and the mines. And in the 1960s, the government forced as many as three million Africans into barren and degrading reservations they called Bantustans, an Orwellian term intended to prop up the sham that these were independent nations. Blacks lucky enough to land a job in a city lived in outlying townships—often, in the early days, with their families. But that changed with the infamous 1964 Bantu Laws Amendments Act, which mandated that new workers live in all-male hostels in the townships. The mining model had become national policy, and the results were disastrous.

"I lived next to a hostel in Soweto, and I would get called to treat someone stabbed or shot," Motlana recalls. "The stench in those places! They were filthy. The hostels bred crime, but it goes beyond that. Children were ill-disciplined because they didn't have fathers. It led to so much human abuse."

It also led to an explosion of AIDS. South Africa has one of the world's fastest-growing HIV epidemics, and many researchers believe that the country's system of migrant labor is one of the driving forces. "If you wanted to spread a sexually transmitted disease, you would take thousands of young men away from their families, isolate them in single-sex hostels, and give them easy access to alcohol and commercial sex," says Mark Lurie, a South African researcher who has studied the effect of migrant labor on HIV. "Then, to spread the disease around the country, you'd send them home every once in a while to their wives and girlfriends. And that's basically the system of migrant labor we have."

In Carletonville, Yodwa Mzaidume works with the hundreds of prostitutes that live in squatter camps by the mining hostels. She trains them to educate each other to use condoms, but it's hard to involve them in anything beyond that. "Take Leeupoort," she says, referring to one of the squatter camps. "People there don't have toilets or running water. If you come to them talking about political activism, they ask, 'What's in it for me?' "

In America, the cry of AIDS activists was simple: "Drugs into bodies!" But in South Africa, the needs are so much more complex. Mzaidume ticks off some of them: "Migrant labor, overcrowding, unemployment, the crime rate. But what are we doing about them? What can we do?" Migrant labor, she notes, has become so ingrained into South African life that "mineworkers don't want their families to stay here. They say, 'Who would take care of my cows back home?' " Mzaidume doesn't dwell on South Africa's past because what's spreading HIV, she quips, "is sex with other people, not sex with apartheid." But with unemployment officially above 30 percent and probably much higher, she says, "There's a lot of anger among the youth. They say, 'Yes, we are in a democratic South Africa, but we still live in apartheid.' "

The result is rage. Njoko, the activist who grew up in KwaMashu, explains: "They'll see me and think, 'She is an HIV-positive woman, how is she doing so well?' And then maybe they'll hurt me or kill me. But when you look deeper you find out the guy has been unemployed for ten years." Some men even take out their anger by infecting other people, she says, echoing a common conviction. "They say they don't want to die alone, they're going to take people with them. I don't support them, but there's absolutely nothing there for the person who is HIV-positive. The message is they're going to die."

Zackie Achmat is one of the architects of the Treatment Action Campaign. He also fought apartheid, organizing student demonstrations and going to jail for it. Although his ancestry is mixed-race, he called himself black, a tactic of solidarity. He is also a leader of South Africa's flourishing lesbian and gay movement, and with his international connections he could get the very latest medication to treat his HIV. But he has publicly declared that he will not take any drug that is not available to all South Africans.

So when he stood up at a meeting this spring, attended by Zuma, then the minister of health, Achmat had credibility. He told her of his longstanding membership in the ANC, pointed out that the AIDS movement supported her opposition to high pharmaceutical prices, and requested a meeting. To the astonishment of most activists, she agreed. And after the meeting, she reversed her policy on AZT for pregnant women.

It was a stunning victory—and it opened the way for much larger advances, especially on drug prices. It was Zuma who pushed through a law that could allow the South African government to bypass pharmaceutical patents and obtain essential medicines at much lower prices—for example, from companies that make generic versions of the drugs. That made South Africa ground zero in a high-profile battle joined by Western AIDS activists and organizations, such as the Nobel-winning Médecins Sans Frontières, to relax patent and trade restrictions that help keep essential drugs unaffordable. Here was a fight AIDS activists and the South African government shared.

But this fall, President Mbeki shocked activists by saying, "There exists a large volume of scientific literature alleging that, among other things, the toxicity of this drug is such that it is, in fact, a danger to health." Never mind that AZT has been evaluated in dozens of trials around the world, that its benefits usually outweigh its side effects, and that countries as strict as Germany and the United States have approved the drug for use against HIV. Indeed, in a study carried out among pregnant women in South Africa, AZT together with another drug showed no more side effects than a placebo. So where did the most powerful person in Africa get the notion that AZT is dangerous? From the Web, one of his spokespeople, Tasneem Carrim, told the Johannesburg *Sunday Independent*. Mbeki's office denied it, but what Carrim said had the ring of guileless truth: "The president goes into the Net all the time," she was quoted as saying. Activists had hoped that Mbeki's new health minister, Manto Tshabalala-Msimang, would correct him, but to their dismay she has staunchly supported him. In the township near Carletonville, the percentage of twenty-five-year-old women infected with HIV is a shocking 60 percent. Most of these women will probably get pregnant. "Why not give a chance to have a baby that is not HIV-positive?" asks Mzaidume. Then she says, bitterly, "It doesn't matter how many presentations doctors make, if politicians don't want it, it will not be." Mbeki did not respond to requests for an interview by the *Voice*.

Because there is scant medical evidence to support Mbeki's opposition to AZT, many South Africans are casting about for what might have motivated him. Perhaps years in the struggle against apartheid imbued him with mistrust of powerful white corporations, such as pharmaceutical companies. Maybe, too, it instilled a stubbornness that won't allow him to admit he erred. But since Mbeki's specialty is economics, much of the speculation has gravitated in that direction.

The popular notion that apartheid was overthrown by the ANC is only part of the truth. What also happened is that the apartheid economy collapsed. Treating workers as wholly expendable was fine when industry needed mainly unskilled labor. But as technological advancements demanded educated, stable workers, apartheid's migrant labor system backfired, as did the policy of giving blacks only rudimentary education. "If those stupid fools had just decided to train one hundred black engineers a year," says Aggrey Klaaste, publisher of the *Sowetan* newspaper, "this country would be phenomenal."

But the country was anything but phenomenal when the ANC took power. GDP was actually shrinking. Inflation was running above 15 percent. Capital was fleeing the country. And wasteful spending on police and defense, required to fight an ever bolder black resistance, had burdened the country with a large debt.

Despite being raised by communist parents, Mbeki has charted an aggressively capitalist course. Even though it burdens the economy, he is reassuring international investors by stoically paying off the apartheid-era debt. He has imposed a strict fiscal discipline to accommodate world financial institutions such as the International Monetary Fund. While such policies may boost South Africa in the long run, they have left the government strapped for cash—and AIDS drugs are expensive. "They're terrified of starting down the slippery slope of treatment," says Achmat, "because they think it will cost too much."

That certainly would be true if the government subsidized the costly drug cocktails that have reduced American AIDS deaths. But there is a middle ground. Some of the opportunistic illnesses that kill people with AIDS can be prevented by taking relatively cheap prophylactic drugs. The reason the government isn't providing such drugs is that it isn't being pushed by "a treatment-literate HIV population that knows its rights," says Achmat. "The level of understanding here is vastly different than in Europe and North America." At the start of the Treatment Action Campaign, he recalls, people thought AZT was a political party.

That is beginning to change, largely because activists have pushed the issue into the media. Two powerful unions have thrown their weight behind the Treatment Action Campaign, and science itself is pushing the government. There is a new drug, nevirapine, which seems to prevent mother-to-child transmission as effectively as AZT, and at a much cheaper cost. It's being studied in South Africa, and the results of that trial are scheduled for release at the huge World AIDS Conference to be held next year in Durban. It will become harder and harder for the government not to act.

Already a groundswell is apparent. People with HIV are more and more visible. Makhalemele, for example, is back from her five-month retreat and cohosting *Beat It!*, a national television show on how to live with HIV. On

World AIDS Day this month, she says, the media was "full of AIDS faces." One of them is the *Sowetan*'s Lucky Mazibuko, the country's first openly HIV-positive columnist. He lives in the township and has become a magnet for people who need someone to talk with. Recently he got a letter that shows how attitudes are changing.

"The letter was from an elderly woman saying she had a son who was HIV-positive, but she had rejected him, chucked him out of house. Now, she was working as a domestic for a white family, and her employer's daughter turned out to be HIV-positive. So as part of her job she has to take care of their daughter—and she only saw her son when he was buried."

In a country with at least 3.6 million infected, an old African proverb has new relevance: "Something with horns cannot be hidden." The sick and dead are forcing South Africans to confront the disease, themselves, and their brutal history.

Research intern: Jason Schwartzberg

MOSCOW DISPATCH
Mental Health

MASHA GESSEN

from The New Republic
| **August 22, 2000** |

"This is what a typical hospital in the area where we were trying to work looked like," the speaker intones heavily as a slide is projected on the screen. The building in the photograph, a medical facility in sub-Saharan Africa, is falling apart: peeling paint exposes blackened concrete, rickety window frames hold cracked glass. The audience at the plenary session of last month's international AIDS conference in Durban, South Africa, lets out a collective sigh. The picture has powerfully dramatized the tremendous difficulties developing nations face in combating the AIDS epidemic.

To me, it just looks like a typical hospital. In fact, it looks a lot like the hospital not twenty miles from Moscow where I had my head sewn up following a car accident a few years back; I will never forget the dry shave, necessitated by the lack of running water. Or the Moscow hospital where I wound up the following year for pneumonia; there, I was offered a broken examination cot as a bed and strongly advised to arrange for my own food. Or the military hospital in Rostov that I visited as a reporter, one of Russia's largest and the one shouldering the heaviest burden from the war in Chechnya. Local military officials assured me the hospital was well equipped and stocked with drugs. But, before I left, representatives of the local Soldiers' Mothers Committee slipped me a list, compiled by the chief doctor, of essential drugs the hospital lacked: aspirin, basic painkillers, vitamins. They also asked me if I knew any foreign journalists who could help obtain a replacement for a long-broken glass part in the hospital's tomography machine, which was itself donated a few years back by some foreigners.

The truth is that, when it comes to health and social services, Russia has joined the developing world. The problem, as the Rostov officers' lie illustrates, is that Russians, or at least Russian officials, won't admit it. Ordinary Russians are bombarded daily with rhetoric aimed at convincing them of their country's continuing accomplishments and power. Otherwise sane Russian journalists proudly referred to last month's economic summit in Okinawa as "the G-8 meeting"—omitting the fact that Russia, whose federal budget equals that of a medium-size U.S. state, was excluded from economic talks (at which, in any case, its representatives would have done little more than ask for debt forgiveness). Despite ten years of collapsing infrastructure, most Russians still foam at the mouth to defend treasured Soviet-era myths—that the country's crumbling education system is the best in the world, for example, or that its battered health-care network, deeply flawed to begin with, is as advanced as any First World country's.

But, national pride notwithstanding, everything said about developing countries at the Durban conference is also true of Russia. The health-care infrastructure is in desperate disrepair, so much so that hospitals and clinics actually pose a threat to the health of their patients. More than half the population lives below the poverty line, and tuberculosis and other diseases afflicting the poor are epidemic. Infant mortality is rising; life expectancy is falling. HIV spreads unchecked.

If you haven't heard much about Russia's AIDS epidemic, you're not alone—most Russians haven't, either. Some of the reasons are common to all countries plagued by the disease: the stigma attached to the ways the virus is transmitted (in Russia, mostly through intravenous drug use), unwillingness to acknowledge the risk, fear. But a more peculiar kind of denial is also to blame. For, though Russia supports a fairly extensive AIDS bureaucracy, none of the country's health officials have raised their voices to say the obvious: Russia doesn't have a First World–style AIDS crisis, it has a Third World–style crisis, and it needs to swallow its pride and learn from countries like Uganda and Thailand.

So far, Russia's response to its AIDS epidemic has been dismal. The country's network of AIDS centers, created during a wave of HIV hysteria that waxed and waned quickly in the late 1980s, serves only one purpose: It attempts to count cases of HIV infection. This effort to catalog cases but not actually treat patients follows a venerable Soviet tradition. Even back when the Soviet Union was creating its now well-publicized epidemic of drug-resistant TB, its epidemiologists were building the world's most extensive TB-surveillance network: everyone was X-rayed, but no one received proper care. Similarly, directors of local AIDS centers now say Russia "has the epidemic under control." When asked what they mean, they explain that they are using a staggering twenty million HIV tests every year to help track cases of infection.

But even the effort to quantify the epidemic is failing. Most tests are effectively administered without consent, and anonymous testing is virtually unavailable. Furthermore, "placing someone at risk of HIV infection" is a criminal offense, and every person who tests positive is forced to sign a document that can later be used against him or her in court. It's little surprise, then, that people who realize they may be at risk for infection do their utmost to stay far away from the testing centers. Equally ominous is that, for at least two years running, official figures have shown that more than 80 percent of the infected are IV drug users. That's ominous because what we know about HIV transmission suggests that the rate of infection among drug users tends to peak quickly, and then other routes of transmission gradually become more common. Russia's AIDS centers know how to find IV drug users—in jail, in detention centers, in detox centers—and test them with or without their consent, but that's about all they know how to do. The centers have no system for locating other infected people, who may by now account for the majority of HIV transmissions. We can only guess at this, of course, because, unlike many other countries, Russia has not undertaken a representative study of HIV prevalence. Still, even its absurdly imperfect system shows that the country has the fastest-growing HIV epidemic in Europe.

The absolute numbers are still small: just over fifty thousand cases of HIV infection are now registered in the country. But health-care officials admit privately that this is an absurd underestimation—some say by a factor of ten, while others say twenty or one hundred. Where prevalence studies have actually been done, the results have been much more dire: in Krasnogorsk, a town in the Moscow region, three percent of people between the ages of fifteen and twenty-five are infected, a rate comparable to that in Angola, Ghana, and Sierra Leone. Moreover, of the fifty thousand registered HIV cases, more than twenty thousand were registered this year alone, which suggests a terrifyingly high rate of transmission. Projections vary wildly, but no one doubts that in a couple of years millions of Russians will have HIV.

And what kind of treatment will Russia offer them? Virtually none at all. In the quality of care available to HIV-positive people, Russia lags behind some of the world's poorest countries. To date, it has not even instituted the common short-term therapy proved most effective in preventing in utero HIV transmission from mother to child—even though the drug required, AZT, is manufactured locally. (Prejudice on the part of many local doctors who believe that HIV-positive women should not become mothers has combined with a lack of initiative at the top to keep the treatment out of the hands of pregnant women.) It is quite likely that other antiretroviral drugs could be made locally as well—Russia retains some First World pharmaceutical technologies—but they won't be: state agencies have already issued licenses to Western drug companies for twelve compounds whose high prices render them out of reach for Russian patients.

Which brings us to a final developing-country malady afflicting Russia: corruption. As it happens, the very pharmaceutical companies granted licenses to make those too-expensive drugs paid to send some highly placed Russian AIDS officials to the Durban conference. And, once there, the officials showed just how much effort they were willing to devote to their country's AIDS crisis. Rather than attend the sessions devoted to drug access for developing or "resource-poor" countries, several members of the Russian delegation used their time to purchase diamonds. The health ministry's AIDS boss, meanwhile, took the opportunity to go on safari.

LOOK AT BRAZIL

TINA ROSENBERG

from The New York Times Magazine

| **January 28, 2001** |

Someday, we may look back on the year 2001 with nostalgia for a time when AIDS was merely a health catastrophe. Soon, AIDS in Africa will be doing more than killing millions every year. It will destroy what there is of Africa's economy and cause further instability and, perhaps, war. In the year 2010, the country of South Africa will be almost one-fifth poorer than it would have been had AIDS never existed. Throughout Africa, the disease has ravaged the young, urban, and mobile. It has robbed schools of their teachers and hospitals of their doctors and nurses. Businesses are depleted by the need to cope with sick and dying employees. AIDS takes the breadwinner, leaving millions of destitute elderly and orphans who will grow up without going to school, many on the streets. As they lose their productive citizens, the nations themselves face collapse.

At the moment, however, AIDS in Africa is only a plague of a severity not seen since the Black Death killed at least a quarter of Europe in the fourteenth century. A fifteen-year-old in South Africa has a better than even chance of dying of AIDS. One in five adults is infected with HIV Hospitals are filled with babies so shriveled by AIDS that nurses must shave their heads to find veins for intravenous tubes. Seventeen million people have died prolonged and miserable deaths from AIDS, and that number is dwarfed by what lies ahead.

While Africa is the region most ravaged, the disease is exploding elsewhere as well. India says it has four million infected; it may well have five times as many. Its AIDS epidemic bears a terrifying resemblance to South Africa's a few years ago—AIDS is widespread in every risk group, and health care is inadequate. The Caribbean has the second-highest rate of infection after sub-Saharan Africa. More than one in fifty adults is HIV-positive, and because the epidemic is primarily spread heterosexually there, most of the population is at risk. In Eastern Europe and the former Soviet Union, the number of infected nearly doubled in the last year.

Until a year ago, the triple therapy that has made AIDS a manageable disease in wealthy nations was considered realistic only for those who could afford to pay $10,000 to $15,000 a year or lived in societies that could. The most that poor countries could hope to do was prevent new cases of AIDS through educational programs and condom promotion or to cut mother-to-child transmission and, if they were very lucky, treat some of AIDS's opportunistic infections. But the 32.5 million people with HIV in the developing world had little hope of survival.

This was the conventional wisdom. Today, all of these statements are false.

The Raphael de Paula Souza hospital sits on the outskirts of Rio de Janeiro. It is a one-story plaster building with peeling blue paint and barefoot boys playing in the parking lot. Nothing in its appearance suggests that it might serve as a model for treating AIDS worldwide.

The AIDS clinic is run by Ademildes Navarini, who spends her days seeing patients like Rogério. He is twenty-six, has tuberculosis as well as AIDS and suffers from an AIDS-related brain infection, toxoplasmosis. The infection has affected his speech, and now he gropes for words. He removes his T-shirt using only his left arm. His right arm and his right leg hang limp.

Rogério is followed by Jerdinete, a forty-six-year-old middle-class woman who came in for tests a year ago because of stomach problems—and was stunned to find she had AIDS. The only way she could have got it, she says, was from her husband, whom she had presumed faithful. When she told him that she was sick, he left her.

Jerdinete is followed by Maura, HIV-positive but asymptomatic, and her seven-year-old son, Emerson, whose HIV was diagnosed ten months ago but has undoubtedly been infected since birth. Emerson, a handsome, curly-haired boy, kisses his mother's cheek, puts his arm around her neck, and caresses her face as she sits on a stool. A year ago, Emerson's hair started to fall out. He got diarrhea and started losing weight. The family went in for testing, and their fears were confirmed. Maura, whose husband also has AIDS and tuberculosis, stopped working to stay home with Emerson. "He's the reason for my life," she says, squeezing her son.

If Rogério, Jerdinete, and Emerson lived in any other poor nation, their future would be achingly foreseeable. But here's the news from Raphael de Paula Souza hospital: each of these patients will walk out with a plastic bag filled with bottles of antiretrovirals—AZT and ddI and the protease inhibitors and other components of the triple cocktail that, for the lucky, have turned AIDS into a chronic disease. Rogério, who started taking triple therapy three weeks before I met him, has gotten much better. He will be scarred by toxoplasmosis, Navarini says, but will improve a little more. Jerdinete and Emerson, on triple therapy for months, are doing fine. And Ademildes Navarini is the happy exception in Third-World medicine, an AIDS doctor who can make her patients healthy again instead of merely holding their hands and watching them die.

Since 1997, virtually every AIDS patient in Brazil for whom it is medically indicated gets, free, the same triple cocktails that keep rich Americans healthy. (In Western Europe, no one who needs AIDS treatment is denied it because of cost. This is true in some American states, but not all.) Brazil has shredded all the excuses about why poor countries cannot treat AIDS. Health system too fragile? On the shaky foundation of its public health service, Brazil built a well-run network of AIDS clinics. Uneducated people can't stick to the complicated regime of pills? Brazilian AIDS patients have proved just as able to take their medicine on time as patients in the United States.

Ah, but treating AIDS is too expensive! In fact, Brazil's program almost certainly pays for itself. It has halved the death rate from AIDS, prevented hundreds of thousands of new hospitalizations, cut the transmission rate, helped to stabilize the epidemic, and improved the overall state of public health in Brazil.

Brazil can afford to treat AIDS because it does not pay market prices for antiretroviral drugs—the most controversial aspect of the country's plan. In 1998, the government began making copies of brand-name drugs, and the price of those medicines has fallen by an average of 79 percent. Brazil now produces some triple therapy for $3,000 a year and expects to do much better, and the price could potentially drop to $700 a year or even less.

Brazil is showing that no one who dies of AIDS dies of natural causes. Those who die have been failed—by feckless leaders who see weapons as more alluring purchases than medicines, by wealthy countries (notably the United States) that have threatened the livelihood of poor nations who seek to manufacture cheap medicine and by the multinational drug companies who have kept the price of antiretroviral drugs needlessly out of reach of the vast majority of the world's population.

But one major reason that only Brazil offers free triple therapy is that, until now, there was no Brazil to show that it is possible. A year and a half ago, practically nobody was talking about using triple therapy in poor countries. Today, it is rare to find a meeting of international leaders where this idea is not discussed. International organizations like the United Nations AIDS agency, UNAIDS, and nongovernment groups like Médecins Sans Frontières are starting to help countries try to replicate Brazil's program. Brazil has offered to transfer all its technology and provide training in the practicalities of treating patients to other countries that want to make drugs and will supply them to patients free. Even the drug companies, hoping to head off more damaging assaults on their patent rights and improve their tattered image, have acknowledged the need to charge less for their products in poor nations. They have begun to make limited offers of cheap drugs.

In other words, the debate about whether poor countries can treat AIDS is over. The question is how.

Pharmaceutical manufacturers argue that many countries are very far from able to administer a program of triple therapy, and they are right. But Brazil shows that poor nations can do it. Others will be able to follow if they get substantial international help.

The drug companies are wrong, however, on how to make AIDS drugs affordable. Their solution—limited, negotiated price cuts—is slow, grudging, and piecemeal. Brazil, by defying the pharmaceutical companies and threatening to break patents, among other actions, has made drugs available to everyone who needs them. Its experience shows that doing this requires something radical: an alteration of the basic social contract the pharmaceutical companies have enjoyed until now.

By the terms of that contract, manufacturers, in return for the risks of developing new drugs, receive a twenty-year monopoly to sell them in some nations at whatever prices they choose. The industry has thrived under this contract. And so have we, the rich. The system has conquered an unimaginable range of diseases. But for billions of people the medicines have remained out of reach. Poor countries, it is now clear, must violate this contract if they are to save their people from AIDS.

Brazil has been able to treat AIDS because it had what everyone agrees is the single most important requirement for doing so: political commitment. At the beginning of 1999, Brazil's economy was skidding into crisis.

President Fernando Henrique Cardoso was under great pressure to cut the budget by abandoning the AIDS program. He rejected that advice, deciding that treating AIDS was a priority.

Such commitment has its roots in the gay community. Although AIDS is now a disease of the poor in Brazil, the first Brazilians infected were gay men. In a country famously open about matters sexual, gays were much more activist and better organized than in most other nations, and AIDS carried less of the stigma that has elsewhere led people simply to deny its existence.

Then the movement found an unlikely ally in José Sarney, Brazil's first civilian president after the country emerged from military rule in 1985 and a conservative who led a pro-military party during the dictatorship. In 1996, scientists at the World AIDS Conference in Vancouver announced that triple therapy with a protease inhibitor could reduce viral load to undetectable levels. Finally, there was a treatment for AIDS. "A doctor friend informed me about what was going on in Vancouver," Sarney told me. "I saw that most of the medicine in the cocktail would not be available to the poor, and I felt that we were talking about the survival of the species."

Sarney proposed a law that guaranteed every AIDS patient state-of-the-art treatment. It passed. At the same time, Brazil was carrying out an aggressive AIDS-prevention program, financed by the World Bank. Activist groups were the keystone, distributing millions of free condoms.

Surveys show that there are about 530,000 HIV-positive people in Brazil. Four-fifths do not know they are infected. Of those who have been identified as needing antiretroviral therapy, however (some 90,000 at the moment), virtually all can get it, even homeless people, even people in the middle of the Amazon, says Paulo Teixeira, who runs Brazil's AIDS program. A slim, elegant man of fifty-two, Teixeira has been an AIDS doctor since 1983 and director of the country's AIDS efforts for a year.

The treatment and prevention programs complement each other—another powerful reason to begin treating AIDS in poor countries. Treating AIDS helps to limit its spread, as people with a lower viral load are less contagious. The availability of lifesaving treatment is also a powerful lure for people to get an AIDS test.

"Treatment brings people into the hospital, where you can talk to them," says Serafim Armesto, a psychologist who works with AIDS patients at the General Hospital of Nova Iguaçu, a major hospital in a working-class town a short drive from Rio. "You can work with them to prevent the spread of AIDS and further disease."

The programs have paid off. In 1994, the World Bank estimated that by 2000 Brazil would have 1.2 million HIV-positive people. In fact it had half that many. The epidemic has stabilized, with some 20,000 new cases each year for the last three years. The treatment program has cut the AIDS death rate nationally by about 50 percent so far, and each AIDS patient is only a quarter as likely to be hospitalized as before.

Treating AIDS also fights other diseases. The incidence of tuberculosis in H.I.V.-positive patients has dropped by half. AIDS has also helped to mobilize people to fight for better health care. "In 1999, the Health Ministry had problems getting its budget passed for AIDS, TB, and other diseases," says Pedro Chequer, Teixeira's predecessor as head of the AIDS program and now the UNAIDS director for the southern part of South America. "There are now six hundred nongovernmental groups that work on AIDS. They demonstrated in the street for a higher budget for all diseases, not just for AIDS, and these protests were covered in the press." The money was restored.

The Health Ministry spent $444 million on AIDS drugs in 2000—4 percent of its budget. The only study of the program's benefits so far shows that the decline in hospitalizations from opportunistic infections from 1997 to 1999 saved the Health Ministry $422 million. But the tally of benefits should also take into account the savings from treatment's contribution to a halving of the expected infection rates and the productivity of those who no longer need to stay home or care for the sick.

"When we started with triple therapy," Teixeira says, "the main criticism from developed countries was that we didn't have the conditions for antiretroviral treatment. They said it would be dangerous for other countries, that we would create resistance."

Antiretrovirals, if taken incorrectly, can indeed create a more resistant strain of virus in the patient—and in anyone to whom it is transmitted. Patients must stick to a rigorous and complicated schedule of pills, some taken with food, some without, and they must keep to this program (at least this is the current thinking) every day for the rest of their lives.

Yet the worries of rich countries that the poor and uneducated will mess things up for the rest of us have proved unfounded. Any nation that provides its AIDS patients with antiretrovirals must also provide them with help and training to take the medicine correctly. Brazil is doing just this, although it has meant turning nurses into organizers of nature hikes and clinics into baby-formula warehouses.

In Ademildes Navarini's clinic at Raphael de Paula Souza hospital, a nurse's aide, Denise Feliciano, spends a large part of her day drawing suns and moons with a purple marker. Today she is preparing Rogério, the patient recovering from toxoplasmosis, to go home with a bag of medicine. Rogério has been taking antiretrovirals for three weeks, and he may or may not be taking them correctly. "What time do you take your pills?" she asks. She waits while he counts. He stops at six, groping for the next number. Seven? she supplies. Eight?

Rogerio makes a noise at eight.

How many pills do you take at eight at night?

"Three," he says, but he is holding up two fingers. It is not clear whether Rogério is confused or merely has trouble expressing himself. The toxoplasmosis has also affected his eyesight; he knows how to read, but he can't see.

Feliciano sits down next to him and takes out his bag of medicine, a sheet of paper, and her marker. "OK, how do you take Biovir?" she says.

They go through each drug, with Feliciano drawing suns and moons on the boxes of pills and making a list on a separate sheet in a large purple hand. She estimates that 30 percent of patients have trouble keeping to their schedules, the same figure I heard from doctors and health workers at other hospitals. Most patients, everyone agreed, eventually understand how to take their medicine.

But that doesn't mean they take it. "Many don't understand the need for treatment, and they abandon it at the first side effects," says Armesto, the psychologist in Nova Iguaçu's clinic. "It can become a vicious circle—no food, no money—so they can't take their medicine properly, so they get opportunistic diseases, so they can't work, they get depressed, and that leads them further away from treatment."

In 1999, the AIDS program conducted a survey of more than 1,000 patients in São Paulo. It found that 69 percent achieved 80 percent adherence, which means they took their medicine properly 80 percent of the time. According to Margaret Chesney, a professor of medicine at the University of California at San Francisco who studies behavioral factors in AIDS treatment, this rate is not sufficient to control the virus—which can kill even people who take their medicine faithfully—but it is no different from adherence rates in the United States. A study in San Diego showed that 72 percent of patients took their medicine 80 percent of the time.

The São Paulo study found that the most important factor in patient falloff was missing a doctor's appointment. Next came the level of instruction and support available at the clinic, followed by a patient's income and education. "Patient adherence depends directly on the quality of the services provided," Teixeira says. "People in bad economic situations have more difficulties, but we can overcome them if we provide good service."

The study reinforced Brazil's attempt to offer patients more sustained and varied help. AIDS officials expanded their training programs for people who work with patients. AIDS sufferers get free bus passes. Clinics ask local churches and Lions Clubs for food and baby formula. They recruit patients to sit in the waiting room and talk with other patients about their problems and to run Alcoholics Anonymous–style groups. The nurse at Nova Iguaçu recently took one group on a nature hike to a waterfall, because the patients seemed to be getting depressed.

"When we realize the patient is no longer coming to appointments, we send a telegram to ask them to come in and tell us why they stopped," says Rosa Maria Rezende, the social worker in Nova Iguaçu's clinic. "Then we try to overcome that. We want them to be more interested in the struggle to live. It is not their attitude toward medicine that matters; it is their attitude toward life."

At first glance, it would seem that Brazil has advantages that are hard to duplicate. It has a well-organized network of civic groups, which were essential to building support for the program, designing it and making it work. It is a big country, with a large market for drugs. It has a health-care system, however patchy. And while it is a poor country, it is a rich poor country.

Some countries will be unable to follow—they are too corrupt or war-torn or venally governed or not governed at all. In many of the African nations most ravaged by AIDS, the annual health budget comes to less than $10 per capita. This reflects the twisted priorities of leaders, many of whom can find sufficient money when they need to buy weapons. And health care is worsening thanks to AIDS itself, as doctors and nurses are among those most ravaged by the disease. But millions and millions of AIDS patients live in countries that could emulate Brazil, although they would need international help. These include virtually all the countries of Latin America and Eastern Europe, most of Asia and the former Soviet Union and at least ten countries in sub-Saharan Africa. Pilot programs in Ivory Coast and Uganda show that at well-run clinics, patients have the same rate of adherence as in Europe and the United States.

Brazil shows how a nation can create an AIDS infrastructure atop an unstable foundation. Fairly good in Brazil's rich regions, health care is bad to nonexistent in poor ones. The country has one of the lowest rates of life expectancy and highest rates of infant mortality in Latin America. "When we passed the bill, we had to rely on a distribution network that didn't exist," former President Sarney says.

It seems absurd to suggest that countries that will not spend 10 cents to cure an infant with diarrhea should spend thousands of dollars on her mother's AIDS drugs. But in Brazil, there has been no trade-off. The program has very likely saved the Health Ministry money, improved the treatment of other diseases, and—very important—fostered a vocal lobby for better health care. For countries with a poor health infrastructure, an internationally financed AIDS program could be a way to develop a network of clinics and trained workers who might also be able to cure diarrhea.

So why have other countries not done it? One reason is indifferent, or even hostile, leadership. Kenya's president, Daniel Arap Moi, only very recently reversed his opposition to condom use. AIDS carries such a stigma that the response of some African leaders has been to deny there is a problem. Other governments are too corrupt or incompetent to organize prevention programs, much less treatment. But for most countries, even middle-income poor countries, the biggest hurdle is cost. Whether AIDS treatment eventually pays for itself is irrelevant; they cannot afford to get started.

Nowhere are the lost opportunities more tragic than in South Africa. According to UNAIDS, South Africa has more than four million infected, and the epidemic is growing geometrically. It is a wealthy country by African standards, with a relatively good health infrastructure and laboratories that could manufacture generic drugs.

But South Africa has done nothing to treat AIDS. The biggest obstacle is President Thabo Mbeki, in other ways a sane and responsible leader, who has inexplicably decided that he is not convinced HIV causes AIDS. Absurdly, it has become politically incorrect to talk about treating AIDS in South Africa—because it would acknowledge that HIV is the cause. Mbeki's musings, as well as an intense political battle in South Africa about the country's AIDS priorities, delayed the institution of even a program to cut mother-to-child transmission.

India, the country that probably has the largest epidemic, is another dismaying example. India does not recognize patents on medicine, and world trade rules do not require it do so until 2005. Indian firms lead the world in the manufacture of generic AIDS drugs. The managing director of Cipla Ltd., an Indian generic manufacturer that meets international quality standards, told me in December that he could make a triple therapy for $500 per year, plus another $200 in packaging costs, "and prices are likely to come down as we improve our techniques." Does India provide its sick with free AIDS treatment? It does not.

But treating AIDS is gradually creeping into the realm of the possible for many countries. AIDS is now bad for business in Africa, and African leaders are hearing a clamor for treatment from the middle class. Several African countries have good prevention programs, which was all they believed possible to do. Now they are starting to think about treatment as well.

While Brazil's ability to reach patients encourages other nations, far more important is its success in lowering the cost of medicine. This is the news that can now allow other countries to dream about treating AIDS.

Eloan Pinheiro is a soft-spoken, ever-smiling fifty-five-year-old chemist who spent the first part of her career as chief of formulation for the Brazilian subsidiaries of two multinational drug companies. Now Pinheiro is tormenting her former colleagues. She is the director of Far-Manguinhos, a government pharmaceutical research lab and factory named for the industrial neighborhood of Rio where it is located. In 1998, with the costs of importing brand-name drugs mounting, Brazil's health minister asked Pinheiro to analyze and copy the world's major AIDS drugs. Far-Manguinhos and Brazil's six other state pharmaceutical factories now make seven of the twelve antiretrovirals taken by Brazilians with AIDS. Pinheiro buys raw materials from India and Korea.

From the drug companies' point of view, the assembly lines below Pinheiro's second-floor office are humming with the violation of intellectual-property rights, forty thousand times an hour. Brazil's 1996 law recognizing patents on medicine, passed to comply with the rules of the World Trade Organization, specifies that anything commercialized anywhere in the world by May 14, 1997, would forever remain unpatented in Brazil. That covers a lot—all the first-generation antiretrovirals like AZT, ddI, d4T, 3TC. It covers nevirapine, one of the nonnucleoside reverse transcriptase inhibitors, which, like protease inhibitors, make up the third drug in the triple cocktail. And by a few weeks, it covers the protease inhibitor indinavir. And at the end of last year, Brazil was causing tremors in the pharmaceutical industry by preparing to produce copies of Stocrin, a Merck antiretroviral that came out after 1996, which is patented in Brazil. Since Brazil started making generics of AIDS drugs, their cost has plummeted. The price of AIDS drugs with no Brazilian generic equivalent dropped 9 percent from 1996 to 2000. The price of those that compete with generics from Brazilian labs dropped 79 percent. But just the credible threat of generic competition is enough to get manufacturers to lower their prices.

There is no legal reason that other countries cannot do the same. Most drugs, including antiretrovirals, have never been patented in most sub-

Saharan African countries, so those countries are free to make or import generics. Even countries that do respect patents on medicines have this possibility. This is important, because every country joining the World Trade Organization must pass laws respecting medical patents—the reason Brazil did. But there is a WTO loophole that allows countries to make copies of patented items in certain situations, including that of a national emergency. According to a WTO official, governments could also choose to import generic drugs instead of making them. They can get what is called a compulsory license—in effect, they seize a patent—and manufacture or import a generic copy of a drug, paying the patentholder a reasonable royalty. Of all the tools available to poor countries, compulsory licensing is what the drug companies fear the most, since it represents the most direct assault on control of their patents. The United States has issued compulsory licenses in situations far less dire than those of AIDS-ravaged poor nations. Recent ones have been for tow trucks, stainless-steel wheels, and corn seeds. Such licenses are common remedies in antitrust cases.

But although trade rules provide legal ways for poor nations to get cheap medicine, there are other obstacles. Many do not even know it is legal. Countries that have tried to manufacture generic medicine have fallen under debilitating pressure from pharmaceutical companies and from Washington.

In Thailand, such pressure kept the government from making cheap antiretrovirals until last year. Thailand has long made zidovudine, the knockoff of Glaxo Wellcome's AZT. But two drugs are needed to slow AIDS, and Thailand was blocked from making the other components of dual therapy—ddI, d4T, and 3TC. Bristol-Myers Squibb sells ddI and d4T under the brand names Videx and Zerit. Glaxo sells 3TC under the name Epivir. None of the three were patented in Thailand because they came out before 1992, when the nation passed patent protections for medicine. Thailand's state drug factory was preparing to produce generic ddI when Bristol obtained a patent on the antacid buffer used to pack Videx into pill form. Krisana Kraisintu, the head of the factory, told me that Bristol also prevented the producers of the raw materials for ddI from selling to her. She was only able to make a generic ddI—in powder form—recently. (Bristol failed to respond to questions despite repeated requests over the course of a month.)

With Zerit and Epivir, Bristol and Glaxo took advantage of a controversial safety monitoring period passed in 1993 at American urging. It gives drugs up to five or six years of market exclusivity while generics undergo special safety tests—a law the World Health Organization and UNAIDS says "unnecessarily delays generic competition." Thailand was able to make generic d4T only when Zerit exited the program last year and is only now beginning to make generic 3TC.

The drug companies' actions are particularly distasteful because neither Bristol nor Glaxo invented these drugs or discovered their use in AIDS therapy. Glaxo's 3TC was discovered and patented for AIDS use by BioChem Pharma, a Canadian company, which licensed the drug to Glaxo. D4T was synthesized by the Michigan Cancer Foundation in 1966, using public funds. Its application for AIDS was discovered at Yale University, which holds the patent, using grants from the federal government and Bristol. In the United States, Bristol's Zerit sells for $4.50 for 40 milligrams. Pharmaceutical manufacturers never disclose their costs, but one indication of Bristol's markup is that Pinheiro can sell her version for 30 cents—and it is possible her costs are higher than Bristol's, since the multinationals have access to cheaper raw materials.

The National Institutes of Health discovered ddI's use as an AIDS therapy. The NIH then licensed the drug to Bristol for a 5 percent royalty, with the stipulation that Bristol's pricing take into account the health and safety needs of the public. But Bristol sells Videx for $1.80 in the United States for a 100-milligram tablet, while Far-Manguinhos in Brazil can sell the generic equivalent for 50 cents. The contract has a fair-pricing clause, but it has never been enforced.

The drug companies' influence has been greatly magnified because the United States trade officials have put the full weight of American trade pressures to work on their behalf. And one official told me that until very recently, "it was pretty rare" that his agency ever considered the health consequences. The statements in the trade representative's annual reports and trade watch lists document a shameful history of successful American efforts to get Thailand to pass patents on medicine, to abolish the pharmaceutical review board that monitored drug prices, to pass the safety monitoring period of market exclusivity, and to refrain from issuing compulsory licenses. Here is one example from the trade representative's 1997 national trade estimate for Thailand: "The Thai legislature is expected in 1997 to consider a bill abolishing the pharmaceutical review board. This measure would advance objectives of American manufacturers."

Numerous countries have been placed on the trade representative's Special 301 Watch List because of pharmaceutical patent disagreements. The list is a precursor to trade sanctions, but simply appearing on it is a form of sanction because it discourages investment. It turns a country's business sector and commerce ministry against generic production—and with such powerful opposition, local health officials lose. "When I wanted to produce generics, I was told, 'Don't move, because we're afraid of trade retaliation,'" Kraisintu says. "All of us know that the reason for all these things is pressure from the United States and multinational companies." Thailand sells a fifth of its exports to the United States.

The drug industry's dominance over American trade policy on pharmaceuticals finally crashed over South Africa. In 1997, South Africa, which does respect pharmaceutical patents, amended its laws to allow compulsory licensing of essential medicines, including AIDS drugs. Pharmaceutical companies sued. The suit is still going on.

Although Clinton administration officials acknowledged that what South Africa proposed was legal under the World Trade Organization, they declared war. President Clinton and Vice President Gore lobbied their counterparts, Nelson Mandela and Thabo Mbeki, then the deputy president. Friends of the drug companies in Congress passed a requirement that the State Department report on Washington's efforts to stop South Africa before the country could receive American aid. It reported in February 1999, that "all relevant agencies of the U.S. government . . . have been engaged in an assiduous, concerted campaign to persuade the government of South Africa to withdraw or modify" the relevant parts of the law.

This was a bizarre policy for an administration that claimed a special relationship with South Africa. But there was no role in the process of decisions about trade pressures for voices that countered those of industry. This resulted in egregious blind spots. In August 1998, I talked with an American trade official who worked on South Africa's medicines act. He told me that until a few months before I spoke to him, he was unaware of the dimensions of South Africa's AIDS problem. "Nobody brought it to my attention that it was a major health crisis," he said.

Today, this official is better informed. The administration changed its policy after activist groups began heckling Vice President Gore at his campaign appearances. When reporters, and later Gore aides, began to take notice, the administration told South Africa it could issue compulsory licenses for essential medicines as long as it stayed within world trade rules. Over the next year, the administration announced that health officials would participate in decisions about pharmaceutical disputes and pledged not to block compulsory licenses in the rest of sub-Saharan Africa and Thailand and in other countries on a case-by-case basis.

But pressure from other parts of the administration continued. In February 2000, William Daley, then the commerce secretary, traveled to Brazil and Argentina with Raymond Gilmartin, the CEO of Merck, and a vice president of Pfizer in tow. Before he went, Daley told students that one purpose of his trip to Brazil was to talk about "serious concerns our companies have" with medical patent laws. In Argentina, he threatened trade sanctions over the issue.

Overall, however, the Clinton administration went through a real conversion. Countries that displease American pharmaceutical manufacturers no longer land on a trade watch list if the trade representative believes they have a health emergency. But this could be reversed in five minutes by President Bush—and probably will be, since the industry is likely to be even more influential in the Bush administration than it has been under President Clinton. Pharmaceutical manufacturers give money to both political parties—$23 million in the last election cycle, according to the Center for Responsive Politics—but 69 percent of it went to Republicans. The drug industry also spends $75 million or so on lobbying every year.

From the beginning of the AIDS epidemic, the major drug makers clung to the idea of one planet, one price. Or worse—some drugs cost more in Kenya than in Norway. The strategy has earned them a public image almost as malignant as that of tobacco companies. By last year, they were also facing the growing threat of generics and the loss of Washington's automatic trade support. Early in 2000, several companies began to discuss the idea of lowering their prices in the Third World.

In May 2000, Glaxo Wellcome, Merck, Boehringer-Ingelheim, F. Hoffmann-La Roche and Bristol announced a program called Accelerating Access, promising to sell drugs at deep discounts to poor countries that met certain standards. The price cuts the drug companies fought until last year have now become their solution to the world's AIDS crisis.

The companies have restricted their discounts, demanding that recipient countries properly administer the medicine. But the restrictions also keep the program small, controlled, and largely secret. Each price cut for each drug in each country is negotiated separately. Glaxo was the only company to specify a price reduction publicly, announcing it would cut Combivir from $16 to $2 a day. And while about twenty countries are talking to the drug companies, only Senegal and Uganda have so far signed agreements to receive cut-price antiretrovirals. The discounts are impressive—Senegal will be able to buy triple therapy for as low as $1,000 per year per person.

But just a few hundred people will benefit, most of them rich enough to pay themselves. In Uganda, about a thousand people will get the drugs, but they will all pay for them.

The pharmaceutical industry argues that collaborative efforts like this one are the way to make AIDS medicine affordable in the Third World. But the program is too crabbed. "Why don't they just lower their prices in poor countries?" asks Ellen 't Hoen, who works in the Médecins Sans Frontières campaign to help poor countries get needed medicines. "Having country-by-country confidential negotiations is not justified. This way, it stays in the charity corner and it hampers the development of more sustainable ways to get medicines to people." The industry's control over the program serves another purpose: the companies can use it to head off the practices they fear most, chiefly compulsory licensing. The document announcing the plan calls on the recipients of their largesse to "respect intellectual property"—code for "stay away from compulsory licensing." And countries are complying, many of them out of ignorance.

Every single drug company executive I spoke with argued that if countries turn to compulsory licensing, new discoveries could eventually slow. "If we are to continue with research and development, then countries that participate in the program must provide conditions basic to innovation," Tadeu Alves, the chief of Merck's Brazil subsidiary, said during a panel at an AIDS conference in Rio. Those conditions, he said, included a free market, price structures that provide incentive to innovation, and respect for intellectual property.

The drug companies' argument is in essence a defense of high profits. Even in the United States, the cost of drugs is provoking questions about whether continued research and development really depends on giving companies a twenty-year monopoly to charge whatever price they choose, especially since they are often marketing other people's discoveries. The manufacturers generally spend twice as much on marketing and administration as they do on research and development. The real threat that Third-World generics pose to pharmaceutical companies is that of blowback in rich nations. They worry that publicity about generic prices will fuel the American demand for cheap imports or price controls. They fear that patent seizures in the Third World could loosen intellectual property rights in the First World.

Innovation would certainly suffer if pharmaceutical manufacturers could not charge high prices in their primary markets, although how high is open to debate. But applying this argument to Ukraine or Uganda is a scare tactic. No manufacturer depends on profits in Africa, which will account for 1.3 percent of worldwide drug sales next year, to motivate the search for new medicines. And companies can sell their AIDS drugs at very steep discounts—some at 90 percent or more off the American price—and still profit.

Once they realized that Brazil was solidly behind its generic drug program, the pharmaceutical companies have made the best of it, and they have not suffered. In fact, the government is buying twenty thousand daily doses of Crixivan (Merck's brand of indinavir), a tenth of the drug's worldwide sales. Merck had to meet Pinheiro's price for indinavir, the generic. But the company can do this and still profit. "The half-million infected today are patients of tomorrow," Tadeu Alves told me.

The same thing may soon happen with Merck's Stocrin, which is patented in Brazil. Pinheiro is threatening to get a compulsory license to make the generic. The threat will most likely force Merck to drop the price or voluntarily license Pinheiro to make the generic or sell Stocrin. And this arrangement will be profitable for Merck, which shows no sign of shutting its labs because of Brazil. Yet the pharmaceutical industry continues to paint the ongoing battle against generics in impoverished nations as Armageddon. Glaxo has even stopped the Indian generic manufacturer Cipla from selling a knockoff of a Glaxo AIDS drug in Ghana. Ghana's share of the international antiretroviral market is virtually zero.

If wealthy countries and the United Nations agencies they influence chose to make AIDS treatment available to every citizen of the earth in the most efficient and cost-effective manner possible, the program would look very much like Unicef's global system of vaccination. When Unicef began a campaign to vaccinate the world's children in the early 1980s, many scoffed. But today vaccination rates top 80 percent, saving three million lives a year and preventing crippling diseases in tens of millions more. This is one of the world's most significant public health victories.

Who pays to vaccinate a child in Angola? We do, without much complaint. Antiretrovirals, of course, do not cost pennies per dose. But they would be a lot cheaper than they are today if the World Health Organization or UNAIDS used a Unicef-like system, which has dropped the price of vaccines to a thirtieth of their American price in some cases. The WHO could buy antiretrovirals for Third-World use from reliable generic suppliers like Cipla in India or brand-name manufacturers if they were willing to lower their prices. The economies of scale and guaranteed markets could drop the price of a year's triple therapy to below the $700 that Cipla could muster today.

This is a price many countries could afford, especially when balanced against the savings in hospitalizations. But everyone agrees that AIDS treatment will require North America and Europe to purchase the medicines and to help set up the necessary health-care network. In my calculus, applying the Unicef system to AIDS would cost $3 billion a year in antiretrovirals alone, assuming five million patients at $600 a year. And the cost will increase as countries reach more patients. This is a large sum of money. It seems somewhat smaller, however, next to the wards of shaven-head babies—or the collapse of a continent.

It is difficult to imagine the Bush administration endorsing such a global plan. There are, however, smaller, worthwhile steps the administration could take if it were so inclined. At minimum, it should bury forever the bad old policy of intimidating countries that want to make or buy generics, especially through compulsory licensing. The administration should also encourage agencies like the World Health Organization and UNAIDS to facilitate these purchases and the necessary training to make them work.

There are also laws already on the books, which the Clinton administration chose not to carry out, that could promote the cheap production of at least some antiretrovirals. One such law allows the government to seize patents of drugs that were discovered at government labs or with substantial public funds if the patent holder is not meeting public health needs—for example, by charging too much. James Love, who runs the Consumer Project on Technology, a Ralph Nader–affiliated advocacy group, argues that it applies to five antiretrovirals. Love would like to see the government license them to a nonprofit corporation that would produce the drugs cheaply for both the First- and Third-World markets.

But the Bush administration is unlikely to be so inclined, because the drug companies have other ideas. "Merck and other companies appreciate that our products need to be more affordable in the developing world," Jeffrey Sturchio, a Merck spokesman, told me, echoing every pharmaceutical maker. "We are willing to sit down and be a constructive partner. Compulsory licensing is unnecessary." But compulsory licensing seems very necessary. Merck would have little interest in constructive partnership in Brazil—or anywhere—if that threat did not exist.

This is the larger lesson of Brazil: AIDS can become a manageable disease in the Third World, but it takes power, in addition to other things. The ability to pull the price of AIDS drugs within reach of those who need them may someday come from the backing of some international organization, or the pharmaceutical industry might find religion. But at the moment, it arises only from the threat to make or buy generic drugs. AIDS is turning the Third World's human landscape into a parched wasteland. Brazil has shown that, armed with the power of competition, a government can do more than sit and watch the desert encroach.

INDIA'S PLAGUE

MICHAEL SPECTER

from The New Yorker

| **December 17, 2001** |

I.

Late on an autumn afternoon a little more than a year ago, a nattily dressed chemist named Yusuf K. Hamied strolled into a conference room at the headquarters of the European Commission, in Brussels. He carried in his briefcase a simple proposition, and, in delivering it to the politicians, health ministers, and international pharmaceutical executives who were gathered there, he dispensed with the pleasantries and dry language so common in conversations about regulation, drug pricing, and global-tariff regimes. "Friends," he began, although he was fairly sure he had none in the room, "I represent the needs and aspirations of the Third World. I represent the capabilities of the Third World, and above all I represent an opportunity." It was time, he said, for the people who control the earth's resources and its capital to face up to their "responsibility to alleviate the suffering of millions of our fellow-men who are afflicted with HIV and AIDS."

Speeches like this one have become standard in the era of globalization. But Yusuf Hamied is not the average do-gooder campaigning for a more equitable world. He is one of India's most successful businessmen. He lives in (among other places) Windsor Villa, the Bombay home where Salman Rushdie was raised, and he earned a Ph.D. from Cambridge at the age of twenty-three. His father, who was also a chemist, and who helped start India's first national university, at Mahatma Gandhi's request, became rich by importing a popular sexual tonic from Germany. In 1935, he used the profits to start Cipla, the giant pharmaceutical house that the younger Hamied now runs.

Yusuf Hamied wasn't in Brussels to talk about money. He was there because he was scared. Over the past few years, he had become convinced that his country was edging into an AIDS apocalypse every bit as severe as the one that has engulfed Africa. With the possible exception of South Africa, there is no country on earth where more people are infected with the AIDS virus than India. By last fall, Bombay, where Cipla has its headquarters, was competing for the dismal honorific of AIDS capital of the world, with more than 250,000 HIV-positive inhabitants.

Hamied laid down a challenge for the officials he addressed that day: start selling drugs at prices that the poor can afford or I will do it for you. It wasn't an empty threat. The Indian government long ago decided that only the *process* used in making a drug could be patented; the final product itself could be copied freely. In the West, Cipla is regarded, with not a little bit of rancor, as one of the great pirate enterprises of the corporate world—a company that flaunts international convention, routinely copies the molecular formulas of new drugs, and then sells for pennies in India what would cost a hundred times as much in Europe or America.

Hamied ended his speech in Brussels by reading a list of drugs that his company makes and the low prices he now intended to charge for them. Soon after returning home, he offered to donate supplies of a drug called neviraprane to the Indian government; when it is taken at the beginning of labor, neviraprane has proved to be remarkably effective at preventing the AIDS virus from being passed from mother to child. The government declined. In December, Hamied made his offer again—of the prime minister personally. This time, he heard nothing.

Then, on the morning of January 26, 2001—India's Republic Day—the state of Gujarat was struck by the most devastating earthquake in the country's history; at least thirty thousand people died, and seven hundred thousand were left homeless. "Somehow, that just really woke me up," Hamied told me when we met in New York this summer, in his suite at the Palace Hotel. It was a muggy day, and from his lounge on the forty-seventh floor we watched as storm clouds danced around the building. "I sent medicine, and I was happy to do it," he went on. "But afterward I sat down with my top managers and I said, 'Look at what the hell is happening in our country. AIDS is the worst tragedy this country could ever experience—

with the possible exception of a nuclear war—and it is a completely foreseen tragedy. Why are we all donating for Gujarat and doing nothing about this great plague?' I decided right then that, if I had to, I would do it by myself. People think this is all about Africa, but it's not. For me, it's about my own home."

So Hamied went out and started a revolution. Thanks to Cipla, a year's worth of crucial AIDS medication that until recently sold in America for more than $15,000 is now available in many parts of the Third World for $350. Multinational pharmaceutical giants condemned Hamied. "Stealing ideas is not how one provides good health care," Shannon Herzfeld, a spokeswoman for the American pharmaceutical industry, said last year.

Yet the big companies have also realized that clinging to patent laws during an international plague is bad for business, and the impact of Cipla's decision has been extraordinary. Entire countries have shifted the focus of their public health systems—simply because AIDS treatment suddenly seems affordable. Led by Secretary-General Kofi Annan, the United Nations this past summer held its first General Assembly meeting devoted solely to a disease. Soon afterward, the heads of the Group of Eight leading industrial nations met in Genoa and committed themselves to spending $12 billion on AIDS, as protesters rioted in the ancient streets around them. This spring, a group of well-known Harvard professors released a lengthy document in which they, too, argued that it is no longer morally permissible for the West to deny patients in the world's poorest countries AIDS drugs that could prolong their lives. From Africa to Brazil, Hamied and his crusade for access to these drugs have been embraced as a symbol of hope by activists who believe they are engaged in a global war against apartheid in health care.

The clamor has been so intense that few public health officials have dared to say publicly what many believe: that it makes far more sense to try to prevent HIV than to focus on treating it. The reasons are obvious: prevention averts the sickness and death that AIDS inevitably causes; many AIDS drugs are not only expensive but complicated, toxic, and difficult to take correctly. In addition, in countries like India—where per-capita spending on health care is about $10 a year, and where the government is committed to using public funds to finance it—placing emphasis on any costly treatment is hard to justify when scores of health problems that could be cured cheaply and easily are so common. Last year in India, there were more than 1.1 million reported cases of malaria; filaria, a parasitic nematode, which blocks the lymphatic system and causes serious swelling, is epidemic; Japanese encephalitis, which is spread by the Culex mosquito, is endemic and kills many children; yaws, a contagious, disfiguring infection, has been prevalent in India for years and is easily cured with a single shot of penicillin. Each year, there are two million new cases of tuberculosis; more than a thousand people die from it every day. India also accounts for 70 percent of the world's leprosy. Statistics like these tend to make Indians weary—and unwilling to listen when they are told that the latest disease to afflict them is the most dangerous.

"In America, there is an endless discourse about risk: which kids are at risk, what are the health risks, how do we guard against them?" says Mark Koops-Elson, an anthropologist at the University of Chicago who is writing his dissertation on India's cultural and financial attitudes toward risk and health. "Which diseases are worse than others? There is no such conversation in India. Given the vastness of the problems that people in India face and the poverty that exists, most people just say our responsibilities lie with those who are closest to us. Trying to fix the entire society is too overwhelming."

II.

I flew into New Delhi at the beginning of June, almost twenty years to the day after the Centers for Disease Control, in Atlanta, published the first words about what would become the AIDS pandemic—an account of five unexplained cases of *Pneumocystis carinii* pneumonia among gay men in Los Angeles. Since then, twenty-two million people have died and forty million live with the infection, most of them too poor to receive even rudimentary palliative care. In its early years, AIDS was an absolute and fairly rapid death sentence. In 1986, however, hope for a prolonged life emerged when the drug AZT, or zidovudine, was shown to delay the degenerative effects that the virus has on the immune system. AZT was the first of a new class of antiretroviral drugs that work by suppressing the ability of HIV to reproduce. This helps maintain the integrity of the immune system and postpones the development of opportunistic infections, which are often the cause of death in people afflicted with AIDS. Among Americans today, the prevailing view is that the AIDS epidemic has begun to wane. That is not true. Each day brings at least sixteen thousand new infections throughout the world. As many as one-quarter of them are in India alone.

The first cases of AIDS in India were not reported until 1986, in Bombay and in the southern industrial city of Madras, and until then there had been every hope that the nation would avoid the devastation that has occurred in countries like Zimbabwe and Botswana, where at least a quarter of the adult population is now infected with HIV. After all, it was said, the Indian family is remarkably close and sustaining. Surveys often show that Indian men, once they are married, are more likely to remain faithful than men from many other cultures; furthermore, half of Indian women marry by the age of eighteen, and more than 90 percent are still virgins when they do. In much of Africa, on the other hand, there is little stigma attached to sexual promiscuity, and the incidence of venereal disease—which is a reliable barometer for the presence of HIV—has always been high. In addition, despite the fact that half a billion people in India live on less than a dollar a day, millions of others are members of a rapidly growing middle class. The streets of Delhi, Madras, and Bombay are not simply overrun with beggars; they are also filled with motorcycles, schoolchildren in crisp blue uniforms, and eager businessmen toting laptops and riding to work in motorized rickshaws.

But prosperity itself—the new mobility, rising income levels, and the excellent system of national highways—has played a role in exacerbating the crisis. During the past twenty years, India has become one of the great migration centers of the world, and migrant populations are at a higher risk for AIDS. They are also more likely to spread the disease. There are at least a hundred thousand long-haul truckers shuttling back and forth across the subcontinent, more than two million prostitutes, 275,000 brothels, and tens of millions of seasonal workers who come to the big cities for a few months each year. AIDS travels along the truck routes as efficiently as white blood cells do along the arteries of the human body—and one can trace the evolution of the epidemic with eerie accuracy simply by comparing traffic patterns moving out of major cities with the rates of infection of people who live along the way. In parts of Nepal, HIV is called Mumbai disease (Mumbai is the Hindi name for Bombay), because the people who contracted it uniformly went to work in the great city and came home sick. And, because there is a lag of many years between infection and any visible sign of illness, the epidemic can grow unnoticed until it is simply too large to control.

Not long after I arrived in Delhi, I stopped by the office of Swarup Sarkar, who is the head of the United Nations AIDS program for South Asia. Sarkar had just returned from a brief visit to Bangladesh, where the epidemic is spreading slowly, and he was planning a trip to the Burmese border, where it is much worse. He gave me a cup of tea and we sat down in front of his computer with a CD full of data, some colorful maps, and a few very disturbing suggestions about the future health of his country. On charts tracing the course of the epidemic as it moved through India, the country was shown in different colors, depending upon the prevalence of infection. A child would have been able to follow the coded patterns: the earliest map, from 1986, was mostly pale, indicating low levels of contagion; by 1990, a bright yellow had begun to appear in abundance. That color represented high-risk groups—gay men, sex workers, drug users—at least 5 percent of whom had been infected. The numbers have been inching upward for years, but studies have shown that once the rate of infection among women who are tested in birth clinics rises above 1 percent, it becomes nearly impossible to keep an epidemic like HIV from seeping into the rest of the population. That is what is now happening in many parts of India. Red represents pockets of infection that have grown beyond that 1 percent figure. The maps that Sarkar showed me from 1986 to 1990 had no red in them; by last year, much of the country, from Manipur, in the northeast, to Kerala, at the southern tip of the continent, was awash in crimson.

The course of the epidemic in India closely resembles the early pattern in Thailand, where infection spread almost exclusively among heterosexuals. Yet the differences in official policy couldn't be greater. In the mid-1980s, HIV hit Thailand with force, and within a few years the government had prepared an aggressive campaign of information targeted directly at the people who were most at risk, preventing hundreds of thousands of new infections. But such success costs money, and requires commitment. Thailand spends more than sixty cents per person on HIV, whereas India spends a little less than six cents, or sixty million dollars a year—in other words, only twice what Thailand spends, although India's population is sixteen times as large. From the king to local village leaders, Thai officials have made many public statements about the dangers of HIV and about how the disease is spread. In India, in part because of a national reluctance to speak publicly about sex, nothing like this has happened. No movie stars appear at fund-raisers, no prominent politicians admit to being gay. No mayor would visit a hospice. India desperately needs a Rock Hudson or a Magic Johnson. "We had very few cases for years," Sarkar said. "It was possible to do something, and all we did was watch." In the nine years between the first cases of AIDS in the United States and the real beginnings of the epidemic in India, fictions and theories evolved to suggest that Indians were immune to HIV, that they had protective genes and simply couldn't get sick in the same way that Africans or Europeans did. By 1994, however, it had become clear that such conjecture was nonsense. Meanwhile, the maps kept getting darker.

Sarkar, who is forty-eight, looks like a middleweight wrestler. His principal job is to help the United Nations formulate and carry out its AIDS policies; but, like virtually all countries that have been seriously affected by AIDS, India has consistently sought to minimize the extent of its problem. Not long ago, Prasada Rao, who runs India's National AIDS Control Organization, complained publicly that the estimate of four million HIV-infected Indians, which is frequently used by the United Nations and the World Bank—a figure that most experts consider very conservative—was "too high and not based on any sound epidemiological evidence." No public health official with experience in India believes that, and most think Rao himself knows better. When I first met Rao, I asked him the question that has so alarmed AIDS experts throughout the world: Did he think India would become another Africa? "I was afraid for a year or two when I began my job," he said. "But I no longer have that fear. We are aware of the problems, and we are working hard to address them. I think it's clear that we have begun to succeed."

When I told Swarup Sarkar about my conversation with Rao, he simply shook his head in sorrowful acceptance. "We have told ourselves so many lies," Sarkar said. "The government says officially that there are 'only' four million infected Indians." He repeated the words. "*Only four million.* Possibly they are correct. But every time we have said the epidemic was limited, or not spreading as fast as in other places, we have been proved wrong. What is scary is that we don't have any reason to say that we are seeing numbers that have reached a plateau. It would be very surprising to think that the AIDS epidemic has stabilized in India, where at least 75 percent of the population gets no education. No intervention. Nothing. Whether it will suddenly have another jump"—as the epidemic did in many places in Africa—"we simply cannot say."

III.

Late one steamy night in the middle of June, I drove to the Pukkenthrui truck stop, which is about an hour out of Madras and just five miles from the spot on National Highway 47 where, in 1991, Rajiv Gandhi was killed by a suicide bomber. The monsoons were about to begin, and the ripe, heavy smell of tamarind rolled across the humid roadway. My guide was Nobin Jos, a thoughtful young man who runs the Trucker-Highway Community Health Project, an AIDS-education program that has such limited resources that the drivers use sawed-off logs by the road for seats during meetings. Steady traffic pounded the battered highway as we passed the city's broad, festering slums. Most Indian cities, because they are extremely congested, don't permit big trucks to enter during the day, so truckers move at night. It was a moonless evening, and as we started to pick up speed I saw a string of women standing by the side of the road, slowly waving red flashlights at the cars driving by. Eighteen-wheelers lined the shoulder.

"They are lonely and ignorant men, but they are desperate for work," Jos told me after we arrived at the truck stop and stood watching his colleagues give a brief lecture on AIDS to the assembled drivers. (There were demonstrations with a wooden penis on how to use a condom, which was cause for great merriment among the startled drivers.) When they are available, a package of three condoms costs less than one rupee (about two cents), but not many men see the point of spending the money. None of the drivers spoke English. But Jos, acting as an interpreter, helped me talk with a few. We sat at a roadside restaurant, next to a military hotel, where flatbread baked in a kiln and we were served a dark, chalky tea in plastic jugs. The men wore turbans, N.B.A. T-shirts, and towels around their waists. Some were toothless, others were barefoot, and all of them were eager to chat. I was surprised by how few had heard of AIDS. None had any basic understanding of the epidemiology of the disease. "I only have sex once a week on the road," a man from north of Bombay told me. Then he added, I think for what he assumed would be my approval, "And I always take a bath with lime water afterward."

During nearly a month spent travelling through cities and towns with a combined population far larger than that of France, I noticed only two posters advertising condoms. One ad on a billboard in Madras, which featured an alluring woman, said simply, "Look before you sleep." (I had no idea that this was an AIDS advertisement until I was told. It could just as easily have been about buying a decent mattress.) The only Indian television commercials that talk about HIV—in Hindi and in English—were paid for by Cipla, not by the government; they are extremely well produced, but they dwell on the fact that new treatments make AIDS a disease that people can finally combat. Explicit messages about how one becomes infected are almost completely absent. Abstinence is neither preached nor practiced. India has a rich sexual history, but outside its biggest cities it remains deeply conservative, and public discourse about sexual conduct is limited.

While I was in Delhi, my driver was a sweet, middle-aged man from a northern hill town. Like tens of thousands of other such men, he returns to his village to see his wife and children no more than three or four times each year. I never had the nerve to ask him what he did about sex the rest of the time. Statistically, at least, the answer is clear: one study of seven hundred Tamil truck drivers showed that the percentage of those infected with HIV rose from 1.5 percent in 1995 to more than 6 percent just two years later. By last year, more than 20 percent of the drivers were infected—a figure with ominous echoes of the early epidemic in Africa, where AIDS made the inevitable leap from groups like truck drivers and prostitutes into the wider population. Many experts find it hard to believe that India can avoid a similar fate. "Even the most conservative government estimates predict that in seven years there will be at least ten million people infected with HIV here," Subhash Hira told me. He is the director of the AIDS unit at the noble, decrepit Sir J. J. Hospital, in Bombay, and a professor of infectious diseases at the University of Texas's medical school, in Houston. "This is a heterosexual epidemic with the potential to destroy this society and decimate our economy. And nobody seems to be terribly concerned."

Perhaps because the epidemic first appeared in Madras and Bombay, those cities have made the best efforts to deal with it. One morning, Suniti Solomon collected me at my hotel and drove me to her bright, tidy clinic on Raman Street in Madras. She is a short, soft-spoken woman, who treated the first AIDS cases in India and has probably seen more patients than any other infectious-disease specialist in the country. I spent most of the morning with her, first talking about AIDS and then sitting in on a counseling session. A barefoot woman with eyes the color of coal, hair coiled to her waist, and rings on nearly every toe crept into the office. She was thirty but looked younger. The woman had been selected randomly to participate in a health survey using residents from 30 of the 945 slums in Madras. In exchange for answering a series of questions about her health and giving blood for research, she would receive free care (paid for by the National Institute of Mental Health, in the United States, which sponsored the studies). The woman's anxiety was obvious. She lived in a slum near the beach that borders the Bay of Bengal. She had been feeling weak and dizzy, and had been unable to make it through her usual eighteen-hour day. "My husband pulls a rickshaw," she told Solomon, an almost preternaturally reassuring woman. "He does not want me to be at this clinic." She said that he had been treated before for sexually transmitted diseases, and had recently become quite ill.

"Do you know whether he has HIV?" Solomon asked.

"What is that?" the woman replied blankly, staring at the wall clock, afraid of what would happen if her husband got home before she did. After she left, the doctor explained that the woman was in a "love marriage"—which among slum dwellers in southern India is still not common. It suggests a certain independence on the woman's part; if the marriage had been arranged, she would probably never have had the resolve to come. "We will know in a day if she is infected," Solomon told me. "But it will be hard to persuade her husband to come in to be tested or to permit her to be treated—even though it will cost him nothing." Doctors have to deal with this problem every day, in every city. Of all the obstacles that physicians and AIDS agencies face in India, nothing is as discouraging as the plight of women. New brides are usually illiterate and are exposed to AIDS by the most highly valued factor in Indian culture: monogamous marriage. "Ninety percent of my women who are HIV-positive have a single partner, and that is their husband," one of Solomon's colleagues, at another hospital in Madras, told me. "I always say to them, 'Don't match your horoscopes for marriage. Please match your blood tests.' But it's hard to enforce. Imagine a girl's parents asking a boy's parents for a blood statement. Not in India; that will never happen."

In many parts of the country, a woman is regarded as a relatively valuable farm animal; her health matters only because she is required to raise children and keep house. "No husband would allow a wife to go alone for an examination outside the immediate slum," the sociologist Radhikha Ramasubban told me. "A woman has to have another woman, an older person, or a man act as an escort." Ramasubban has been studying the health of women in the slums of Bombay for years. "Nobody is willing to free them from household duties, child-minding duties. And what is that one visit going to do? Even if you can get them to go, they won't make the follow-up. And then the test, and the confirmation for the test. And going back for consultation. With tuberculosis, social workers used to go to their houses to find out if they had taken their medicines. With HIV, the treatment is far more complicated, and it must go on for life. Who is going to attempt that here? It's such a hopeless task."

IV.

It is only after spending some time in India's government hospitals that one can fully understand that the debate about access to the most advanced

AIDS therapy, though good-hearted, is beside the point. The hospitals are depressing because they are filled with dedicated, well-trained doctors who don't have enough money to do their jobs properly. At several facilities that I visited, needles are routinely bleached and used more than once, medical instruments are sterilized in giant soup pots, and patients had better hope that a family member or friend will bring them food if they want to eat. At the Hospital of Thoracic Medicine, just south of Madras, a former tuberculosis clinic that has become a vast government holding pen for hundreds of people infected with HIV, antiretroviral drugs are not offered or discussed; neither is aspirin. The patients are treated with as much compassion as an overburdened staff can muster, and that's about it. As one nurse explained to me, "In America, you may do an MRI scan every time somebody has a headache. We can't even take X-rays when somebody breaks a bone."

Suniti Solomon's Y.R.G. center, in Madras, presents a different and more complex picture. Y.R.G. is the biggest AIDS clinic in southern India, and it is probably the best one in the country. So far, eleven thousand patients have passed through it (not all of them HIV-positive). With the help of foreign aid money and many donated drugs (from Cipla and other companies) and grants for research, patients receive counseling, testing, nutritional guidance, and what palliative care there is to offer. Doctors treat the many infections that HIV can cause; they also explain the more fundamental powers of antiretroviral drugs, which are often available to those who can afford to pay up to $2,000 a year. Only about one patient in ten attempts to use the medicine.

In the past five years, the treatment for AIDS has had to become more complex in order to match the sophistication of the virus, which quickly learns to evade the effects of a single drug. Standard care has moved far from the days when AZT was the drug of choice; each patient must now take an assortment of medicines, which work together to suppress the virus. The therapeutic cocktail is called haart (highly active antiretroviral therapy), and a patient has to take at least three drugs a day; it also requires constant monitoring and medical attention. The treatment can dramatically improve an infected person's prospects for a healthy future, but it must be fine-tuned frequently and taken for life. For many of Solomon's patients, it is simply not an option.

Y.R.G. also has a ward at a local hospital. The day I was there, the staff was struggling to deal with a long line of emaciated people waiting for help. N. Kumarasamy, who works with Suniti Solomon, keeps his medicines in metal gym lockers in the hallway—they serve as his pharmacy. In order to provide AIDS drugs, he takes whatever he can get; the occasional grant from a pharmaceutical firm or a few dozen doses of AZT brought back by a friend from an international conference. Kumarasamy was educated at Johns Hopkins, among other places, and when Solomon asked him to direct the health-care clinic he agreed without hesitation. "Lots of our patients come from other, pretty good clinics," he told me. "Doctors see them as a liability and a waste of time. They are going to die, it's an expensive disease to treat, so why bother? You have no idea how many famous people fly from Delhi so that they don't have to be treated in their own town. The first thing they ask is 'Do you recognize me?' We always say no."

The clinic—a former leprosy center that had been abandoned—is open and warm, but, even here, the stigma that surrounds AIDS in India remains. If you ask for Y.R.G. at the hospital reception desk, the clerk will look at you differently than if you were to ask for any other ward. This is typical. In Delhi, I had spent a morning in a leafy suburb at an AIDS group home owned by a prominent politician. It was lovely—light and filled with children, mothers, and the smell of curry coming from the communal kitchen. The man who owns the house has no idea that it is used as an AIDS-care center. If he did know, he would undoubtedly evict the group at once. Still, there is plenty of suspicion about the house in the neighborhood. No laundry man will go there, nor will fruit venders or trash collectors. Children steer clear of it. "They all look away when we walk down the street," one HIV-infected mother told me when I visited. "Nobody will even look at our faces."

The stigma of the disease makes it hard for doctors and aid workers to do their jobs, but the obstacles that confront the patients themselves seem almost biblical in their severity. "One day, this man came to see me," Solomon told me. "A nice man, caring. He is a landlord and owns acres and acres. His only son is positive. Of course, people came to him and sought to arrange a marriage, and he kept telling everyone, 'No, no, my son has to study and isn't ready for marriage.' And finally his own sister brought her daughter, which in south India is very common. She said, 'You can't do that, my brother, you have to marry your son to my daughter. It's only right.' So he told her the truth: 'My son has HIV, and I don't want your daughter to get sick.' He saw the change in his sister's face, and she walked away without a word. His wife, who had been hiding behind the door, heard what he said, and she told their son. The mother and child dressed in their best clothes and went out and bought poison powder in bulk. They drank it together and got into the car. Then the son drove as fast as he could into a big tree and killed them both. After that, the father came to me—his life was ruined. He said, 'All I have done is try to save my niece from getting HIV, and now I have lost everything.'

"It was a very, very hard moment for me. I just left the office and went home. I have a dog, and I tell him things I would never say to a human being. So through my tears I told him all about the man who tried to save his niece."

For Solomon and her staff, the stress is almost unbearable. She spends half her day fighting denial; the rest of the time, she must explain to her patients why drugs so commonly available in other countries remain too expensive for them. It is a difficult and often contradictory task: she knows as well as anyone that while drug treatment won't solve India's AIDS problems, it could help focus more attention on the implications of the epidemic. Indeed, one of the strongest arguments for providing expensive treatment to poor countries is that without it people will have no reason to learn if they are infected and no reason to change their behavior. But a simpler and cheaper approach would save more lives.

"I hear these people in the West talking about what we should have all the time," Solomon said. "For us, it's not about patents and pharmaceutical giants and money. It's about our poverty, which is profound. If I were offered drugs or food, I would take the food, because I know it will give my patients a better quality of life. I would do that even if the drugs cost nothing. You have to distribute drugs, and they need to be used by the right date. You have to take eight glasses of water a day with some of them. You have to store some of them in a refrigerator. Nobody has a refrigerator here. On top of all this, there will be resistance developing to the drugs. People will take them as long as they can afford them, then they will stop."

Resistance develops when patients fail to complete the full course of treatment, and that can cause more harm than not taking a drug at all. (It is for this reason that tuberculosis has returned to such deadly prominence throughout the world.) Resistance makes it possible for any virus to gain resilience and power. "Look at penicillin," Solomon said. "In 1949, if you took one hundred strains of staph, penicillin killed them all. Every one. Today, if you take the same one hundred strains, ninety-nine of them will survive because of indiscriminate use. You think that won't happen with HIV?" In fact, in America it is already happening. One recent study, based in San Francisco—which has some of the world's most sophisticated medical facilities, experienced AIDS doctors, and motivated patients—predicts that by 2005 nearly half of all HIV patients in the city will fail to respond to the drugs they currently use to treat the disease. When resistant strains of HIV are passed on to others, the people who have been infected have a much harder time from the start and are less likely to respond to conventional treatment. "People will become resistant, and the disease will redouble its power," Solomon continued. "All the while, people will be getting the message that there is a cure, and they will carry on having sex without condoms. Drugs used the wrong way kill people—and they are used the wrong way all the time. We have to get more training. Food. Clean water. Give us condoms, for God's sake. Teach women to read. But keep your drugs. They really won't help us now."

V.

The most important question about Yusuf Hamied's personal revolution has also been the most difficult to confront: Is the movement for affordable AIDS treatment, which Cipla almost accidentally came to represent, actually pulling attention and money away from the vaccines and preventive strategies that in India are most likely to save millions of lives? More than five times as much money is spent treating sick people as is spent keeping them healthy in the first place. And much of that money is spent on people who are on the verge of death. Can that be fair? One reason the debate between prevention and treatment has always been so difficult is that sick people are easily identified, they have names, and their suffering can be acute. Who would want to ignore such pain? Money spent on prevention, on the other hand, is often used to protect people we don't even know. The public is vast and vulnerable, but it does not have a face or a name. (This is one of the reasons that AIDS-prevention efforts are so often weak. In the United States, for example, several hundred million dollars in federal funds is dedicated each year to prevention and education programs, whereas seven billion dollars annually is allocated for AIDS treatment.)

One is not supposed to make calculations like these, because they explicitly attach a cost to a human life; such thinking is considered callous and particularly unfair in an age of global wealth beyond measure. Nevertheless, we attach costs to human lives every day; in the United States, we know that lowering the speed limit by ten miles an hour would save thousands of lives each year, yet, as a society, we feel it's worth that price to travel that much faster; we also know that alcohol and tobacco are responsible for much sickness and death. We don't ban them, because we are willing to pay the price for the pleasure they provide.

AIDS activists insist that the potential devastation of the illness is so great that we cannot afford to make a choice between preventing the disease and treating the sick; whatever the cost, we must do both. But an essential question is often left unasked: What approach would help people in the poorest countries most? The Harvard economist Jeffrey Sachs has argued, for example, that if Americans contributed $3 billion dollars a year to combat AIDS in Africa, it would solve many problems and amount to only "about $10 a year for every American, the cost of a movie ticket with popcorn."

But would it? The idea that a small sacrifice from wealthy Western countries can alleviate much misery in places like Africa and India is comforting, of course, and it has become a first principle for the world's many health politicians. "These distinctions between preventing AIDS and treating it are criminal," Siddharth Dube, who has consulted for UNAIDS and the World Health Organization, told me. Dube was raised in Calcutta and has frequently written about AIDS and the health problems of India. "We are not living in the medieval ages, where a continent can be wiped out by the plague and nobody knows about it anywhere else. That we can know all this and yet do nothing is the most remarkable fact of our time. . . . AIDS is not watches or jewelry or software. People are dying. There are drugs, there is unimaginable wealth in this world, and the people who have the money are refusing to help. It's that simple."

Nothing about AIDS is simple, though. Providing treatment for even a minority of sick people comes at the expense of preventing many others from falling ill. It is true that many countries now permit local pharmaceutical firms to ignore patents and make some medicines more cheaply. But discussing any price reductions of these drugs is meaningless in countries like India, where poverty is so acute that the government can't afford them. When I was in Delhi, for example, Indian officials were debating whether to add the hepatitis-B vaccine to their program for children—because it costs sixty-five cents a shot, and not ten cents, like other vaccines. How can you argue about whether it's worth spending fifty-five cents to save a life and then begin to talk about spending immense sums on an extremely complicated treatment for a disease that cannot be cured?

The reality that the spread of AIDS could be greatly reduced through governmental effort has been routinely ignored by politicians in nearly every country. To focus on AIDS is to acknowledge the potential devastation the epidemic can cause, and politicians have rarely done that. What elected leader would wish to associate himself with a national calamity, particularly if it occurred on his watch or could largely have been avoided? This was as true in the United States in the 1980s and in Kenya and Zimbabwe in the 1990s as it is in India, China, or Cambodia today. "At all stages of the AIDS epidemic, politicians find reasons not to invest in prevention," Martha Ainsworth, a World Bank economist, told me. Ainsworth, along with her colleague Mead Over, wrote *Confronting AIDS,* the best book on making economic decisions about handling the epidemic. "At the beginning, you take countries like India or Russia, and nobody is really sick. They have tens of thousands dying of tuberculosis every year. Nobody wants to spend scarce resources on AIDS, because it takes years to go from infection to illness. And then you get later into the epidemic"—when millions of people can be visibly, disturbingly sick "—and everyone is demanding treatment. It is much less controversial to treat somebody who is sick than to talk about homosexuality, drug abusers, prostitution, sexual habits, or social mores.

"In parts of the world today, millions of people need treatment," Ainsworth continued. "When you then say, 'We are going to protect you by making sure that prostitutes and their clients use condoms and that drug users have clean needles,' people say, 'Don't spend money on them. They cause the problem.' "

Yet the effect of focusing prevention efforts on high-risk groups like prostitutes and truck drivers cannot be disputed. It costs three hundred rupees to avert one trucker's infection in India with targeted education programs and the distribution of condoms. That is about $6. For sex workers, the cost is less than $3. No treatment approach makes as much sense. Not long ago, Andrew Natsios, the Bush administration's chief of USAID, said that it wouldn't pay to buy a complicated set of antiretroviral drugs for Africans, because they are people who "don't know what Western time is" and thus cannot take the drugs on the proper schedule. His comments were patronizing and untrue, and he was condemned for them. If, however, he had said that most Africans shouldn't use the drugs because they are so toxic that they are difficult to take regularly and, if not taken regularly, might create increased resistance and actually *worsen* the epidemic, he would still have been condemned. But he would have been right. Indian officials and Western health philanthropists have been forced into a nearly impossible position by the increased availability of cheaper AIDS drugs. Nobody has been placed more squarely in this vise than Prasada Rao, the director of the Indian AIDS program. "In a just world, there would be enough money available so that you wouldn't have to pick and choose between prevention and treatment," he told me. "But today that world does not exist, and that money is not available. When it comes to treatment with antiretrovirals, we don't have a thousand dollars for a patient. We don't have a hundred dollars. We don't really have ten dollars. This is something that doesn't seem to register in the West. The model of Brazil"—where the government will pay for antiretroviral drugs—"doesn't work here." Brazil's per-capita income of $5,029 is eleven times India's, and Brazil spends twenty times as much per person on health care. India has a much bigger AIDS problem than Brazil does, and significantly fewer resources.

"They are wasting their money," Rao said. "They are spending three hundred million dollars every year to treat one hundred thousand people. This is ridiculous. This is a figure nobody quotes. You may think I am unkind to say this, but it would be wrong, it would be even criminal, to take that money and spend it on one hundred thousand Indians. If you spend for some on antiretroviral drugs, whom do you choose? Do you save the mothers so they can spend more time with their children? Do you go for the élite class, who run the cities? When you spend money on these people, you are implying that others can die. Because that is what this drug movement is all about. This talk of denying people treatment. Look outside my window." His office is on the grounds of the government health complex, in Delhi, a grim park filled with families looking for miracles that doctors can't provide. "They are dying of malaria, of diarrhea, of leprosy. There are thousands of the blind. And AIDS is important, even more important. But you can't tell me we should ignore everyone so that we can serve a few people. Not in this country."

Almost as an afterthought, Rao added, "What we need is a vaccine. We need attention paid to the 995 million Indians who are not infected with HIV." Vaccines are among the world's most effective health interventions. Millions of lives are saved each year by a standard package of cheap vaccines that reach three-quarters of the world's children. However, there is little incentive for companies to invest in them. As the Harvard economist Michael Kremer has written, "Despite recent scientific advances which have increased the feasibility of developing malaria, tuberculosis, and AIDS vaccines, global R&D on these vaccines is woefully inadequate."

Vaccine development is hampered not only by science—or even principally by science—but also by market forces and liability issues. When I asked Seth Berkely, the president of the International AIDS Vaccine Initiative, about the scientific obstacles that stand in the way of developing a vaccine, he acknowledged that there were many, but then said, "What would happen if tomorrow we had an HIV mutation that started to spread by the respiratory route in the United States? Well, we would all work 24/7, and we would throw a ton of money at the problem." AIDS primarily affects poor countries, however, and, twenty years into the epidemic, there has been no such all-consuming effort to produce a vaccine. Most pharmaceutical companies believe that they will have a hard time selling enough vaccine in places like Africa or India to recoup their research costs. There is an irony here: research suffers because it is a global public good—and an extremely costly one—in which no single country has sufficient incentive to invest. As desperate as South Africa, India, and China are, it's not realistic to expect the governments of these countries to put up $5 or $10 billion for vaccine research, particularly before it's possible to know whether this research will succeed. Kremer has been the most eloquent advocate of creating a global system that would allow countries to buy vaccines in advance—in other words, of guaranteeing companies a market for their investment. That way, there would be a reason for them to take the risk.

"We must treat those who are sick with compassion and with whatever medicine we can provide," Rao told me before I left his office. "But the answer has to be in the form of a vaccine. After all these years, I can't think of anything more profoundly frightening than spending billions of dollars on drugs and making the epidemic worse."

VI.

"I make drugs," Yusuf Hamied told me when I asked him whether it made sense to focus so heavily on treatment rather than on prevention. "I can only do what I do."

With a billion people living in Hamied's principal market, it is natural to wonder if the potential sale of HIV drugs, and the profit it would bring in India, interests him. "We have four hundred products, and the AIDS drugs are twelve of them," he told me. "You must understand my philosophy in life. For the year ending March 31st, our turnover was $227 million. A profit of $33 million net, after tax and after everything, you see. It's just my wife and I. We have no children. We are very rich. Even in the first six months of this year, our sales were up 25 percent over last year. I'm not a revolutionary. I'm a businessman. But, really, how much money do you think I need?"

Hamied is an unlikely person to call himself an Indian nationalist, but he often does. His father, who died in 1972, was a Muslim from Aligarh, and his mother was a Lithuanian Jew. They met in Germany in 1925, while

Hamied's father was studying chemistry. Hamied has a place in Mauritius, is fond of Hong Kong, and travels frequently to New York. But he spends most of his time in a quiet, sun-drenched apartment not far from the center of London.

When I went to see Hamied, he was eager to share the yellowed treasures of his life—pictures of his Lithuanian grandparents, who died in the gas chambers, and one of the day, in 1939, when Gandhi came to visit Cipla in Bombay. There was a picture of Zakir Husain, who was India's third president and one of Hamied's father's closest friends. There were also many pictures of Hamied, his younger brother, Mohammed, who helps him run the business, and the conductor Zubin Mehta, with whom he grew up, in Bombay. For more than fifty years, he and Mehta have remained as inseparable as two men who live mostly on airplanes and different continents can be. It was after riots erupted between Muslim and Hindu residents of Bombay, in 1984, that Hamied and his wife decided to find a place in London, though they are still tax-paying citizens of India.

"People who grow up in Bombay can never give up the vision of what it was," Hamied told me during lunch at his favorite Chinese restaurant, near Hyde Park. "But that changed for me completely after the second round of riots, in 1992. In the thirties, my father often worked with this Jewish-run medical company in Germany. In 1938, he went with my mother to Berlin. One day, he was on a train and the Nazis came on and they started to talk to him; they thought he was a Jew and said, 'Shut up, you bloody Jew.' He saw what was happening maybe in a way that people who lived there could not, and he begged all his Jewish friends to get out. They laughed and said, 'We are the intellectual élite.'

"My mother told me this story over and over—how the Jews of Berlin told my father they were safe because they were the intellectuals, the people who made the nation work. She said to always keep that in mind. And in 1992 I felt exactly as if it were 1938 in Berlin. In my own home. Because my name was Hamied. Everything in India is your name. A reporter rang me in the middle of the rioting and asked, 'As a so-called eminent Indian Muslim, what are your views of what is going on in Bombay?' I said, 'Why are you asking me as a Muslim? Why not ask me as an Indian Jew? I am a Jew.' I said, 'Forget Hindu, Muslim, Jew. Let us talk about Bombay. Eight million of sixteen million below poverty. Seven million living on the streets. No water. No home. No sanitation. This is not religious. This is haves and have-nots. That is what is happening in Bombay, in India, and in the Third World. That is our future.' "

After weeks of torrential rains, the sun came out on my last day in India. I left Bombay early in the morning and drove north to one of Cipla's factories, in Patalganga. The slums were alive with people taking advantage of the clear, dry air: kids, soaped up by their mothers, were enjoying their baths in rainwater that had been carefully collected the night before. Barbers with straight razors were at work by six; so were hawkers, prostitutes, and men selling mangoes by the side of the road.

It takes only an hour to ride from some of the world's most crowded slums to the factory, which is filled with antiseptic rooms where hoods and gloves must be worn at all times. Cipla manufactures nearly every major type of antibiotic, as well as nasal sprays, iron chelators, cardiovascular drugs, and antidepressants. The company's factories export to more than a hundred countries. The workers are well paid. Morale is high. I watched the stamping machines as they churned out as many as four thousand tablets every minute. Yet, at the end of each day, Cipla ships its AIDS drugs in bulk to Russia, Africa, Europe, and even to the Gulf of Oman, when, only miles away, people are infected (and will soon be dying) in numbers recorded almost nowhere else. Hamied told me it was his greatest shame. "Our first batch of AZT we had 200,000 pills, and we couldn't even give them away in India," he said; the drugs reached their expiration date before the government approved their use. This is just one of many bureaucratic problems facing even someone who has the money and the will to donate drugs in large quantities. Back at the main office, in Bombay, I sat with some of Cipla's scientists and with Hamied's younger brother, Mohammed. He handed me a bottle of pills that contained something called Triomune. It is a combination of three main AIDS drugs—mixed into a single tablet that can be taken twice a day.

Triomune can't be manufactured in Europe or America, because each drug is made and patented by a different company. In those places, this pill, which eliminates much of the complication of the antiretroviral regimen, would clearly prolong some lives and ease the suffering of many patients. But is it the answer for countries like India, China, and Africa? Of course not. Even the increased efficacy of the pills does not change the economic facts: the Indian government can't afford them. The simple cost of shipping the drugs around the country and storing them could equal the money the government spends on treating all other infectious diseases combined. A society that lacks a sophisticated health-care system, and one in which tens of millions of people do not even have access to clean drinking water, needs to focus on prevention. It simply can't afford to start with the most expensive drugs for its most complicated disease.

Hamied understands all that; he told me so more than once. Yet he is a drug manufacturer, and he feels compelled to make his stand. "Maybe it's just a prayer to cling to, but we need the prayer," he said with a sad shrug the last time we met. "What else do we have to offer?"

CAN AIDS BE STOPPED?

HELEN EPSTEIN AND LINCOLN CHEN

from New York Review of Books

| **March 14, 2002** |

During the past two decades, while virtually all Western countries experienced more or less constant economic growth, much of the rest of the world suffered a series of financial catastrophes—from the international debt crisis of 1982, to the Mexican peso crisis of 1994, to the Asian financial crisis of 1997, to the Russian default of 1998. The social consequences of these economic disasters—including impoverishment, mass unemployment, and ill health—have been felt almost entirely outside the West: in Africa, much of Asia, Latin America and the Caribbean, and the former Soviet bloc.

While the causes of these crises were complex, much public criticism has been directed at some of the institutions that are attempting to establish rules for economic globalization—the World Trade Organization, the World Bank, and the International Monetary Fund. Protest movements have emerged, involving many different, sometimes conflicting, constituencies—from labor unions to environmentalists to college students to nongovernmental organizations involved in health, social justice, and human rights. Their grievances more or less converge on a common theme: as Western governments, backed by multinational banks and corporations, push economic liberalization to extremes, they are exacerbating, and even exploiting, the vast social and economic inequalities that exist in the world.

Recently, George Soros, the financier and philanthropist, seems to have joined this chorus. In his new book *George Soros on Globalization*, Soros concludes that international finance and trade have outstripped the capacity of sovereign states to manage the politics of globalization. Especially neglected has been the provision of global public goods, things needed by everyone but not produced by the marketplace, such as clean air and disease control. Instead of proposing to dismantle the WTO, the World Bank, and the IMF, Soros would like to see them strengthened, and complemented by stronger global institutions in social fields like health, such as the World Health Organization, and labor standards, such as the International Labor Organization. Successful globalization, he argues, requires effective global institutions devoted not only to finance and trade, but also to public health, human rights, environmental protection, and other public goods.

At the top of Soros's list of global social problems in need of attention is HIV/AIDS. Public concern over the global AIDS epidemic, particularly in Africa, has grown enormously in recent years, but there is considerable debate about what the international community can and should do about it. Especially controversial has been the high cost of antiretroviral drugs used to extend the lives of people with AIDS. The pharmaceutical companies that make these drugs price them beyond reach of the world's poor, but in November 2001 at the WTO meeting in Doha, Qatar, these companies were forced to accede to pressure from developing-country governments, nongovernmental organizations, and activists, and allow poor governments to adjust certain rigid patent rules applying to vaccines and drugs in order to protect public health. Despite this apparent triumph of international pressure, far more needs to be done. A coalition of governments and nongovernmental organizations, led by the UN, recently launched the Global Fund Against AIDS, Tuberculosis, and Malaria (referred to here as the Global Fund), and its performance will test how well such a global institution can confront the most serious health crises of our time, and perhaps in all of human history.

1.

To date, an estimated fifty million people have contracted HIV; about twenty-five million people in sub-Saharan Africa are infected, and about three million of these people die annually. In some countries, average life expectancy has fallen by more than a decade because of HIV/AIDS. Unfortunately, it has been only in the past two or three years that the gravity of the AIDS problem in Africa and other parts of the developing world has been fully recognized by those in the best position to do something about it, including many African presidents and prime ministers and such Western government leaders as Secretary of State Colin Powell, former President Bill Clinton, and the G-8 heads of state at meetings in Okinawa and Genoa in 2000 and 2001.

Yet by 1985 many epidemiologists were already warning about the scale of the global AIDS epidemic. Perhaps it should not surprise us that the AIDS crisis in Africa in particular has taken so long to become a matter of concern at such high political levels. In 1999, the UN Security Council declared AIDS in Africa an international security issue, because it further destabilizes already politically fragile African nations. But how much does this really matter to the West, particularly the United States? The postwar history of the West's relationship with Africa suggests that when millions of Africans die, or when African states collapse, Western leaders often look away.

Diseases like malaria, respiratory infections, measles, and diarrhea, all preventable or curable and largely controlled in the West, continue to kill millions of African children, and yet U.S. overseas bilateral aid to Africa fell by half in the 1990s. During the Cold War, the United States actively supported regimes in Liberia, Zaire, and South Africa that were responsible for the deaths of thousands more. The United States and Western Europe failed to intervene during the Rwandan genocide, and had it not been for a group of rock stars, Americans and Europeans might well have ignored the Ethiopian famine in the 1980s. Throughout the 1990s, U.S. funding for HIV prevention in developing countries averaged some $70 million per year, about the same as the U.S. military allocated for Viagra when this medication first became available. Why did AIDS in Africa at last grab the rich world's attention? Why haven't similar deadly scourges of the Third World done the same? One possibility is that when Western leaders, activists, corporation heads, and the general public look at the problems of the developing world, they mainly see reflections of problems in their own societies.

For many reasons, the suffering of African AIDS patients may draw international sympathy in a way that the suffering of malaria and diarrhea victims do not. For one thing, AIDS is a manifestly "global" disease; by the time it was first recognized in the early 1980s, HIV had already spread to nearly every continent. It has killed people of all races and classes, from the economically flourishing gay neighborhoods of San Francisco and New York to the poorest slums in Africa, Asia, Latin America, and the Caribbean.

Other infectious diseases were once as widespread and devastating as AIDS. Five hundred years ago, measles and smallpox introduced by Old World explorers and settlers decimated indigenous people in the New World. In 1918, "Spanish flu" killed millions around the world. Until the early twentieth century, malaria and typhoid claimed lives not only in the tropics, but also in Minnesota, England, and Arkhangelsk, Russia. During the past half-century, however, deaths caused by infectious diseases, particularly those common in childhood, became increasingly rare in industrialized countries. This led epidemiologists to associate certain patterns of disease with different stages of economic development. They classified communicable, nutritional, and reproductive problems such as malaria, tuberculosis, malnutrition, and death in childbirth as "diseases of poverty."

A second generation of diseases—which includes heart disease, stroke, diabetes, and cancer—were classified as "diseases of affluence," common in industrialized countries (although many people in developing countries, especially the well-to-do and middle class, also suffer from these chronic and degenerative diseases).

AIDS is part of a "third wave" of infectious, environmental, and behavioral pathologies that have accelerated in recent years. Some of these may be seen as "diseases of globalization" because they affect all countries and their ultimate control will require unprecedented global cooperation. During the past two decades, more than two dozen new infectious agents have been identified, including the prions that cause new variant Creutzfeldt-Jakob disease and the measles-like virus that killed fourteen horses and their trainer in Australia in 1994—along with new environmental health problems like global warming and ozone depletion. In addition, health problems associated with hazardous behavior, such as drug abuse, unsafe sex, traffic accidents, and violence, have also increased, particularly in societies undergoing rapid social change. The global distribution of these emerging diseases may explain why AIDS in particular is no longer seen as just another "Third World" problem that people in the West feel they can largely ignore.

AIDS also raises troubling issues surrounding the global influence of private markets and the spread of infectious diseases. The collision between these two trends has created a kind of moral riptide with momentum of its own. Since 1996, HIV-positive patients in rich countries have had access to "cocktails" of drugs called antiretrovirals that can slow the progression of AIDS. These drugs are designed to attack the HIV virus, allowing the patient's immune system to repair itself and fight off opportunistic infections. Although the drugs do not cure AIDS, can have serious side effects, and do not work for all patients, their use has added many healthy years to the lives of thousands of people living with HIV in rich countries. There are now on the market around twenty antiretroviral drugs developed in the past fifteen years by pharmaceutical companies, the U.S. National Institutes of Health, and university laboratories.

Partly because they are so expensive, these lifesaving drugs are largely inaccessible to the world's poor, especially the millions of HIV-positive people in Africa. One reason they are expensive is that international trade rules allow pharmaceutical companies a twenty-year patent, which effectively grants them a monopoly. During this time, the companies can charge whatever the market will bear. Until recently, patents on Western pharmaceuticals were valid only in a few countries, but that is now changing.

In 1994, Western governments concerned about protecting intellectual property pushed for an agreement on Trade-Related Aspects of Intellectual Property Rights (TRIPS) linked to membership in the World Trade Organization. TRIPS aims to extend patent protection to all WTO members, so that someone who produces a new CD or computer program, or invents a new pharmaceutical drug, will have the rights to that invention protected not only in the country in which it was first developed, but also in every country that joins the WTO. TRIPS was partly a response to the accelerated globalization of information which has made it easy for music and video pirates in China and generic drug makers in India, Thailand, and Brazil to copy Western inventions and products. Not all countries have signed on to TRIPS, but most have or will do so within the next decade.

Patenting drugs that could, if they were cheaply available, extend the lives and postpone the suffering of thousands or even millions of poor people in developing countries raises serious ethical concerns. The development of antiretroviral drugs owes a great deal to gay HIV activists in rich countries, particularly in the United States, who, beginning in the late 1980s, picketed the U.S. National Institutes of Health (NIH) demanding that more money be spent on AIDS research. They also demanded that the Food and Drug Administration accelerate the regulatory approval process for promising drugs. In the late 1990s, many of these same activist groups, including ACT UP, began to ally themselves with campaigns led by such international development organizations as Médecins sans Frontières, Oxfam, and CARE. They claimed the pharmaceutical industry set exorbitant prices to enrich their shareholders while ignoring the plight of the world's poor. Why, they asked, were these lifesaving drugs, now finally available, so expensive? Could they not be sold more cheaply to HIV-positive people in poor countries?

The debate over access to AIDS drugs in poor countries has taken place at the same time as an even larger debate about the mysteries of pharmaceutical pricing policies in general. There is some parallel between the AIDS drug debate and the debate over the high cost of prescription drugs for Americans, including Medicare patients. Drug companies are increasingly having to confront growing discontent among their customers in rich countries where they make most of their profits. These customers may be particularly sympathetic to poor Africans with AIDS because they share their concerns. Increasingly, Americans are asking: Why are drugs so expensive? How much profit is fair? Shouldn't moral standards apply to drug pricing for all people, poor Africans with AIDS as well as ourselves?

Concerns about the high cost of drugs in general have led to increased public scrutiny of the pharmaceutical industry, and this is beginning to pay off. Activists calling for greater use of generic drugs in poor countries with serious public health problems recently won a number of concessions. Generic drug companies in Brazil were already producing an antiretroviral cocktail before the country joined the WTO in 1996, and these drugs now form the basis of an exemplary treatment program, which offers free antiretrovirals to all Brazilians who need them. However it is not clear how easily Brazil's program could be reproduced in Africa, since Brazil's per capita income is ten times that of most African countries affected by AIDS, and only 0.5 percent of its citizens are HIV-positive, compared to between 5 and 35 percent in most countries of sub-Saharan Africa. The obstacles to distributing AIDS drugs in much of Africa are therefore much greater than they are in Brazil. Nevertheless, last April, the government of South Africa won a court case allowing it to manufacture its own generic versions of some patented drugs, and if Thabo Mbeki, South Africa's president, were to revise his idiosyncratic views on AIDS, a similar program could be launched there in the near future.

At the recent WTO meeting in Doha, Qatar, poor governments were given permission to issue compulsory licenses, permitting local pharmaceutical manufacturers to produce generic versions of patented drugs for the local market in order to protect public health. Negotiations are underway to determine whether some countries might also be permitted to import patented drugs made by generic producers in other countries. In this way, a country such as Uganda that does not have the capacity to manufacture its own antiretrovirals might be permitted to purchase them from the Brazilian generics companies. To reduce the din of negative publicity, multinational pharmaceutical firms have been forced to offer AIDS drugs to a limited number of health institutions in developing countries at reduced prices under the Accelerated Access program, endorsed by the United Nations. However, this program offers only a limited number of drugs, and critics believe that only global generic competition will bring AIDS drug prices low enough so that they will reach a significant number of poor people in developing countries.

2.

Indignation over the high cost of AIDS drugs has helped focus international attention on the global AIDS epidemic and by the end of 2001, an antiretroviral drug cocktail could be obtained in some developing countries for $300 to $500 per year, many times less than the price in the West. However, for a variety of reasons, including the sluggishness of government bureaucracies, the stinginess of drug companies, and the fact that even at these low prices the drugs are still too expensive and difficult to distribute, few AIDS patients in developing countries are actually receiving these drugs or, for that matter, any modern medications at all beyond the cheapest antibiotics. With this larger dilemma in mind, the UN recently launched the Global Fund for AIDS, Tuberculosis, and Malaria. But despite the fact that it is greatly needed and holds great promise, the Global Fund still faces great challenges. Kofi Annan originally proposed that between $7 and $10 billion per year was needed, to be met by contributions from rich governments, corporations, and private donors. Thus far, however, the pledges total about $1.7 billion. Despite the rhetorical concern of Western donor governments, the commitments have been astonishingly stingy. The U.S. government has promised only $500 million over three years, setting off a series of correspondingly disappointing commitments by other rich countries.

Difficult decisions will have to be made about how to allocate these limited resources to prevent and treat these three diseases. Opinions vary, for example, about how much of the Global Fund should go to pay for AIDS treatment. Last year, a group of Harvard academics proposed that some of the money be spent on buying discounted antiretrovirals from Western pharmaceutical firms. They cited various small-scale AIDS-treatment programs including one based at the Clinique Bon Sauveur in Haiti and

Médecins sans Frontières' Khayelitsha Project near Cape Town, South Africa, as evidence that administering antiretroviral drugs to poor AIDS patients in developing countries is feasible. The greatest obstacle, say the directors of these programs, is the cost of antiretroviral drugs.

These small pilot projects are admirable and offer many practical lessons and hope, but there are grounds to question whether they could easily be extended throughout sub-Saharan Africa. Both the Bon Sauveur and Khayelitsha projects are currently administering antiretrovirals to only around one hundred patients each, while there are millions of people in Africa alone who might benefit from antiretrovirals. But experience shows that distributing even relatively simple drug regimens on such a large scale poses formidable obstacles. Programs in developing countries that aim to treat people with syphilis and tuberculosis, or even to distribute vitamin A supplements to children, show how difficult it is to deliver health care in such countries, even if the drugs are free or nearly so. An estimated 1.6 million women who give birth every year in those countries have syphilis, a disease that puts their newborns at high risk of deformity or death, even though the tests and drugs to treat it cost only about twenty-five cents. Hundreds of thousands of children go blind every year, and more than a million die, because they are deficient in Vitamin A. Vitamin A supplements, which need to be taken only twice a year, are virtually free. Of course some treatment and vaccination programs have been very successful, for example those for smallpox, polio, and onchocerciasis ("river blindness"), but vaccines for polio and smallpox need to be administered only a few times in a lifetime, while the oral dose to prevent the onset of onchocerciasis symptoms is taken once a year; and the recipients of such treatment, unlike AIDS patients, do not require ongoing care. And even these relatively simple programs have required enormous donor commitment and funding over long periods.

The failure to deliver some even very cheap, simple treatments in developing countries is largely owing to the lack of sufficient trained and motivated health personnel, inadequate management and administrative capacity, and insufficient supplies of vehicles, refrigerators, lab reagents, and other basic equipment. For example, syphilis screening and treatment in antenatal care requires adequate staffing, an efficient referral system, reliable supplies of testing materials and drugs, an on-site rudimentary laboratory with quality control, and other resources that a great many health centers in poor countries simply do not have.

Treating AIDS patients is far more complicated than testing for syphilis or administering Vitamin A drops. AIDS patients need counseling, laboratory tests, and ongoing clinical care to treat opportunistic infections and monitor drug side effects. Even if the drugs and other necessary supplies were available, and in most cases they aren't, antiretroviral treatment programs require considerable effort on the part of public-sector health workers. But because of political instability, economic stagnation, and misguided health-sector reform policies mandated by donor institutions such as the World Bank, the health workforce throughout sub-Saharan Africa has been collapsing. Doctors are severely underpaid, earning sometimes as little as $100 a month. Nurses and other staff earn far less. Low staff morale and moonlighting by government workers already severely undermine health services. During the past year, frustrated health workers in Zimbabwe and Uganda went on strike, and throughout sub-Saharan Africa trained doctors and nurses are leaving the public sector to seek better pay in the private sector, or migrating to other continents.

Any effective AIDS treatment program must endeavor to strengthen the health care system generally, especially the human infrastructure of front-line health workers, as well as meet the concerns of people affected by AIDS. The Harvard group proposed spending an additional $150 per year for the extra clinical work associated with each patient on antiretrovirals; but this may not be sufficient because adequately trained and motivated staff and organized health systems require many years of sustained investment. The antiretroviral treatment program at Clinique Bon Sauveur in Haiti, like many similar small-scale antiretroviral treatment programs in developing countries, is carried on through a health center that has long been well funded by foreign donors. Since Clinique Bon Sauveur was established fifteen years ago, it has always provided a far higher standard of care than is generally available in the public sector in Haiti, even before it began dispensing antiretroviral drugs to people with AIDS. Staff are paid regularly and decently, and know they have the resources, in drugs and supplies (in addition to antiretrovirals), to do their jobs well.

While antiretroviral drugs are important, they are not a panacea for the AIDS crisis in Africa. Indeed the debate over the high cost of the drugs has made AIDS in Africa appear to many to be merely a medical problem, when it is in fact far more than this. When an American or European becomes ill with AIDS, it is often mainly a matter for the patient and his doctor. Friends and family may grieve; but the effect of AIDS on an African family is of an entirely different order. This is because AIDS kills and weakens the adults who grow the food and earn the money that supports everyone else. The dependency ratio in Africa is much higher than it is in the West, not only because there are so many young children, but also because there are so many unemployed people, and most countries have no social safety net. Most sub-Saharan African workers are farmers, but because of inequitable land distribution and declining prices for Africa's agricultural products, farmers increasingly depend on relatives who are migrant workers or casual laborers in urban areas.

Migrant workers are particularly at risk of HIV, because of their youth and because of the loneliness and social anomie in the hostels and urban slums where many of them end up. When a South African mine worker, for example, becomes sick or dies of AIDS, he may leave behind in his rural home village as many as ten or twenty destitute dependents, including children, wives, in-laws, brothers and sisters, parents and grandparents. Antiretroviral drugs could help some of the mine workers stay healthy longer, but the drugs have side effects of their own, they don't work for everyone, and they are certainly not a cure. Eventually, the family will need other kinds of help, including money for children's school fees and seeds, small loans, or help finding jobs and business advice, so that survivors can start small enterprises.

Because the economies of so many African countries are in such a bad state, many small enterprises fail, so families affected by AIDS also require some sort of financial safety net to tide them over while they try again. In addition, families affected by HIV need education about their legal and human rights, especially regarding property rights and HIV-related employment discrimination, which is widespread in developing countries. Since laws protecting the rights of people with HIV currently exist almost nowhere in Africa, mechanisms must be found to create and enforce them at local and national levels. Communities affected by HIV also need information about how people can protect themselves from the virus, and they will also need reliable supplies of condoms, which are still, twenty years into the AIDS epidemic, not easily and cheaply available everywhere.

Overemphasis on the medical aspects of AIDS in Africa probably arises from the tendency to see the problems of the developing world as reflections of problems in the West. But many small African AIDS groups see AIDS quite differently. They provide a wide range of social support and HIV-prevention services, in addition to rudimentary care for AIDS patients. Most of these projects rely at present on dedicated volunteers and shoestring budgets, and there are not nearly enough of them to help everyone. Emphasizing access to AIDS drugs alone risks bypassing much of the very good work that these groups are already doing.

A strong case can be made that the pharmaceutical companies should either donate their drugs to Africa entirely for free or permit the use of generics, in exchange for some guarantee that their markets in industrialized countries will be protected. The companies can well afford to do this. A similarly strong case can be made that projects like the Faraja Trust in Morogoro, Tanzania, or the Friends of Street Children Project in Kampala, Uganda—to name just two of thousands of such groups in East Africa alone—should get most of the support from the Global Fund. Antiretrovirals could then be part of such programs whenever feasible.

The governing board of the Global Fund seems to recognize the importance of both national health systems and nongovernmental programs that strive to meet the complex and specific needs of particular communities. Under the fund's guidelines made public at the end of January 2002, National AIDS Coordinating Councils, quasi-governmental bodies that include members from nongovernmental organizations, will submit proposals to the fund, and the money will be disbursed to the government, usually the Ministry of Health, which will then pass the money on to nongovernmental entities. However, there are already concerns that many groups will be overlooked. Cronyism and corruption, perennial problems with international aid in general, will also have to be addressed, but as yet, it is not clear how this will be done, or how the spending will be monitored.

Addressing the AIDS crisis in Africa will require an emphasis on more than antiretroviral drugs alone, important as they are. What sub-Saharan Africa seems to need even more than it needs AIDS drugs is the improvement of its health-care systems, the creation of livelihoods for families impoverished by AIDS illnesses and deaths, and the alleviation of the loneliness, poverty, and despair that are likely to motivate risky sexual behavior. The Global Fund cannot deal with all this on its own. Until scientists discover an effective vaccine to prevent HIV infection, sustained relief from the African AIDS epidemic may depend on the subcontinent's social and economic stability, which in turn will depend on better governance by Africa's leaders. But it will also depend critically on greater support for Africa from the international community, which could begin by establishing fairer terms of trade for African farmers and debt-relief programs that are not tied to the same harsh conditions—such as underinvestment in

African institutions, especially those devoted to health and education, and reduced government support for nascent African business enterprises that need to be nurtured—that have combined with local corruption and mismanagement to undermine African development.

Nevertheless, it is of enormous importance that the Global Fund succeed, not only because it could reduce much human suffering, but also because it could advance the credibility of new mechanisms to manage the negative consequences of globalization. If the fund's performance were to generate cynicism, it could undermine similar efforts in other areas. If successful, it could become a model for global governance in the future.

INFECTED CELLS:
As HIV Epidemic Hits Russia, Crux of Problem Is Jail

MARK SCHOOFS

from The Wall Street Journal

| **June 25, 2002** |

ST. PETERSBURG

When Alexander Multanovskiy was locked up in Kresty jail, a squalid, overcrowded brick complex built in the late nineteenth century, he blocked out the misery with heroin.

The twenty-five-year-old Russian believes that's how he contracted HIV, the AIDS virus, from one of his fellow inmates. "We were using the same needle," he says.

Prisoners like Mr. Multanovskiy are helping make the former Soviet bloc home to the world's fastest-growing HIV epidemic, according to a report last year from the United Nations' AIDS program and the World Health Organization. Between 1996 and 2001, the number of registered new HIV infections in Russia annually surged to more than 87,000 from about 1,500.

The rapid increase in infections and the huge number of Russians using injection drugs have fueled concern that the country could soon be host to one of the world's worst AIDS crises. But Russia faces an enormous challenge containing the disease, as harsh drug laws send droves of HIV-positive patients into prisons, where treatment is minimal and the disease spreads through shared needles and sexual contact.

Drug use soared in Russia amid the social disintegration following the collapse of the Soviet Union. Enforcement of harsh drug laws, largely unchanged since Soviet times, has helped flood Russia's jails and prisons with HIV carriers. About a sixth of the country's roughly 195,000 registered people with HIV are currently in jail, and many others who are now free have previously been incarcerated. At Kresty, which had fewer than ten inmates with HIV in 1997, more than 1,000 have the AIDS virus today, out of a total of about 7,800 prisoners.

HIV prevalence is far higher in prisons than in the general population, but health officials fear the figures are poised to rise both inside and outside prison. Russia's drug users number as high as 4 million of the country's 145 million people, according to some estimates. Intravenous drug use is the principal source of HIV infection in the country. Draconian drug statutes mean possession of even a minute amount of heroin can bring years behind bars. With the prevalence of needle sharing in prison and the tendency of drug users to be jailed more than once, some experts project ever-rising infection rates across Russia through infected drug users moving in and out of prison.

Andrei Kozlov and Vadim Pokrovskiy, two of Russia's leading HIV researchers, fear the infected prison and drug-using populations could provide the opening the virus needs to work its way into the general population. Judging from Russia's high rates of sexually transmitted diseases such as syphilis and gonorrhea, HIV could spread rapidly from drug users through sexual contact.

Prison officials acknowledge that the disease could spread unnoticed. Usually, inmates are tested only when they enter prison or if they get sick. Prison officials say they have no reliable estimate for how often HIV is transmitted in prisons.

The Ministry of Justice, which runs the country's prisons, has pushed to reduce overcrowding and to reform the legal code so that fewer addicts are sent to prison. "We want to improve our legislation to protect young people committing their first, not-very-serious crime," says Yuri Kalinin, deputy justice minister. The prison leadership has won praise from AIDS advocates for piloting new approaches to HIV control. But change has been slow and piecemeal.

A visit to Kresty reveals the magnitude of the problem and the obstacles to solving it. Located on the Neva River in St. Petersburg, Kresty is the largest of the country's SIZOs, from the Russian for "pre-trial detention center." With the surge in drug crimes, these jails have become severely overcrowded in recent years because all suspects, innocent and guilty, are held in SIZOs until their trial verdict—a process that usually takes months and can take more than a year.

Each cell measures about ten square yards. Crammed into that space are two three-tier bunk beds and as many as ten prisoners. They sleep in shifts. Inmates and even some prison officials say the crowding makes controlling contraband such as drugs and syringes nearly impossible. Guards are underpaid and susceptible to bribery. Inmates pass drugs and syringes, along with innocuous messages and cigarettes, through what they call the "internet": black ropes they dangle down the exterior brick walls or fling from one barred window to another.

Like most Russian prisons, Kresty tightly restricts access to condoms, because sex isn't allowed. It also restricts bleach, which can sterilize needles and tattooing instruments but can also be used to attempt suicide or attack other prisoners, officials say.

Prisoners are supposed to be given an HIV test when they arrive. As in most Russian penitentiaries, Kresty's main defense against the spread of HIV is keeping infected inmates and uninfected ones in separate cellblocks. But as the case of Mr. Multanovskiy shows, segregation doesn't always work, and it can even promote the spread of the disease by making inmates feel they know who is infected and who isn't.

Mr. Multanovskiy, broad-shouldered and blond, offers an incongruously clean-cut appearance in his black prison uniform. A drug user before he came to the SIZO, he says he tested negative for HIV upon arrival in March of last year. A senior prison doctor, who reviewed his medical record, could only confirm that Mr. Multanovskiy was placed in a cell with inmates who were all supposed to be free of HIV infection.

After eight months, during which time Mr. Multanovskiy says he and his cellmates thought it was safe to share needles, he tested positive for the AIDS virus and was transferred to the block for infected prisoners.

Prison medical authorities say lapses are rare. But evidence of mistakes isn't hard to find. Penal Colony Three in the small town of Dimitrograd conducts its own HIV tests on all prisoners arriving from SIZOs, because officials of the institution say the SIZOs often run out of money to perform the tests. Through June 7 of this year, the tests turned up five previously undetected HIV carriers, according to Sergei Tskhmistrenko, chief of the colony. Eight such cases turned up last year and three the year before. All of these inmates were probably held with HIV-negative prisoners in SIZOs, Mr. Tskhmistrenko says.

In interviews, four HIV-infected prisoners who stayed in various SIZOs said they spent from one month to six months incarcerated with prisoners who weren't supposed to have the AIDS virus—a fact confirmed by prison officials. One of the four prisoners said he knew he was HIV-positive and told fellow inmates but not prison authorities, for fear they might mistreat him. But the other three said they didn't know they were infected. One of these men admitted to sharing needles with his cellmates, and another said he shared his shaving razor.

At Kresty, two HIV-negative prisoners—Dmitri Vasiliev and Alexander Lotzman—said three infected prisoners were plucked from their midst at various times. These cases weren't confirmed by Kresty officials, but they acknowledged that HIV testing was sometimes delayed for lack of money, syringes, test tubes, or fuel for the car used to deliver blood samples to the laboratory.

Infected inmates also can slip through a biological hole in the net. The test detects antibodies to HIV, not HIV itself. Since it can take the immune system as much as several months to generate those antibodies, inmates can test negative when they actually have an HIV infection.

Perhaps the most dangerous aspect of the segregation policy is that it encourages prisoners to believe they can safely share needles. A 2000 survey of 1,200 Russian prisoners conducted by the humanitarian group Doctors Without Borders found that about 8 percent of inmates admitted to injecting drugs in prison. Of those, almost two-thirds said they shared syringes.

"The striking thing is the risk-taking behavior," says Murdo Bijl, director of AIDS Foundation East West, an organization created by Doctors Without Borders to deal with AIDS in Russia. "If there is HIV in this group, it will be fairly quickly transmitted."

Some critics say change must begin outside the jails, with Russia's tough criminal code and its hard-line medical establishment. The drug laws practically guarantee that anyone caught with any quantity of heroin, the most popular injection drug in Russia, can expect to spend a long time behind bars. Possession of up to five one-thousandths of a gram—a gram is 1/28 of an ounce—can draw as much as three years' imprisonment. Possession with intent to sell or process, a charge that nets many addicts who sell small amounts to support their habit, can bring a decade in prison.

Russia's medical establishment has largely opposed reforming the penal system and treatment of drug addiction. Many doctors who hold influential positions today were educated under the authoritarian Soviet public health system. They disagree with Western methods of treating heroin addiction and controlling HIV, especially needle-exchange programs, which provide addicts with free clean syringes, and methadone therapy.

Some doctors, such as Alexei Mazus, director of the Moscow AIDS Center and one of the most prominent AIDS physicians in Russia, oppose needle-exchange programs. They fear the practice lures youths into addiction. Studies show that such programs have been effective in other countries in reducing HIV infection without encouraging drug use.

Methadone is illegal in Russia. Prisoners suffering from withdrawal rarely receive any treatment and may resort to used needles and whatever is available to cope with the wrenching physical and psychological stress of withdrawal. "Unfortunately, we don't have methadone, so [prisoners] use home-made drugs," says Pytor Prokopenko, commander of Matrosskaya Tishina, Moscow's main SIZO.

An alliance of prison authorities, the Russian drug-control police and human-rights advocates has put forward a bill to overhaul the drug law. It would increase penalties for big-time dealers but reduce them for small-time users. One major change would be to raise the official recommendation on the amount of heroin that could lead to a serious prison term. The earliest this bill could take effect, however, would be the end of this year.

Russian prison reform has been fitful, as well. Last year, a law took effect that limited to six months the time suspects could be held in a SIZO after their trials began. But on July 1, that reform will be stricken from the books, allowing authorities to hold prisoners for the duration of their trial. SIZO overcrowding is likely to worsen.

Under U.S. federal law, possession of one hundred grams of heroin will earn a first-time offender a mandatory five-year sentence. It's unlikely that a federal prosecutor would take a case involving five one-thousandths of a gram, and a state court probably wouldn't sentence a first-time offender to jail for that amount. In the U.S., many experts consider the incarceration of drug users one of the main contributing factors to the spread of HIV among African-Americans, the hardest-hit group in America. Most U.S. prisons also don't distribute condoms or needles in prison.

A few of Russia's penal colonies have started selling condoms. In an effort to improve its AIDS-prevention programs, the Ministry of Justice is collaborating with various Western aid organizations, such as the French doctors' group Médecins du Monde and the Open Society Institute, funded by financier George Soros. There are some signs of progress: Education has reduced HIV risk behavior among inmates, according to surveys by AIDS Foundation East West. The foundation has also started a pilot program with the Justice Ministry to distribute bleach and condoms. But the program began only this spring and doesn't operate in all prisons.

These efforts could help limit the spread of the virus, but they can't help those already infected.

The vast majority of Russians with HIV were infected in the past few years. But because HIV typically takes more than five years to reach full-blown AIDS, the country has not yet been hit with an onslaught of sick people who require the expensive cocktails of so-called antiretroviral AIDS drugs.

Despite their high numbers among the infected, prisoners will almost certainly be the last to get those drugs. The prison system can barely afford the most basic health measures. Prison officials recently reported that almost a quarter of inmates in St. Petersburg SIZOs lacked their own bedsheets. Released prisoners are referred to specialized AIDS centers, but they also are strapped for funds. The richest, in Moscow, has funds to give antiretroviral drugs to just five hundred patients.

Some leading AIDS doctors frankly say they won't treat HIV-infected addicts, whom they see as unlikely to stick with the demanding regimen of antiretroviral pills. Since prisoners overwhelmingly acquire the virus by injecting illegal drugs, many won't qualify for treatment. "Homeless people and drug addicts will be at the end of the list," says Dr. Mazus, of the Moscow AIDS Center.

AIDS activists say the Russian health establishment has stacked the deck against drug users by denying them methadone and other therapies that could stabilize their lives and help them adhere to the complex AIDS regimens. The prevailing attitude, charges Kasia Malinowska-Sempruch, who coordinates AIDS-prevention programs for drug users in the former Soviet bloc for the Open Society Institute, is that "HIV and drug use will take care of each other."

PERMISSIONS

Excerpt from *Burning Desires* by Steven Chapple and David Talbot. Copyright © 1990 by Steven Chapple and David Talbot. Reprinted by permission of Ellen Levine Literary Agency.

"AIDS and Politics: Transformation of Our Movement" from *Women, AIDS, and Activism, 1990* by Maxine Wolfe. Copyright © 1990 by Maxine Wolfe. Reprinted with permission of South End Press.

"A Manhattan Project for AIDS" by Larry Kramer. Copyright © 1990 The New York Times Agency. Originally appeared in *The New York Times*, July 16, 1990.

"Esthetics and Loss" from *The Burning Library* by Edmund White. Copyright © 1994 by Edmund White. Used by permission of Alfred A. Knopf, a division of Random House, Inc.

"Stop the Church" and "Seize Control of the FDA" from *AIDS Demo Graphics* by Douglas Crimp with Adam Rolston. Copyright © 1990 by Douglas Crimp. Reprinted by permission of Douglas Crimp.

"Going for the Gold" from *Surviving AIDS* by Michael Callen. Copyright © 1990 by Michael Callen. Reprinted by permission of HarperCollins Publishers.

"Sex, Drugs, Rock-n-Roll, and AIDS" from *Women, AIDS, and Activism* by Iris de la Cruz. Copyright © 1990 by Iris de la Cruz. Reprinted with permission of South End Press.

"Love Story" by Judith Valente. Copyright © 1992 by Dow Jones & Company, Inc. All Rights Reserved Worldwide. Originally appeared in *The Wall Street Journal*, March 16, 1992.

Address on AIDS at the Democratic National Convention, 1992, by Bob Hattoy. Reprinted by kind permission of Bob Hattoy.

Address on AIDS at the Republican National Convention, 1992, by Mary Fisher. Reprinted by kind permission of Mary Fisher.

"Roy Cohn" by Paul McCarthy from *A Promise to Remember: The Names Project Book of Letters*, 1992.

"How Illness Has Affected Me As a Woman and a Wife" by Dambudzo from *Positive Women*.

"Eloquence and Epitaph" from *Writing AIDS* by Phillip Brian Harper. Copyright © 1993 by Columbia University Press. Reprinted by permission of the publisher.

"Whatever Happened to AIDS?" by Jeffrey Schmalz. Copyright © 1993 by The New York Times Agency. Originally appeared in *The New York Times Magazine*, November 28, 1993.

"Letters to the Dead" by Marlon Riggs.

"To My Readers" by Harold Brodkey. Copyright © 1993 by The Estate of Harold Brodkey. Reprinted with kind permission of The Estate of Harold Brodkey. Originally appeared in *The New Yorker*, 1993.

"Political Funerals" from *Queer and Loathing* by David B. Feinberg. Copyright © 1994 by the Estate of David B. Feinberg. Used by permission of Viking Penguin, a division of Penguin Putnam, Inc.

Excerpt from *My Own Country* by Abraham Verghese. Copyright © 1994 by Abraham Verghese. Reprinted with the permission of Simon & Schuster Adult Publishing.

"The Ninth Dive" from *Breaking the Surface* by Greg Louganis with Eric Marcus. Copyright © 1995 by Greg Louganis. Used by permission of Random House, Inc.